OFFICE DERMATOLOGY

OFFICE DERMATOLOGY

Henry H. Roenigk, Jr., M.D.

Professor and Chairman of Dermatology
Department of Dermatology
Northwestern University Medical School
Chicago, Illinois

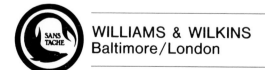

WILLIAMS & WILKINS
Baltimore/London

Made in the United States of America

Reprinted 1982

Library of Congress Cataloging in Publication Data

Main entry under title:

Office dermatology.

 Includes index.
 1. Skin—Diseases. 2. Dermatology. I. Roenigk, Henry H., 1934–   [DNLM: 1. Skin Diseases. WR140 0291]
RL71.035   616.5   80-16590
ISBN 0-683-07316-8

Composed and printed at the
Waverly Press, Inc.
Mt. Royal and Guilford Aves.
Baltimore, Md. 21202, U.S.A.

PREFACE

There are many textbooks of dermatology which are available to the practicing physician who wants to expand his knowledge. Many large detailed textbooks are designed mainly for the dermatologist or the resident in training in dermatology. Other textbooks are simplistic, shorter, and designed specifically for the family physician or internist who must handle a large amount of skin disease in their daily practices.

The original intention of the editor was a dermatology textbook for primary care physicians. Most of the chapters are written with the practical aspects and treatments as the main goals. Very little basic science is presented and only general references are given since both of these can be obtained from larger textbooks on dermatology. We also hoped to cover the types of treatments that can be done in the office with a strong emphasis on surgery. Certain chapters could not be kept small because of the tremendous amount of new research in these fields (i.e. lupus erythematosus and blistering disorders).

In the past 5 to 10 years, there has been an increased interest in dermatologic surgery.

One of the goals of this book was to place more emphasis on surgery of the skin than is usually presented in general dermatology textbooks. Chapters on excisional surgery, hair transplants, dermabrasions, and Mohs' chemosurgery are examples. Some of these procedures require special training, but all can be done in the office and therefore reduce the overall cost of medical care.

This book on *Office Dermatology* has multiple authors and I am grateful to the many members of the faculty of Northwestern University Medical School for their contributions. There were many areas in which we did not have expertise and we have relied on faculty from other medical centers for certain chapters. The secretaries of the Department of Dermatology, especially Mary Ann Theberge, shouldered the burden of preparing the manuscript and the index. I wish to express deep gratitude to my wife and family for their interest and encouragement during the period of preparation of this book.

Henry H. Roenigk, Jr., M.D.

CONTRIBUTORS

Wilma F. Bergfeld, M.D.
Head, Section of Dermatopathology, Department of Dermatology, Cleveland Clinic, Cleveland, Ohio

William A. Caro, M.D.
Associate Clinical Professor of Dermatology, Department of Dermatology, Northwestern University Medical School, Chicago, Ill.

Susan Chappe, M.D.
Resident in Dermatology, Department of Dermatology, Northwestern University Medical School, Chicago, Ill.

Frank E. Dunlap, M.D.
Assistant Clinical Professor of Dermatology, Northwestern University, Chicago, Ill.

Nancy B. Esterly, M.D.
Professor of Pediatrics and Dermatology, Northwestern University Medical School, Head, Division of Dermatology, The Children's Memorial Hospital, Chicago, Ill.

Ruth K. Freinkel, M.D.
Professor of Dermatology, Department of Dermatology, Northwestern University Medical School, Chicago, Ill.

Nancy L. Furey, M.D.
Assistant Professor of Dermatology, Department of Dermatology, Northwestern University Medical School, Chicago, Ill.

Richard Giacobetti, M.D.
Resident in Dermatology, Department of Dermatology, Northwestern University Medical School, Chicago, Ill.

Mark Gordon, M.D.
Assistant Professor of Clinical Dermatology, Northwestern University School of Medicine, The Hammond Clinic, Munster, Ind.

Junji Hasegawa, M.D.
Professor of Dermatology, Department of Dermatology, Northwestern University Medical School, Chicago, Ill.

Alfred D. Hernandez, M.D.
Assistant Professor of Dermatology, Department of Medicine, University of Tennessee, Center for the Health Sciences, Staff Physician, Dermatology Section, Veterans Administration Medical Center, Memphis, Tenn.

Paul Lazar, M.D.
Clinical Professor of Dermatology, Northwestern University Medical School, Chicago, Ill.

Peter McKinney, M.D., F.A.C.S.
Associate Clinical Professor of Surgery, Northwestern University School of Medicine, Chicago, Ill.

James E. Rasmussen, M.D.
Associate Professor of Dermatology, Department of Dermatology, University of Michigan School of Medicine, Ann Arbor, Mich.

June K. Robinson, M.D.
Assistant Professor of Dermatology and Surgery, Department of Dermatology, Northwestern University Medical School, Chicago, Ill.

Henry H. Roenigk, Jr., M.D.
Professor and Chairman of Dermatology, Department of Dermatology, Northwestern University Medical School, Chicago, Ill.

Richard K. Scher, M.D.
Clinical Professor of Dermatology, Department of Dermatology, New York University Medical School, New York, N.Y.

vii

Bryan C. Schultz, M.D.
Instructor, Department of Dermatology, Northwestern University Medical School, Chicago, Ill.

Chester Raymond Zeiss, M.D.
Assistant Professor of Medicine, Department of Allergy, Northwestern University Medical School, Chicago, Ill.

Charles Zugerman, M.D.
Assistant Professor of Dermatology, Department of Dermatology, Northwestern University Medical School, Chicago, Ill.

CONTENTS

Plate I

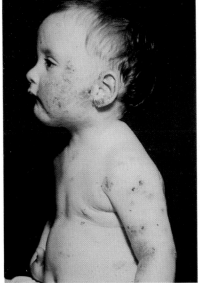

Fig. 4.1

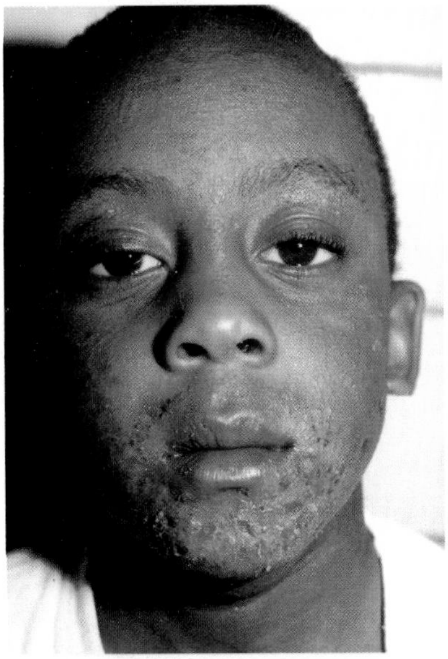

Fig. 5.4

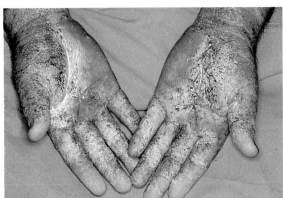

Fig. 6.3

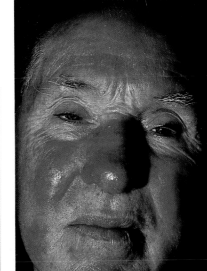

Fig. 7.2

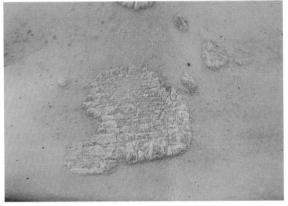

Fig. 8.1

Plate II

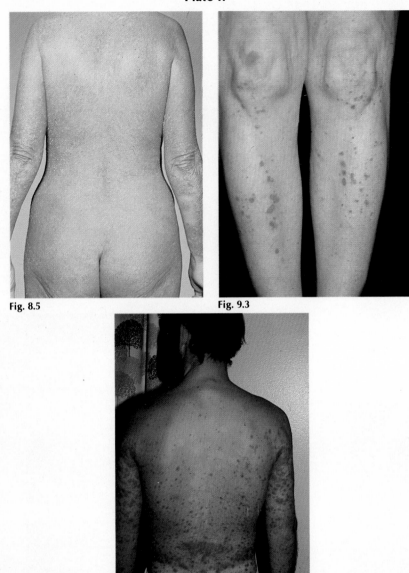

Fig. 8.5

Fig. 9.3

Fig. 9.9

Fig. 8.5. Generalized erythroderma due to psoriasis vulgaris.

Fig. 9.3. Lichen planus with papular lesions over both legs.

Fig. 9.9. Extensive lesions of pityriasis rosea.

Plate III

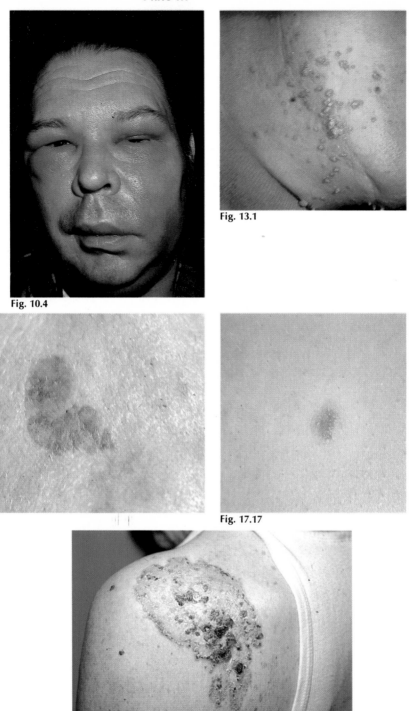

Fig. 10.4

Fig. 13.1

Fig. 17.2

Fig. 17.17

Fig. 18.4

Fig. 10.4. Erysipelas of face.

Fig. 13.1. Multiple warts in bearded area. These are spread by shaving. Eradication is difficult.

Fig. 17.2. Seborrheic keratosis. Stuck on, or glued on, appearance of lesion.

Fig. 17.17. Halo nevus. Central lesion is an intradermal nevus.

Fig. 18.4. Large superficial basal cell epithelioma. Irregular, somewhat elevated border, erythema with scaling, crusted, superficial ulceration.

Plate IV

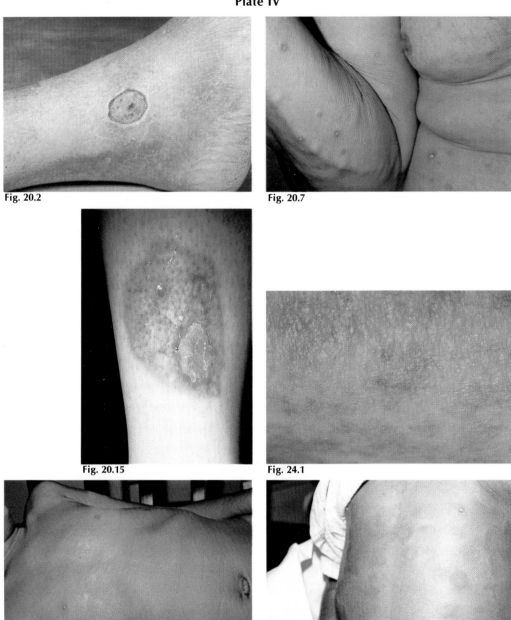

Fig. 20.2

Fig. 20.7

Fig. 20.15

Fig. 24.1

Fig. 24.2

Fig. 24.3

Plate V

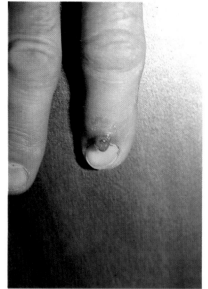

Fig. 27.13

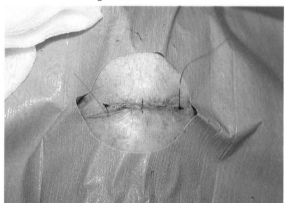

Fig. 28.7

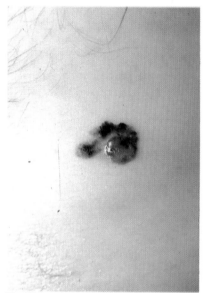

Fig. 28.8

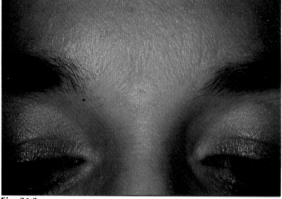

Fig. 31.3

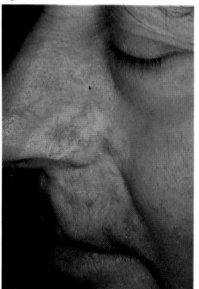

Fig. 32.8

CHAPTER 1

GROSS MORPHOLOGIC DIAGNOSIS OF SKIN DISEASES

JUNJI HASEGAWA

In an era of sophisticated laboratory diagnosis, physicians may forget the essential first step in the diagnosis of skin diseases—the interpretation of the morphology of the lesion. Scientific dermatology began when Plenck of Vienna first advocated in 1776 the classification of skin diseases based on the morphology of the lesion and not the distribution pattern. The diagnosis of a cutaneous lesion or a disseminated eruption is a three-step procedure: 1) the examination of the lesion, 2) the classification of the lesion, and 3) the interpretation. Admittedly, in some cases, the procedure must be repeated at other levels. For example: biopsy examination, classification, and microscopic interpretation, or examination for bacteria and fungi, classification, and interpretation with respect to the lesion are two common procedure cycles on levels other than gross morphology. In this chapter, however, we will restrict the discussion to the intial cycle of gross morphologic examination, classification, and interpretation of cutaneous eruptions.

EXAMINATION

The examination of a cutaneous eruption, like any other part of the physical examination, ordinarily follows a careful history and requires a good light source for an even illumination. Frequently, a magnifying lens may be necessary. The examiner notes 1) the color, 2) reactive surface changes, 3) the level of the lesion, 4) the shape of the lesion, 5) the number and distribution pattern (Figs. 1.1–1.3), 6) the consistency or feel of the lesion, 7) other signs confirming the symptoms in the history, and 8) extracutaneous signs noted from the remainder of the physical examination. The number and distribution pattern can only be determined by examining the entire skin surface. The discipline of examining all of the cutaneous surface may also reveal the variability in the morphology of the lesions and aid in assessing the evolution of the eruption.

Color

The color of a lesion when it differs from that of the surrounding skin may be due to surface cellular changes, vascular reactions, or pigment deposition, natural or foreign. Tan, brown, or black usually indicates deposits of melanin although reactive iron deposits following purpura or hemochromatosis may contribute to the brown color, and certain types of fungus infection may produce black or

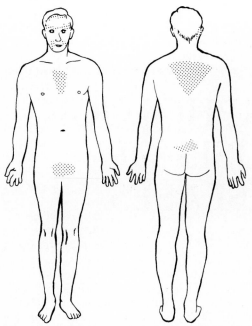

Fig. 1.1. Seborrheic distribution pattern. (Reproduced with permission from R.M. Caplan, A.W. Kopf, and M.B. Sulzberger: *A Brief Course in Dermatology. Skin Lesions Depicted and Defined, Part 1, Primary Lesions.* Institute for Dermatologic Communication and Education, San Francisco, 1980.)

Erythema appears in infinitely varying shades of red, the color of the blood in the subpapillary plexus being modified by the thickness of the stratum corneum, stratum granulosum, melanin, and the oxygenation of the hemoglobin in the microcirculation of the skin. A violaceous red hue is characteristic of lichen planus, the magenta or heliotrope color of the face of dermatomyositis, a dusky opaque red of psoriasis, and a cyanotic blue-red of stasis dermatitis and many tumors of the reticuloendothelial system. A red color that does not blanch on pressure suggests purpura. A yellow-red shade can be seen in xanthomas and necrobiosis lipoidica, icterus, and carotenemia.

Yellowish and off-white colors may be seen in many lesions with extracellular deposits like lipids (xanthomas), colloid degeneration, solar elastosis, pseudoxanthoma elasticum, su-

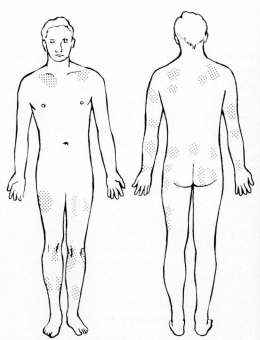

Fig. 1.2. Dermatitis herpetiformis—clusters over extensor areas and pelvic girdle areas. (Reproduced with permission from R.M. Caplan, A.W. Kopf, and M.B. Sulzberger: *A Brief Course in Dermatology. Skin Lesions Depicted and Defined, Part 1, Primary Lesions.* Institute for Dermatologic Communication and Education, San Francisco, 1980.)

brown pigment. Increased melanin production and deposition frequently follows injury and inflammation of the skin, and postinflammatory melanosis is a common cutaneous change. Melanin pigmentation, of course, can appear in a multitude of noninflammatory lesions such as chloasma of pregnancy, freckles, nevi, café au lait spots, and mastocytosis.

Similarly, the pale color of a lesion is commonly due to a lack, or total absence, of melanin and, paradoxically, postinflammatory depigmentation is a common type of cutaneous change. The pallor, due to a lack of melanin, also occurs in noninflammatory diseases such as vitiligo, albinism, and some patients with tinea versicolor. The pale color may also be due to edema of the upper dermis (lichen sclerosus et atrophicus), fibrosis (morphea), or permanent vasoconstriction of the subpapillary plexus of vessels (nevus anemicus).

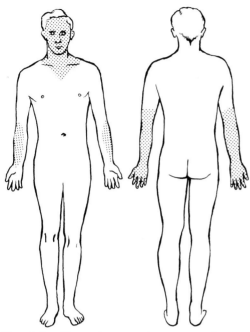

Fig. 1.3. Photodermatosis—exposed areas (modified by clothing other than average fashion). (Reproduced with permission from R.M. Caplan, A.W. Kopf, and M.B. Sulzberger: *A Brief Course in Dermatology. Skin Lesions Depicted and Defined, Part 1, Primary Lesions.* Institute for Dermatologic Communication and Education, San Francisco, 1980.)

perficial cysts, and collagen (scar and perforating collagenosis). Foreign pigments are capable of producing colors of much greater range than those of natural pigments, and bizarre colors may be seen in accidental or deliberate tatoos. The diagnosis of brightly colored lesions is ordinarily not a problem.

Reactive Surface Changes

Reactive surface changes consist of 1) vesicle, bulla, crust, and erosion; 2) scale; 3) keratosis; 4) lichenification; 5) pustule; 6) atrophy; and, paradoxically, 7) absence of surface changes. Vesicles are lesions filled with clear fluid and represent an acute cutaneous reaction. A bulla is a fluid-filled lesion larger than an arbitrary diameter of 1 cm. Crusts are straw-colored, dried, tissue fluid and in-

dicate concomitant or antecedent gross or microscopic vesicles that have ruptured. Erosions are superficial loss of tissue or shallow ulcers frequently suggesting a preexisting vesicle or bulla. Scales are stratum corneum desquamating in lamellar fashion as flakes and usually accompany mild inflammatory reaction of the skin or a subsiding stage of an inflammation. Keratoses are rough surfaced lesions with a dense adherent compact stratum corneum and differ from the loose flaking stratum corneum comprising scales. Lichenification is the thickening of the epidermis and appears grossly as increased skin surface markings much like the surface of the leather in a basketball. Pustules are lesions filled with pus. They frequently harbor microorganisms, but some of the chronic pustulosis show no organisms with current laboratory methods. Atrophy may appear as 1) a depressed lesion indicating diminished tissue volume (example, linear scleroderma), 2) fibrosis usually with shrinkage of the tissues but occasionally without visible depression of the surface of the lesion (example, discoid lupus erythematosus) and 3) pallor (example, lichen sclerosus et atrophicus). Finally, the lesions with no reactive surface changes comprise a large group usually with a smooth surface but occasionally a wrinkled one. Such lesions indicate a minimum of epidermal inflammatory reaction (example, basal cell carcinoma without ulceration) or a deeper dermal or subcutaneous pathologic process. Microscopic tissue examination is usually indicated in this group of lesions although a presumptive diagnosis is often possible on gross morphology alone. The wheal of urticaria is a common but especially easily recognizable lesion in this group.

Level

The level of the surface of the lesions (Fig. 1.4) determines the classification into raised lesions (papule, nodule, tumor—terms applied to lesions of increasing size), lesions with the surface level to the surrounding skin (macule) and therefore dependent on differences in color for detection, and depressed lesions (Fig. 1.5) (one form of atrophy). For the neophyte, it is preferable to try to classify lesions as raised when he is torn between minimally

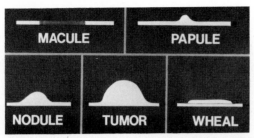

Fig. 1.4. Classification based on the level of the surface of the lesion. (Reproduced with permission from R.M. Caplan, A.W. Kopf, and M.B. Sulzberger: *A Brief Course in Dermatology. Skin Lesions Depicted and Defined, Part 2, Secondary and Special Lesions.* Institute for Dermatology Communication and Education, San Francisco, Calif., 1980.)

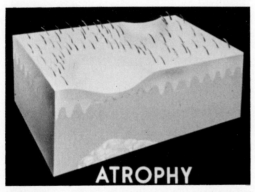

Fig. 1.5. A depressed lesion is one form of atrophy. (Reproduced with permission from R.M. Caplan, A.W. Kopf, and M.B. Sulzberger: *A Brief Course in Dermatology. Skin Lesions Depicted and Defined, Part 2, Secondary and Special Lesions.* Institute for Dermatologic Communication and Education, San Francisco, Calif., 1980.)

raised and flat classifications. Similarly, classification as a depressed lesion is preferable when in doubt about minimally depressed and flat lesions.

Shape

Cutaneous lesions frequently have distinctive shapes that aid in morphologic diagnosis. The polygonal papule of lichen planus, the linear inflammatory reaction of contact der-

matitis to plants, the pigmentation resembling whip marks in bleomycin therapy, the ovoid lesions of pityriasis rosea, and the corymbose or satellite lesions resembling petals on a daisy occasionally seen in secondary syphilis are just a few examples.

Number and Distribution Pattern

While the classification and diagnosis of skin diseases based primarily upon the distribution pattern is extremely treacherous, it is a useful observation in conjunction with other observations in the interpretation of the pooled data. A bilateral symmetrical eruption usually favors diseases in which the inciting agents are disseminated by the blood stream. Localized or bizarre asymmetric distribution pattern usually indicates inciting agents of external origin. The exception to these rules is the fixed drug eruption. A dermatome pattern suggests diseases related to the nervous system. Lesions along the lymphatic channels suggest centripetal spread of infectious agents.

Consistency

Frequently, the palpation of the lesion yields clues to the diagnosis. The absence of resistance to the palpating fingers in a lesion is almost diagnostic of neurofibromatosis. The unexpected hardness of a nodule suggests bony tumors, granular cell myoblastoma, massive calcium deposition, and hard foreign materials. A cheeselike consistency suggests a cyst. Fibromas and lipomas have a firm consistency and are usually freely movable on the underlying structures. Painful and tender tumors suggest glomus tumor, neuroma, eccrine spiradenoma, angiosarcoma, leiomyoma and, occasionally, foreign body reactions. The crepitus of gas in the skin is unusual but is easily classified.

Signs Confirming Symptoms

When patients speak of severe itching, the physician looks specifically for excoriations, lichenification, surface inflammation, or abrasions of rubbing. Such signs permit some objective assessment of the severity of the itch-

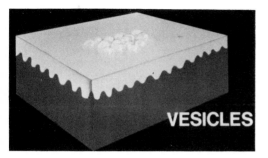

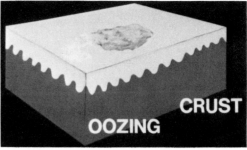

Fig. 1.6. Vesicles imply acute inflammation. (Reproduced with permission from R.M. Caplan, A.W. Kopf, and M.B. Sulzberger: *A Brief Course in Dermatology. Skin Lesions Depicted and Defined, Part 2, Secondary and Special Lesions.* Institute for Dermatologic Commmunication and Education, San Francisco, Calif., 1980.)

Fig. 1.7. Oozing and crusting imply inflammation. (Reproduced with permission from R.M. Caplan, A.W. Kopf, and M.B. Sulzberger: *A Brief Course in Dermatology. Skin Lesions Depicted and Defined, Part 2, Secondary and Special Lesions.* Institute for Dermatologic Communication and Education, San Francisco, Calif., 1980.)

Table 1.1
Classification of the Lesion

Lesion	Classification

Vesicle-bulla-crust-erosion
  Erythema
  Itching
	Acute inflammation

Lichenification
  Erythema
  Itching
	Chronic inflammation
	  (Fig. 1.8)

Rough surfaced, compact, adherent stratum corneum	Keratosis (Fig. 1.9)
Depressed lesion, minimally depressed but palpably fibrotic lesion, or minimally depressed but palpably pale lesion of subepidermal edema	Atrophy (Fig. 1.10)
Pustule or pus	Pyoderma
Lack of surface reactive changes Palpable or raised lesion	Dermal lesions including subcutaneous lesions
Macular erythema disappearing on pressure and no surface reactive changes	Erythema
Macular erythema persisting after application of pressure and no surface reactive changes	Purpura (Fig. 1.11)
Tan-brown macule and no surface reactive changes or palpable resistance	Hyperpigmentation
Pale macule and no surface reactive changes or palpable resistance	Hypopigmentation (Fig. 1.12)
Loss of tissue including the epidermis and no evidence of specific surface reactive changes or dermal changes at the margins	Ulcer (Fig. 1.13)

ing. In a pigmented eruption, rubbing a small area of the lesion may be followed by urticaria (Darier's sign) and confirms the diagnosis of mastocytosis. Painful and tender nodules may be palpated gently to confirm the changing shape of a contracting smooth muscle tumor. An history of massive shedding or breaking of scalp hairs without visible alopecia may be checked by traction of hairs on representative areas of the scalp.

Extracutaneous Signs

The diagnosis based on gross morphology of the skin eruption must be tempered by the physical examination of the patient as a whole. An eruption which may be classic dermatitis herpetiformis may prove to be a vesicular eruption secondary to a gastric carcinoma. A presumptive drug eruption at the beginning of the examination may be modified to an eruption secondary to a leukemia at the end of the examination. By assembling all of the data of the examination, the physician may begin the process of classifying the reaction pattern of the eruption.

CLASSIFICATION OF THE LESION

While bright unnatural colors of lesions imply foreign pigment deposits, the various shades of erythema due to the vasodilatation of the dermal vasculature are relatively nonspecific changes induced by an endless list of

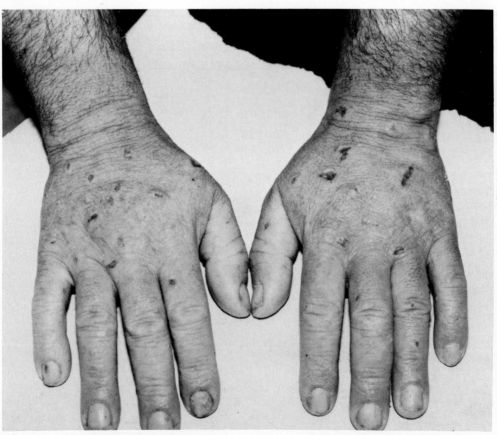

Fig. 1.8. Chronic Dermatitis. (Reproduced with permission from R.M. Caplan, A.W. Koipf, and M.B. Sulzberger: *A Brief Course in Dermatology. Skin Lesions Depicted and Defined, Part 1, Primary Lesions.* Institute for Dermatologic Communication and Education, San Francisco, 1980.)

cutaneous diseases. A more rewarding classification begins with the consideration of reactive surface changes. The combination of erythema, itching, and vesicle-bulla-crust-erosion imply acute inflammation (Figs. 1.6 and 1.7). Lesions manifesting lichenification, itching, and erythema classify as chronic inflammation. The classification of some other features of lesions is summarized in Table 1.1.

INTERPRETATION

An acute inflammation may be interpreted as evidence of an acute dermatitis or some of the specific vesiculobullous diseases that may manifest itching and erythema. The minimum prerequisite for interpretation beyond this point is familiarity with the gross morphology of at least five vesiculobullous diseases: 1) the fragile blister of pemphigus and the easy separation of the epidermis adjacent to the blister (Nikolsky's sign), 2) clustered

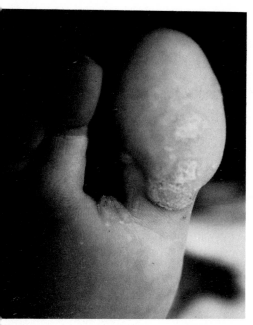

Fig. 1.9. Keratosis (verruca). (Reproduced with permission from R.M. Caplan, A.W. Kopf, and M.B. Sulzberger: *A Brief Course in Dermatology. Skin Lesions Depicted and Defined, Part 1, Primary Lesions.* Institute for Dermatologic Communication and Education, San Francisco, 1980.)

lesions of dermatitis herpetiformis and their distribution over the extensor surfaces of the extremities and the shoulder and pelvic girdle areas, 3) the lesion within a lesion (iris and target lesion) or erythema multiforme, 4) the vesicles and bullae in patients over 60, and 5) the blisters on the exposed areas—upper extremities, face, and neck—in prophyria cutanea tarda. If the physician can place these diseases low on the list of possible diagnoses, he can consider the category of acute dermatitis. The shape and distribution pattern frequently aids in arriving at a more specific diagnosis. A dermatitis affecting 95–100% of the cutaneous surface is exfoliative dermatitis; dermatitis affecting the cubital and popliteal fossae, neck, wrists, and/or ankles, is a flexural dermatitis (usually atopic dermatitis); dermatitis affecting the face, V-area of the neck and chest, and the distal parts of the upper extremities, is probably a photodermatitis; and a dermatitis of the scalp, face (especially the nasolabial folds) and eyebrows, sternal, and/or interscapular areas, is a seborrheic dermatitis. Differential diagnosis of exfoliative dermatitis, photodermatitis, atopic dermatitis, seborrheic dermatitis, and dermatitis with other distribution patterns will be discussed in appropriate chapters.

Similarly, a chronic inflammation may be interpreted as evidence of chronic dermatitis or some of the specific papulosquamous diseases that may have itching and erythema. The minimum prerequisite for interpretation beyond this point is familiarity with the gross morphology of at least three papulosquamous eruptions: 1) the sharply outlined lesion with a dusky opaque red base frequently covered with abundant scales—psoriasis vulgaris, 2) bilateral symmetrically tan, finely scaling, ovoid lesions with the long axis parallel to the lines of skin tension—pityriasis rosea, and 3) shiny-surfaced polygonal violaceous-red papules of lichen planus. In conjunction with these three, it is useful to consider the eruption of secondary syphilis which can be confirmed by serologic testing and tinea which can be confirmed by potassium hydroxide preparation of the scales examined under the microscope and by fungus culture. If these five can be placed low on the list of possible diagnoses, the physician may consider chronic dermatitis and follow the same procedure described

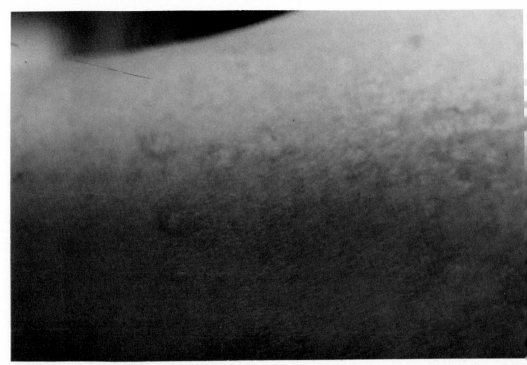

Fig. 1.10. Lichen sclerosus et atrophicus. (Reproduced with permission from R.M. Caplan, A.W. Kopf, and M.B. Sulzberger: *A Brief Course in Dermatology. Skin Lesions Depicted and Defined, Part 1, Primary Lesions.* Institute for Dermatologic Communication and Education, San Francisco, 1980.)

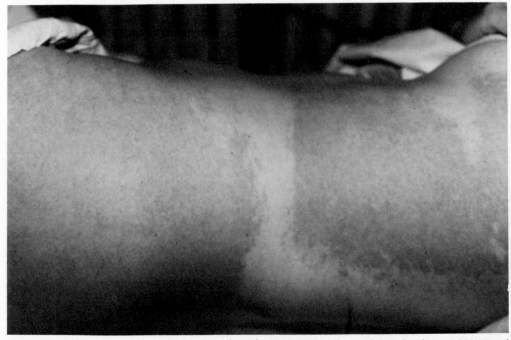

Fig. 1.11. Drug eruption. (Reproduced with permission from R.M. Caplan, A.W. Kopf, and M.B. Sulzberger: *A Brief Course in Dermatology. Skin Lesions Depicted and Defined, Part 1, Primary Lesions.* Institute for Dermatologic Communication and Education, San Francisco.)

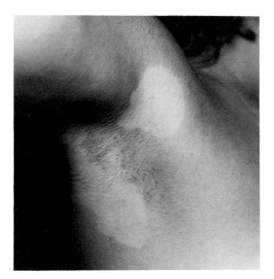

Fig. 1.12. Vitiligo. (Reproduced with permission from R.M. Caplan, A.W. Kopf, and M.B. Sulzberger: *A Brief Course in Dermatology. Skin Lesions Depicted and Defined, Part 1, Primary Lesions.* Institute for Dermatologic Communication and Education, San Francisco, 1980.)

above, using the distribution pattern as an aid to diagnosis.

The interpretation of keratosis leads to verruca, seborrheic keratosis, actinic keratosis, keratoacanthoma, keratosis follicularis, and many others that may be listed in the index of the major texts of dermatology. Atrophy may be interpreted as a manifestation of morphea, lichen sclerosus et atrophicus, macular atophy, acrodermatitis chronica atrophicans, discoid lupus erythmatosus, and others. Pyoderma (Fig. 1.14) may be interpreted as any of a multitude of cutaneous infections discussed in texts on bacterial, viral, and rickettsial diseases; "sterile" pustules of palmoplantar pustulosis, acropustulosis, pustular psoriasis, or the cutaneous lesions of Reiter's disease; or infectious eczematoid dermatitis. Dermal lesions frequently require biopsy and microscopic examination even when a presumptive diagnosis is possible. The classification of erythema is restricted to those erythematous lesions that cannot be classified on the basis of surface reactive changes. This definition is necessitated by the observation that vasodilatation is a relatively nonspecific reaction occurring in most cutaneous diseases. This re-

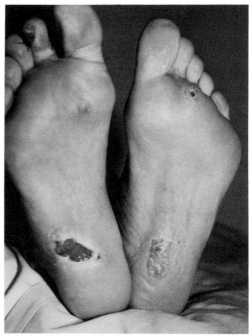

Fig. 1.13. Diabetic ulcer. (Reproduced with permission from R.M. Caplan, A.W. Kopf, and M.B. Sulzberger: *A Brief Course in Dermatology. Skin Lesions Depicted and Defined, Part 1, Primary Lesions.* Institute for Dermatologic Communication and Education, San Francisco, 1980.)

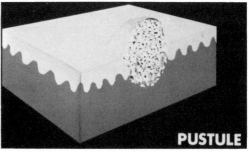

Fig. 1.14. Pustules imply a pyoderma. (Reproduced with permission from R.M. Caplan, A.W. Kopf, and M.B. Sulzberger: *A Brief Course in Dermatology. Skin Lesions Depicted and Defined, Part 2, Secondary and Special Lesions.* Institute for Dermatologic Communication and Education, San Francisco, Calif., 1980.)

striction makes it possible to tap the index of textbooks on dermatology. A similar restriction applies to hyperpigmentation and hypopigmentation and allows the physician to con-

sult the section on the diseases of pigmentation or melanin formation. The restriction is
also applied to the classification of ulcers. A
multitude of lesions ulcerate and the discipline of examining the margins for clues on
the essential morphology is more rewarding
than the evaluation of all lesions which ulcerate.

Acquiring the ability to interpret the gross
morphology of the skin requires repetition
and practice, much like attaining facility in
understanding and speaking a foreign lan-
guage. For those physicians who do not have
the time for protracted or intense training, the
application of the procedure of examination,
classification, and interpretation of cutaneous
lesions in their practice with the aid of a
major textbook in dermatology will lead to
some facility in the diagnosis of cutaneous
diseases.

CHAPTER 2

PROCEDURES AND TECHNIQUES IN DERMATOLOGY

CHARLES ZUGERMAN

Diagnostic as well as therapeutic techniques and procedures are employed routinely by the dermatologist. Therapeutic techniques include surgical diathermy, cryosurgery, ultraviolet light therapy, radiation therapy and surgical curettage, hair transplantation, and dermabrasion. Diagnostic techniques include the cutaneous biopsy, the Tzank smear, Wood's light examination, phototesting, patch testing, diascopy and potassium hydroxide preparations. There are a few procedures such as the cutaneous punch biopsy which may be employed diagnostically as well as therapeutically. The following chapter deals primarily with diagnostic techniques commonly employed by the dermatologist.

BIOPSIES

The cutaneous biopsy is a benign but important adjunct to the diagnosis of skin disease. It is most useful if both the type of lesion as well as the site of the lesion are carefully selected. Biopsies of diseases and conditions such as chronic dermatitis, acne, impetigo, striae, insect bites, pityriasis rosea and pyoderma are usually not important in making the correct diagnosis. In these cases, the disease can be diagnosed by history of physical or laboratory examination. On the other hand, biopsies of processes such as vasculitis, bullous disease, malignant tumors, lichen planus, granuloma annulare, adnexal tumors, and cutaneous granulomas are of paramount importance in making the correct diagnosis.

Selection of the appropriate biopsy site is equally important in making the appropriate diagnosis. Primary lesions are the most useful for biopsy while secondary lesions such as excoriations, fissures, or ulcerations are not helpful. The biopsy should be performed on unaltered fresh lesions in order to avoid these secondary changes. A new and fully developed lesion is considerably more useful than is an old, healing one. When biopsing a blister, it is important to include with the biopsy specimen a surrounding rim of normal tissue.

Once a correct site is selected, the area should be cleansed and locally anesthetized with either lidocaine or procaine.

Dermatologists use a number of techniques in performing a cutaneous skin biopsy including the cutaneous punch, the excision, curettage, shave biopsy, or incisional biopsy. A few of these methods will be described briefly in the following paragraphs.

Cutaneous Punch

In using the cutaneous punch (Fig. 2.1) the instrument is driven through the skin with a

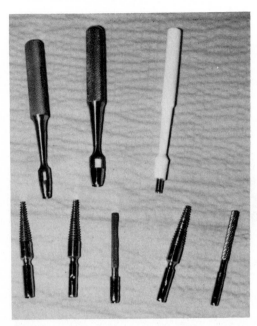

Fig. 2.1. Disposable punch (*upper, right*), reusable punches (*upper left*), and hair transplant punches (*bottom*) are shown.

rotary motion to a depth of approximately 4 mm (Fig. 2.2). The physician must go deep enough with the punch to include areas of pathology. If the pathologic process is deep, superficial punch biopsy may be inadequate. When performing a punch biopsy, tension is provided on the skin perpendicular to normal skin lines. In this manner, when the tension is released, the skin biopsy site will form an oval in the direction of the skin lines, giving the patient a more suitable cosmetic effect. A disposable punch is now available and punch biopsy sets can be obtained in all sizes from 2–10 mm. At completion of the biopsy procedure, the skin can be closed with a suture which is removed in 5–10 days or the wound left open to heal secondarily.

Excisional Biopsies

Excisional biopsies are useful for larger lesions that cannot easily be removed with a punch (Fig. 2.3). This procedure is somewhat more difficult and requires a more extensive area of anesthesia. It is useful to outline the lesion to be biopsied with a dye such as gen-

tian violet in order to localize the lesion before anesthesia obscures normal markings. The excision is made along skin lines with a No. 15 scalpel blade in order to give the patient the most cosmetically pleasing effect (Fig. 2.4). At completion of the biopsy procedure, the skin is again closed with sutures (Fig. 2.5).

Curettage

Curettage can also be used as a biopsy technique, but it is usually reserved for tumors whose architecture is unimportant (Fig. 2.6). Because curettage fragments the lesion, this technique is performed only on lesions such as basal cell carcinomas and seborrheic keratoses. If the correct diagnosis is uncertain at the time that the procedure is undertaken, a punch biopsy may be performed prior to curettage and desiccation. The area to be curetted is anesthetized and a small ring-shaped curette is applied to the lesion. A scraping or digging motion is used to remove a clump of tissue which is then sent to the pathologist for examination. If a basal cell carcinoma is suspected, then the technique is repeated two or three times in order to remove the entire mass of tissue. This allows for both the diagnosis and treatment of a suspected basal cell carcinoma or seborrheic keratosis at the same patient visit.

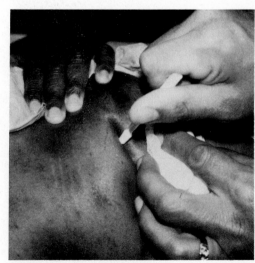

Fig. 2.2. A Keye's punch is being driven through the skin with a rotary motion.

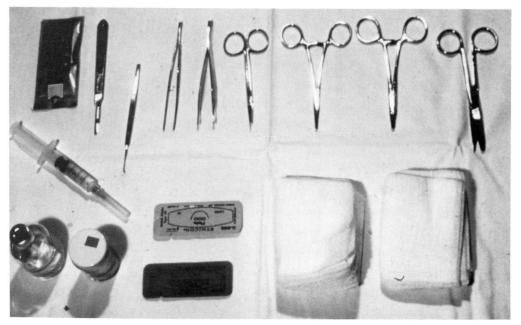

Fig. 2.3. Instruments necessary to perform an excisional biopsy.

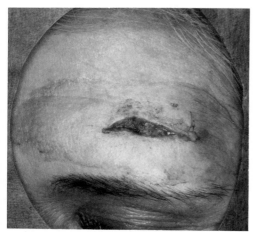

Fig. 2.4. An elliptical excision prior to closure. (Courtesy of Dr. June K. Robinson.)

Shave Biopsies

Shake biopsies are usually performed on superficial lesions such as seborrheic keratoses. The lesion is anesthetized and is raised up by pressure between the thumb and the first finger. A single-edged razor blade or No. 11 blade can be used to shave the lesion off while

hemostasis is obtained by using either a hot-tipped cautery or trichloracetic acid.

Incisional Biopsies

A dermatologist occasionally employs an incisional biopsy technique. This is reserved

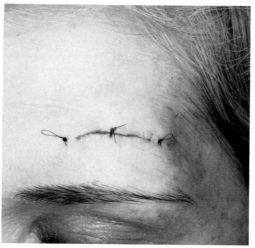

Fig. 2.5. An elliptical excision after closure. (Courtesy of Dr. June K. Robinson.)

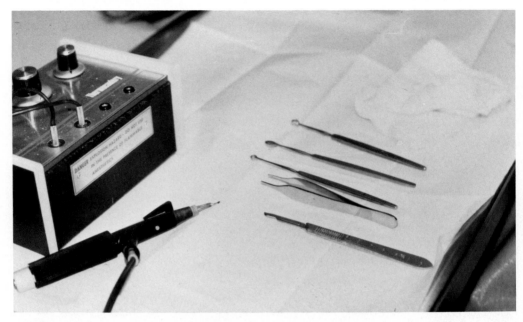

Fig. 2.6. Different sized curettes are available.

for lesions such as the keratoacanthoma which may be too large to excise. An eliptical incision is made into the lesion, including normal tissue on each side. In this way, an adequate biopsy specimen may be obtained without causing an unnecessarily extensive cosmetic defect.

After the biopsy is performed, the specimen must be correctly handled. It should not be squeezed with the forceps so that distortion of the tissue occurs. It must be carefully removed from the normal skin and placed in a bottle containing 10% formaldehyde. The bottle should be labeled as to the type of lesion, the name of the patient, and the area of the body from which the lesion was obtained. Detailed information both about the patient and his lesion should be included for use by the pathologist.

POTASSIUM HYDROXIDE MOUNT

The potassium hydroxide (KOH) mount is useful for the identification of hyphae and spores (Fig. 2.7). Consequently, KOH preparations are vital in the diagnosis of candidiasis, tinea and, in some cases, deep fungal disease such as blastomycosis. In addition,

some dermatologists find KOH preps useful in the diagnosis of scabies.

Dry scaly lesions are usually scraped with a No. 15 blade or the edge of a microscope slide. Vesicular lesions are examined first by removing the roof of the vesicle with a No. 11 blade and then placing the overlying skin on a microscope slide. It is useless to examine vesicle fluid in these infections. In cases of scabies, KOH or mineral oil is placed on the skin over a burrow or vesicle and the entire lesion is scraped. The tissue to be examined is placed on a microscope slide and is covered with 1 or 2 drops of 10–20% KOH in water or glycerin. A coverslip is placed over the specimen and the slide is gently heated for a few seconds in order to dissolve the keratin. It is important not to boil the tissue since this can destroy hyphae making diagnosis impossible. The specimen is then examined under a high dry microscope objective looking for fungal hyphae, spores, or mites (Fig. 2.8).

DIASCOPY

Diascopy is a technique that is helpful in delineating purpura from erythema secondary to vascular dilatation. The diascope is any

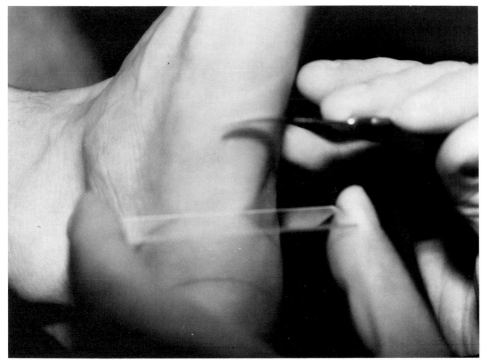

Fig. 2.7. Scales being removed from the patient for examination with potassium hydroxide KOH.

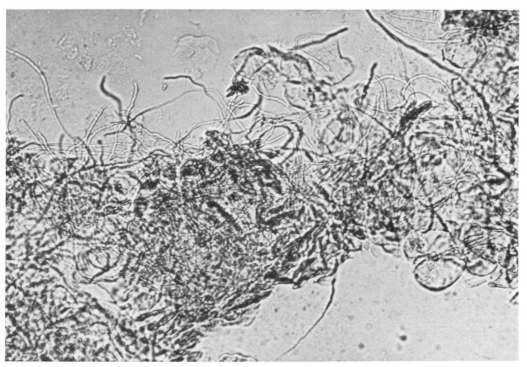

Fig. 2.8. A positive potassium hydroxide (KOH) mount demonstrating fungal hyphae. (Medium magnification).

clear piece of glass and often microscope slides are used for this purpose. The slide is placed against the lesion and slight pressure is applied. Blanching indicates that the vessels are intact while lack of blanching suggests purpura. This technique is used in the diagnosis of vasculitis.

WOOD'S LIGHT EXAMINATION

The Wood's light is an ultraviolet light containing a filter which transmits light at a wavelength of 365 mm. The patient is placed in a darkened room and the lesion in question is examined under the Wood's light. This technique may be used in the detection of a number of diseases including ringworm, tinea versicolor, erythrasmas, vitiligo, and porphyria. Ringworm caused by the organisms *Microsporum canis* and *Microsporum audouinii* fluoresces blue-green whereas tinea versicolor fluoresces a golden color. Erythrasma, a disease caused by a bacterium *Corynebacterium minutissimum*, fluoresces red because of porphyrins produced by the bacteria. Vitiligo, which is a depigmenting disease, shows up under Wood's light because the lack of pigmentation causes light to be reflected. The Wood's light is also useful in the detection of the presence of certain drugs in the skin. For example, tetracycline is used in the treatment of acne, and it is occasionally necessary to determine whether the patient is correctly taking the drug. If yellow fluorescence of tetracycline, especially in the mouth and around the hair follicles, is evident under Wood's light, the patient is probably taking the medication correctly.

PATCH TESTING

Patch testing entails placing test material in a standard form under an occluded patch on a patient's back or arm in an attempt to reproduce an allergic contact dermatitis similar to the patient's eruption.

Role of Patch Testing in Clinical Diagnosis

Allergic contact dermatitis will be described fully in Chapter 6. Determination of the etiology of contact dermatitis is made possible by an accurate medical history, physical examination, and patch testing. It is important to remember that once the patient becomes allergic to a cutaneous hapten the entire skin surface is sensitized. The eczema appears, however, only in areas where the contact is made, but patch testing is possible because the entire skin surface will react.

Patch testing is indicated in order to confirm the diagnosis of allergic contact dermatitis. Since allergy may be simulated by other types of eruptions, patch testing is useful in ruling out the diagnoses of psoriasis, atopic dermatitis, tinea, seborrheic dermatitis, and lichen simplex chronicus. Patch testing is also indicated in situations in which an allergic contact dermatitis is superimposed upon an irritant contact dermatitis or a dyshidrotic eczema.

Several countraindications to patch testing should be discussed. First, when the patient has acute dermatitis of any etiology, patch testing may cause a flare of the dermatitis. Second, if the composition or the degree of irritancy of the material that is to be patch tested is unknown, patch testing should not be performed. Finally, patch testing with potent allergens such as *Rhus* oleoresin may lead to iatrogenic sensitization.

Techniques of Patch Testing

NATURE OF THE ANTIGEN

The material to be tested can be in either solid or liquid form. Before patch testing is performed, the content of the material should be known. Liquids and solids should be in a chemically pure state. If the material to be tested is a textile, it can be applied directly to the skin and covered with an occlusive tape. Larger solid material such as plastic, wood, or bark should be pulverized to a very fine powder. Excess pressure from jagged edges or thick rough surfaces may cause a false positive reaction. If one is testing material from shoes, a small curette is useful in digging out the antigen. Cosmetics, underarm deodorants, and emollient creams can be tested by applying the liquid material directly to the patch which is then applied to the patient's skin. When dealing with an irritating compound such as nail polish, the solvent can be removed from the nail polish by allowing it to evaporate prior to application, leaving intact the substance you wish to test. No material should ever be tested when the content or general nature of it is completely unknown. If the material is extremely toxic, it can cause a severe contact dermatitis or, even worse, it may be absorbed percutaneously causing a generalized reaction.

Another factor to consider is the vehicle in which the test substance is placed. An irritating vehicle such as chloroform or turpentine is totally inadequate. Allergenic materials such as lanolin are also inadequate as patch test vehicles. The best vehicle for a liquid or powder is petrolatum, because it does not evaporate, protects against oxidation, and stabilizes the substance to be tested. The concentration of the material in the vehicle is extremely important. The correct concentration of specific materials can be obtained from some of the books which are listed at the end of this chapter. In general, the concentration must be great enough so that the allergy can be elicited and not so great that the material to be tested is irritating.

The antigens most likely to cause contact dermatitis have been prepared at the correct concentration in the correct vehicles. This is called the standard patch test series, and its content depends upon several factors. First, as antigens are shown to be more or less irritating, they are added to or deleted from the standard patch test series. In addition, as the antigen is shown to be less prevalent as a cause in allergic dermatitis in the population concerned, it may be dropped from the standard test series. Finally, the standard patch test series may vary from one geographic location to the next.

Standard patch test materials are available from several sources (Table 2.1). Johnson & Johnson Pharmaceutical Company, in association with the American Academy of Dermatology and the North American Contact Dermatitis Group have put together a standard patch test series which is periodically modified. This currently includes 23 substances most of which are dispersed in petrolatum. This series includes allergenic medications, preservatives, perfumes, emollients, metals, and rubber compounds. Trolab, in Denmark, has an extensive list of patch test

Table 2.1
Patch Tests Materials

Substance	%
Medications	
Neomycin sulfate	20
Ammoniated mercury	1
Caine mix	8
Preservatives	
Parabens mix	15
Benzyl alcohol	5
Quaternium 15	2
Imidazolidinyl urea	2
Captan	1
Formaldehyde (aqueous)	2
Perfumes	
Balsum of Peru	5
Cinnamic alcohol	5
Hydroxycitronellal	4
Stabilizers and emollients	
Ethylenediamine dihydrochloride	1
Wood alcohols	30
Lanolin	100
Metals	
Potassium dichromate	0.5
Nickel sulfate	2.5
Rubber compounds	
Mercapto mix	1
Mercaptobenzothiazole	1
Thiuram mix	1
Naphthyl mix	1
p-Phenylenediamine mix	0.6
Carba mix	3
Others	
p-Chloro-m-xylenol	1
p-tert-Butylphenol	2
Epoxy resin	1

[a] All in petrolatum except as noted.

materials. These materials can be ordered individually and include a European standard of 28 chemicals similar to that which is produced by Johnson & Johnson. Hollister-Stier Laboratories in the United States also manufacturers several excellent screening test trays. The addresses for these companies are mentioned at the end of this chapter.

If it is necessary to patch test with non-standard materials, the chemical composition or the nature of the chemical should be known to the physician. One can look carefully at the description for normal use of the material in order to get an idea about its usual concentration and its solubility in oil or water. A solvent which is itself irritating should never be used to dissolve the material. In addition,

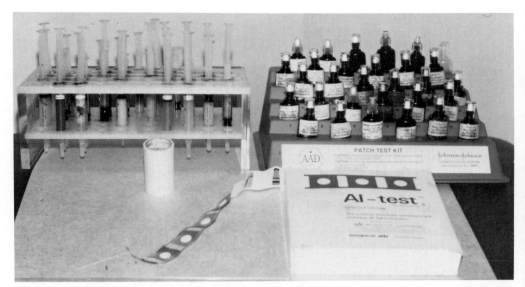

Fig. 2.9.   Materials necessary for performing a patch test. These include standard antigens, cellulose discs and occlusive tape.

the label on the bottle will give the physician an idea as to the overall strength and toxicity. A bathroom cleaner, for instance, is usually less dangerous to test than is an industrial cleanser. Most chemicals can be tested safely at 0.5%–1% concentration in petrolatum. Several exceptions to the rule include cosmetics, perfumes, antibiotics, lanolin, and preservatives which can be used at either a 10% or a 100% concentration.

APPLICATION OF THE ANTIGEN

The standardized patch test technique developed in the 1960s requires the application of the specific amount of material at a specified concentration in a suitable vehicle (Fig. 2.9). An occlusive tape is used to make the patch airtight. This is removed after 48 hours and readings are performed at 48, 72, or 96 hours. The usual site of application of the patch test is the upper or lower back but the lateral side of the arm can also be used. Other sites are unsuitable because of excessive trauma with premature loss of the patches or because of inadequate or irratic absorption of the material into the skin.

A cellulose disc on an aluminum strip is available commercially (Fig. 2.10). The material to be tested is placed on the proper vehicle and is applied to the cellulose strip

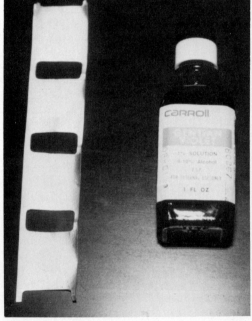

2.10.   An aluminum strip used for patch testing is shown along with gentian violet which is employed to mark the position of the patches on the patient's back.

(Fig. 2.11). If the standard patch test set is used, this material is applied to the strip. The test strips are placed in vertical rows on the

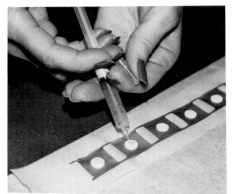

Fig. 2.11. Application of the test material to a cellulose patch.

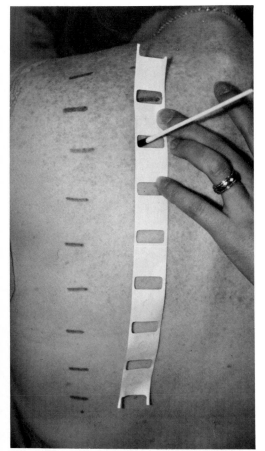

Fig. 2.12. The position of the patches is being carefully marked with gentian violet on the patient's back.

upper back with two to eight tests being applied per row (Fig. 2.12). The entire row is then taped in place using an occlusive tape

(Fig. 2.13). It is best to avoid placing the rows in areas where bending occurs such as on the midback or the lumbar area, since bending in these areas will cause the strips not to adhere properly. The rows are carefully marked and the location of each of the test materials is recorded on the patient's chart. The patches are then removed by the patient after 48 hours, and the physician interprets the test 48, 72, or 96 hours after application.

Reading and Interpreting Patch Tests

One of the most difficult problems in interpretation is deciding whether the result represents an irritant reaction or whether it demonstrates a true allergy. In several instances, it is impossible to determine whether the reaction is irritant or allergic. One reason for

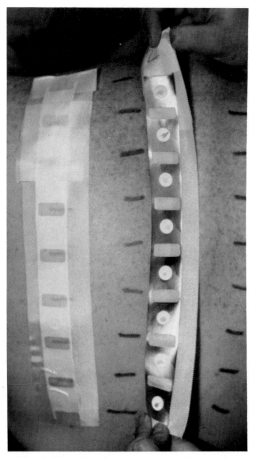

Fig. 2.13. Patches are taped in place.

reading the patch test on several days is that often an irritant reaction will fade rapidly after the patches are removed whereas a true allergy develops more slowly and reaches its peak at 48 or 96 hours after removal. The interpretation key that is currently employed by the North American Contact Dermatitis Group is as follows:

NT,	Not Tested
?,	Doubtful
1+,	Weak nonvesicular eruption, macular erythema
2+,	Strong edematous or vesicular eruption
3+,	Extreme spreading bullae or ulcer reaction
IR,	Irritant reaction
-,	Negative

In general, weak reactions are not significant except in cases of mild cosmetic allergy. Most allergens should yield 2+ or 3+ reactions in order to be considered positive (Fig. 2.14).

PITFALLS OF INTERPRETATION

There are several pitfalls encountered by the physician in the interpretation of a patch test (Table 2.2). False-positive reactions occur because the tested chemical is too irritating, either because of an excessively high concentration, because it is placed in an irritating vehicle, or because the skin surface is made irritable by the presence of other diseases such as atopic dermatitis. If the patient's contact dermatitis is in the acute phase, or if there is dermatitis close to the test site, a false positive reaction may result. Finally, false-positive reaction may occur secondary to excessive pressure at the site of application.

There are many causes of false-negative patch tests including an inadequately low concentration or the use of an incorrect vehicle. If the patch test fails to reproduce the conditions which prevail during the actual use of the test substance, then a false-negative result may result. Finally, a patient who is immunosuppressed may not react to a patch test.

The final major question which must be answered by the physician is that of relevance. Since there are many sources of exposure to

Fig. 2.14. A strongly positive patch test reaction to *p*-phenylenediamine in a patient with hair dye dermatitis.

**Table 2.2
Causes of False-Positive and
False-Negative Patch Tests**

False-Positive Reaction
  Material is irritating
    Because of vehicle, concentration, solvent
    or presence of irritating chemical in the
    patch-test compound
  Threshold of irritation of the patient's skin is
    low
    Because of concomitant disease such as
    acute dermatitis or atopic dermatitis, or
    because of dermatitis near the test site
  Readings are taken at the wrong time
  There is a *pressure* effect

False-Negative Reaction
  Material does not cause allergy
    Because of *improper application*, wrong
    vehicle, wrong concentration or
    application to wrong area of the body
  Reading is done at the wrong time
  The patient is unable to react to the material
    Because of drug therapy (e.g.
    corticosteroids) or because of
    immunosuppressive disease
  Conditions of exposure are not reproduced
  You are dealing with a *photoallergy*

---

specific chemicals in our environment, a positive patch test may simply indicate prior exposure and may have little to do with the current problem. In addition, cross-allergies and concommitant allergies can occur. There are instances when a patch test relates well to the patient's eczema and can explain the patient's problem. These are called relevant positive patch tests. In other situations, however, the patch test may simply be a "red herring" and may have little relevance to the problem.

Addresses for Patch Test Materials

1. Trolab
   6 B.A.N. Hansens Alle
   2900 Hellerup, Denmark
2. Hollister-Stier Laboratories
   P.O. Box 14957 Dept F74
   Atlanta, Ga. 30325
3. American Academy of Dermatology
   820 Davis Street
   Evanston, Ill. 60201

References

1. Epstein, E.: *Skin Surgery*, Ed. 4. Charles C Thomas, Springfield, Ill., 1977.
2. Caplan, R.M.: Medical uses of the Wood's lamp. JAMA *202:* 123, 1967.
3. Fregert, S., and Bandmann, H.J.: *Patch Testing*. Springer-Verlag, New York, 1975.
4. Malten, K.G., Nater, J.P., and Van Ketel, W.G.: *Patch Testing Guidelines*. Dekker and Van de Vegt, Nijmegen, The Netherlands, 1976.
5. Fisher, A.A.: *Contact Dermatitis*, Ed. 2, Lea & Febiger, Philadelphia, 1974.

CHAPTER 3

SPECIAL PROBLEMS IN PEDIATRIC SKIN DISEASE

NANCY B. ESTERLY

Most of the common skin diseases occur in individuals of all ages although the incidence of a particular disorder may vary considerably in different age groups. Certain problems, however, are limited to pediatric patients and will thus be encountered frequently by those physicians who care for infants and young children. The conditions to be discussed in this chapter are conveniently grouped under the headings of 1) Transient Lesions of the Neonate, 2) Nevoid Lesions (Birthmarks), and 3) Diaper Area Eruptions.

TRANSIENT LESIONS OF THE NEONATE

Skin lesions in the newborn infant, even when minor or evanescent, are a source of considerable concern to parents. Some of the most common entities that affect this age group are discussed below. Arrival at a specific diagnosis will often alleviate anxiety and permit nonintervention since many of these conditions are self-limited and are best managed expectantly.

Sebaceous Gland Hyperplasia and Milia

Minute, profuse, light yellow papules are frequently found on the forehead, nose, cheeks, and chin of the term infant. These lesions are frequently confused with milia, also seen in some newborns, but actually represent enlarged sebaceous glands which become visible at the site of the pilosebaceous duct pore. Since the hyperplastic glands are the result of maternal androgen effect, they gradually diminish in size and disappear during the first few weeks after birth. An occasional infant may have coexistent lesions on the mucosal surface of the lower lip. (Fig. 3.1).

In contrast, milia are usually larger, white in color, and more randomly distributed. Sites of predilection are the cheeks, nasolabial folds, forehead, chin, and periorbital areas. These firm papules are caused by an invagination of epithelium which forms a keratin-producing inclusion cyst. Similar lesions may also form in the mucosa (Epstein's pearls) and most frequently affect the midline palate or the gingivae. These lesions are innocuous, whether cutaneous or mucosal, and exfoliate spontaneously within the first several weeks of life.

Acne Neonatorum

This condition is also benign and self-limited and may be extremely perplexing diagnostically. Onset occurs during the first few weeks of life, and affected infants are usually male. The lesions are those of adolescent acne; open and closed comedones, inflammatory

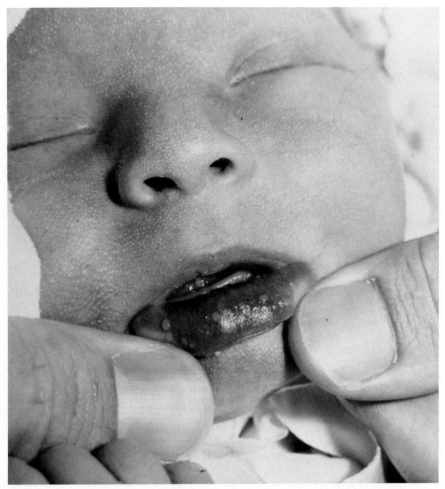

Fig. 3.1. Numerous tiny yellow sebaceous glands representing sebaceous hyperplasia of the newborn visible on the nose, cheeks, and chin. Enlarged glands in the labial mucous membrane are also present.

papules and, only rarely, nodulocystic lesions. Cheeks, nose, and chin are the preferred sites of involvement (Fig. 3.2).

Although neonatal acne is often attributed to maternal androgen effect, the postpartum onset and persistence throughout early infancy makes that explanation untenable. It may be that maternal androgen can be implicated in the initial event, but it is difficult to avoid the conclusion that the infant's hormones must be at least partially responsible for the eruption. A genetic component may be involved since a strong family history for acne is said to be present in these instances, and one could speculate that a genetically

determined end organ hyperresponsiveness to androgen in the male infant might account for the condition. Certainly, no known overt endocrine disturbances have been detected in these infants.

If tolerated, mild neonatal acne may be ignored since it resolves spontaneously. If treatment seems indicated, a mild benzoyl peroxide lotion or gel (5%) is appropriate for initial therapy. Alternatively, a sulfur and/or salicylic acid-containing lotion (e.g. Komed Mild Acne Lotion) may be applied once daily. If a comedonal component predominates, Retin-A Brand Tretinoin 0.05% cream in a once daily application may suffice. It is desirable

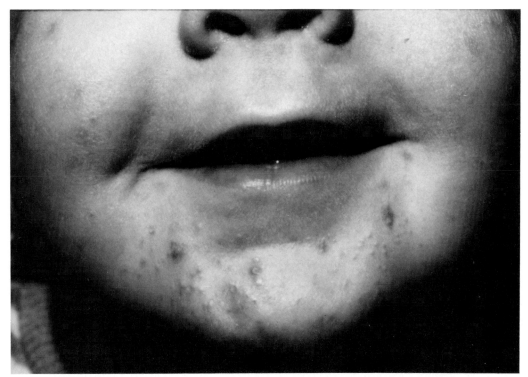

Fig. 3.2.   Multiple inflammatory papules and comedones on the cheeks and chin of an infant with acne.

to avoid harsh or abrasive soaps and washes or stronger preparations of benzoyl peroxide and vitamin A acid since they may cause undue irritation, erythema, and desquamation. Topical corticosteroids are never indicated and may, in fact, induce an acne rosacea mimicking neonatal acne. Parents should be informed that scarring is rare, therefore, aggressive management is inappropriate. Although it has been stated that these infants have severe acne as adolescents, more data is needed to support that contention.

Erythema Toxicum

This benign inflammatory cutaneous eruption occurs in approximately 50% of term infants and less commonly in preterm infants. Lesions appear most frequently during the first 3 days of life but may occur as late as 2 weeks of age. There is no predilection for sex, race, season, or geographic location.

The lesion of erythema toxicum is a small (1–3 mm) papulopustule which is firm, ivory or yellow in color, and surrounded by a broad erythematous halo (Fig. 3.3). Occasionally, only a splotchy erythema is present. These lesions erupt in crops, and may be sparse or profuse affecting any area of the body except palms and soles. Individual lesions persist from a few hours to a couple of days. The infant is otherwise well, and the lesions appear to be asymptomatic.

Erythema toxicum lesions may be confused with pustular melanosis, staphylococcal folliculitis, candidiasis, and other infectious eruptions. However, erythema toxicum is readily differentiated from these disorders by a Wright-stained smear of intralesional contents which demonstrates a monomorphous infiltrate of eosinophils. Cultures of the vesicopustules are always sterile. A peripheral eosinophilia of varying degree may be present as a transient phenomenon.

The etiology of erythema toxicum remains obscure despite attempts to incriminate chemicals, transplacentally acquired substances,

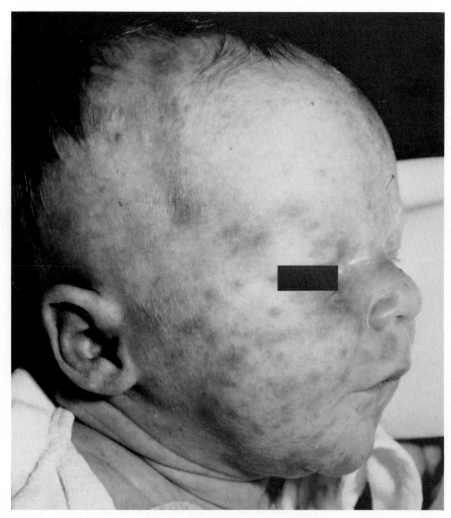

Fig. 3.3. Florid erythema toxicum on the face of a newborn.

and exogenous irritants. Histologically, the inflammatory response is confined to the area of the pilosebaceous follicle. Speculation that erythema toxicum represents a hypersensitivity reaction is based solely on the finding of eosinophilia and lacks further supportive evidence. Treatment is not indicated since the course is brief and the eruption harmless.

Transient Neonatal Pustular Melanosis

Pustular melanosis can be regarded as another eruption peculiar to the neonate which, like erythema toxicum, is benign and self-limited. The disorder is characterized by three types of lesions, not all of which are necessarily present simultaneously: 1) superficial pustules lacking a substantial erythematous base; 2) ruptured pustules represented by a collarette of fine scale which, at times, surrounds a central hyperpigmented macule; and 3) hyperpigmented macules (Fig. 3.4). One or all types of lesions are present at birth and lesions may be few or numerous involving all surfaces including the palms and soles. The pustules are evanescent lasting only a few hours and seem to represent the early phase of the disorder; they usually evolve into hyperpigmented macules. This eruption is more common in dark-skinned infants suggesting that the hyperpigmented macule may represent a

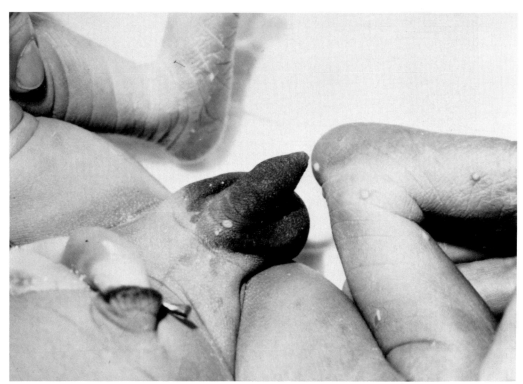

Fig. 3.4.   Lesions of transient neonatal pustular melanosis on the genitalia and legs.

postinflammatory response to the preceding intraepidermal pustule. Since the pustules are relatively brief in duration and are often ruptured at the time of the first bath, their presence may be missed, particularly in white infants who lack the postinflammatory pigmentary change.

The cause of this disorder is unknown, and affected infants are otherwise well. Smears of intralesional material demonstrate varying numbers of polymorphonuclear leukocytes, a few eosinophils, and amorphous debris. Cultures are sterile. The pustular phase may persist for 2–3 days; the macules may last for as long as 3 months but always fade eventually.

Miliaria

Morphologic interference with the function of the eccrine sweat glands may result in one of the forms of miliaria. Although this eruption may occur at any age, it is frequently a problem in infants and young children since they are often unable to convey their discomfort in an overheated environment. Miliaria was a regular occurrence in infants before the advent of air-conditioned nurseries and thermally controlled isolettes and it is now usually seen only in the neonate with hyperpyrexia.

The major forms of miliaria occurring in the infant and young child are miliaria crystallina and miliaria rubra. In the former, small, noninflammatory, thin-walled, superficial vesicles filled with crystal-clear fluid appear abruptly, often fusing to form bizarre-shaped loculations (Fig. 3.5). The blisters are the result of sweat retention within the stratum corneum and are easily ruptured even with gentle pressure. The underlying skin appears normal. Miliaria rubra consists of grouped, inflammatory papulopustules on an erythematous base and results from rupture of the intraepidermal portion of the sweat duct, sweat retention, and the subsequent inflammatory reaction. In a humid environment, the skin may become macerated and boggy promoting occlusion of the sweat duct pore.

Miliaria often occurs in the intertriginous

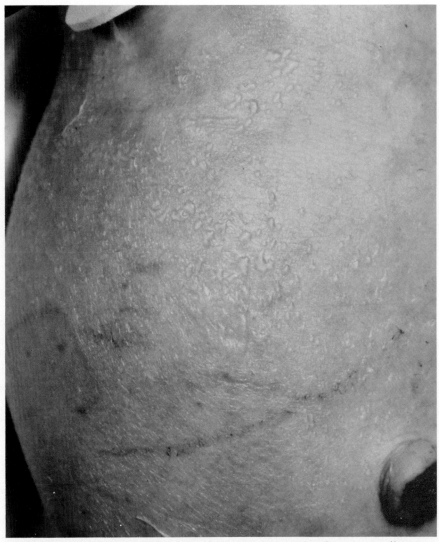

Fig. 3.5. Tiny irregularly shaped clear vesicles of miliaria crystallina.

areas but may also erupt on the face, trunk, and proximal limbs. Differential diagnosis includes all of the vesiculopustular eruptions of the newborn and infant. Treatment of miliaria should be conservative. The infant should be dressed in light, loose clothing and placed in a cooler environment. For the pruritus associated with miliaria rubra, a soothing bland shake lotion such as calamine will alleviate itching and dry the lesions. Miliaria crystallina is usually asymptomatic.

Subcutaneous Fat Necrosis

Subcutaneous fat necrosis is uncommon but may be alarming when it develops in the newborn infant. Onset is usually during the latter part of the first week of life but onset earlier or later is not infrequent. The lesions are sharply demarcated nodules or plaques, stony hard in consistency, and skin colored or of a dusky red-purple hue (Fig. 3.6). Sites of predilection are the cheeks, buttocks, back, thighs, and upper arms. Most of the infants are otherwise well although increased irritability may be associated with pressure on the lesions which often seem to be painful. Rarely, there is associated fever, failure to thrive, hypercalcemia, and soft tissue and visceral calcification.

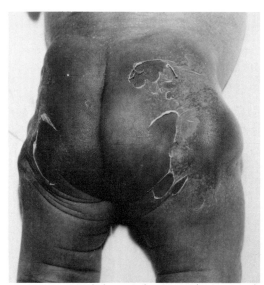

Fig. 3.6. Nodular violaceous lesions of subcutaneous fat necrosis on the buttocks and thighs of a neonate.

The cause of subcutaneous fat necrosis is unknown although it is often ascribed to obstetrical trauma or hypothermia. Nevertheless, many infants sustain such insults and do not exhibit fat necrosis; likewise, a history of these complications is often absent in affected infants. It is possible that susceptibility varies and that minor degrees of trauma, perhaps unappreciated, may elicit such a reaction in selected infants. The diagnosis can often be made clinically but can certainly be verified by histologic evaluation of a skin biopsy which shows a granulomatous reaction in the subcutaneous fat with thickening of the fibrous septae. The necrotic fat cells display characteristic clefts produced by dissolution of crystals during the process of fixation and embedding.

The usual course of subcutaneous fat necrosis is several weeks to several months duration. Most of the lesions resolve spontaneously without residual atrophy or scarring but, occasionally, there is massive deposition of calcium resulting in ulceration and extrusion of liquified material. In general, the lesions of subcutaneous fat necrosis should be managed expectantly. Careful needle aspiration of fluctuant areas may reduce the possibility of rupture and scarring, however, the hazard of introducing an infectious agent is considerable.

Transient Vascular Lesions

Harlequin color change is an evanescent but dramatic vascular event characterized by reddening of one-half of the body and simultaneous blanching of the other half. The body is longitudinally bisected by a line of demarcation into a pale upper half and a suffused lower half. Occasionally, the line of demarcation is incomplete, sparing the face and genitalia. This phenomenon appears when the infant is lying on his side and may be reversed by a change in position.

Harlequin color change occurs more frequently in low birth weight infants and is most common on the 3rd or 4th day of life. Duration of an episode ranges from minutes to hours but the color difference rapidly becomes obliterated by sudden activity or crying which causes generalized flushing. Multiple episodes may be noted up to 3 weeks of age. Harlequin color change is unaccompanied by changes in respiratory rate, reflexes, or muscle tone; however, it is thought to reflect vascular instability due to the immaturity of the autonomic nervous system. It may be regarded as an insignificant vascular event requiring neither investigation nor therapy.

Salmon patch is the term used to describe the very common light pink macular hemangiomas that are most often found on the upper eyelids, glabella or upper lip. Unlike the port wine stain (nevus flammeus) with which it can be confused, the salmon patch is usually relatively small with an indistinct border (Fig. 3.7).

Deepening of color is noted with temperature change or crying, but the overall course is one of progressive fading until the lesion is imperceptible, usually by 1–2 years. Similar lesions occurring on the nape are more often fixed and permanent, persisting in up to 40% of affected infants. Nevertheless, they are of no consequence and, once covered by hair, usually forgotten. An occasional nuchal nevus will periodically scale excessively. This minor skin change usually responds to conventional treatment for seborrheic dermatitis.

Cutis marmorata is a normal physiologic event during which the entire skin acquires a mottled or netlike bluish pattern. Exposure to cool environmental temperatures usually evokes this response which may occur throughout the early childhood years. This

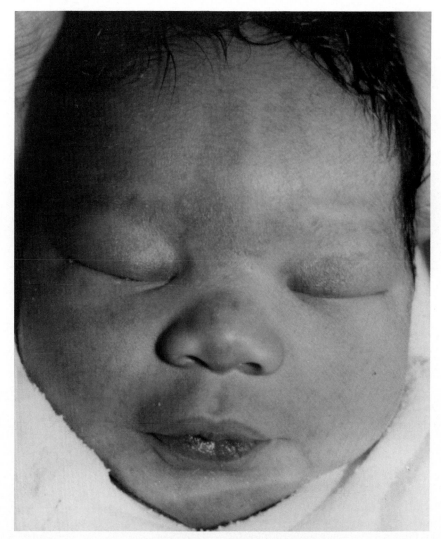

Fig. 3.7.   Salmon patch on the glabella.

accentuated vascular pattern is more prominent in some infants than in others. It should not be confused with a more pronounced and fixed nevoid vascular anomaly called cutis marmorata telangiectatica congenita.

Mongolian Spot

Poorly defined, macular, blue or slate-gray marks are found in the presacral area of more than 80% of black, oriental, and Indian infants and less than 10% of white newborns. Solitary or multiple lesions may be present and, less commonly, similar macules are located on the posterior thighs, legs, back, and shoulders. The color of these lesions is due to the dermal location of melanin-containing melanocytes presumably arrested in their migration from neural crest to epidermis. Mongolian spots usually fade gradually during childhood but may not disappear completely. Unusually dark or sharply demarcated lesions and those in atypical sites may not involute at all (Fig. 3.8).

NEVOID LESIONS (BIRTHMARKS)

Through common usage, the term nevus has acquired a variety of meanings, some of

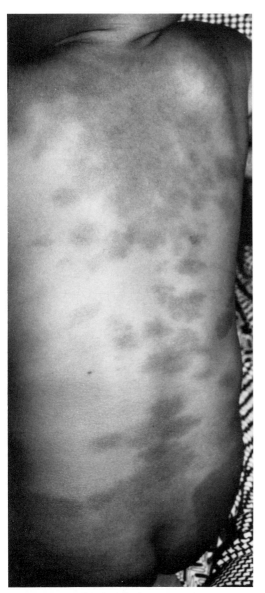

Fig. 3.8. Multiple dark mongolian spots over the entire back of a young child. Lesions this dark and extensive are less likely to fade.

well defined cell types normally found in skin. Hence, there are vascular nevi (hemangiomas), pigmented nevi (moles), connective tissue nevi, epidermal nevi, and nevi of various sorts derived from the cutaneous appendageal structures. The pathophysiologic mechanisms responsible for the development of the lesions are not known. Psychologic and physical trauma to the fetus were cited as playing a role in early hypotheses; thus, these lesions were often referred to as birthmarks. Although this concept is obsolete, physicians currently have no alternative explanation to offer parents. Genetic factors may be implicated in some instances, but large gaps still exist in our understanding of the pathogenesis of these lesions.

Hemangiomas (Vascular Nevi)

Localized vascular anomalies may occur as isolated developmental defects or as part of a syndrome complex for which the cutaneous lesion serves as a visual marker. Hemangiomas are the most common of the nevoid vascular conditions and, with rare exception, occur sporadically and without genetic predisposition. Hemangiomas can be macular or elevated; the raised types can be subdivided into superficial or capillary lesions (65%), subcutaneous or cavernous lesions (15%), and mixed lesions (20%). The terms capillary and cavernous describe the histologic pattern which does not always correspond exactly to the clinical appearance. Capillary hemangiomas are composed of dilated capillaries with or without endothelial proliferation, whereas cavernous hemangiomas consist of large blood-filled cavities that have a compressed single-layered endothelial lining and a fibrous wall of variable thickness.

Nevus Flammeus (Port Wine Stain, Macular Hemangioma, Telangiectatic Nevus)

These lesions are composed of dilated mature dermal vessels, are always present at birth and, in general, should be regarded as permanent lesions. The typical nevus flammeus in the newborn is flat, sharply demarcated, and pink to purple, occasionally appearing

which deviate considerably from the original definition of the word. Nevertheless, it is still a useful general term for a spectrum of cutaneous lesions that are basically benign and that represent circumscribed malformations of congenital origin. Although the words nevus and mole are often used interchangeably, in fact, the term nevus can be used to describe any growth characterized by a collection of

almost black in deeply pigmented infants. Lesions may involve any surface of the body including the mucosa, however, the face is a site of predilection where the distribution is often unilateral (Fig. 3.9). With maturation, port wine stains may become slightly raised and pebbly in consistency; alternatively, paler lesions may fade until they are almost imperceptible.

The facial nevus flammeus should be distinguished from the common salmon patch. Macular hemangiomas in the nuchal region have an unpredictable outcome; some persist for life like the port wine stain while others fade completely like the salmon patch. When a facial port wine nevus is localized to the trigeminal area, the diagnosis of Sturge-Weber syndrome (seizures, mental retardation, hemiparesis contralateral to the facial lesion, ipsilateral intracranial calcification) must be entertained. It is critical to consider this possibility in the young infant since associated glaucoma or other ocular defects may cause irreparable damage if not diagnosed and treated promptly. Glaucoma is more likely to

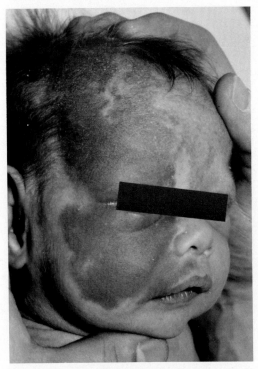

Fig. 3.9. Nevus flammeus in the trigeminal area, the most common site.

develop if the nevus flammeus involves the area of the face supplied by both the first and second sensory branches of the trigeminal nerve. Rarely, Sturge-Weber syndrome may occur in association with a bilateral facial nevus flammeus or with macular hemangiomas elsewhere on the skin. If the diagnosis of Sturge-Weber is under consideration, the infant deserves a careful ophthalmologic and neurologic examination. Nevus flammeus also occurs as a component of several other rare syndromes including the Klippel-Trenaunay-Weber, and Cobb, syndromes and with variable frequency in trisomy 13, Rubinstein-Taybi syndrome, Wiedemann-Beckwith syndrome, SC (pseudothalidomide) syndrome, and the epidermal nevus syndrome.

Capillary Hemangioma

Also known as strawberry marks, these nevi are bright red, protuberant, compressible, and sharply delineated and may occur as solitary or multiple lesions anywhere on the integument. Approximately 25% are present at birth, but most have appeared by 2 months of age. Early lesions often resemble a bruise or scratch or, alternatively, may present as an area of pallor that develops a delicate telangiectatic pattern prior to the growth phase.

Capillary hemangiomas undergo rapid expansion for several weeks or months and then enter a stationary phase which may persist for several months. Eventual spontaneous involution is usual, occurring in 90–95% of patients. Regression is heralded by the appearance of grey areas of fibrosis on the surface of the hemangioma (Fig. 3.10). The course of a particular lesion is unpredictable, but 60% may be expected to have involuted by approximately age 5 and 90% by age 9. Involution cannot be correlated with size or site of involvement; however, lip lesions are said to persist more often than those in other sites. Complications include ulceration, secondary infection, and hemorrhage, which is rarely life threatening in the absence of thrombocytopenia.

The treatment of choice for uncomplicated capillary hemangiomas is expectant observation. Parents of these infants require repeated reassurance and support. Before and after

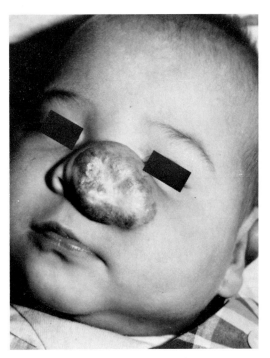

Fig. 3.10. Involuting strawberry hemangioma showing gray fibrotic areas on the surface. This patient was treated with oral prednisone.

photographs of other children with hemangiomas often provide a satisfactory means of allaying anxiety. Minor complications such as bleeding can be managed with simple compression, and ulceration and infection by administration of appropriate antibiotics topically or systemically as well as a protective ointment. Ulceration is a relatively benign complication but may result in scarring. In selected patients, surgical excision of the hemangioma may be advisable, but the decision to operate should be tempered by consideration of the amount of scarring that will result. Radiation is hazardous causing damage to local organs and impairment of bone growth and, therefore, is rarely indicated. Elastic bandages provide constant compression and are useful in certain patients to reduce the amount of tissue distortion from rapid growth of the hemangioma. Following spontaneous resolution, approximately 5–10% of patients are left with minimal cosmetic defects such as puckering of the skin, telangiectasia, or areas of pallor. These defects can be managed with

the aid of a cosmetic to match the normal skin tone (Covermark) or by judicious plastic repair.

Cavernous Hemangiomas

The cavernous hemangioma differs clinically from the strawberry hemangioma in that it is more deeply situated and, therefore, appears more ill defined. The overlying skin may be normal in color, have a bluish hue or, occasionally, is a deep livid purple (Fig. 3.11). On palpation, some lesions feel cystic, others firm, and large lesions may present as a massive swelling with no definable borders. Mixed lesions have a cavernous hemangioma at the base with a superimposed capillary hemangioma.

Like strawberry hemangiomas, cavernous lesions have a growth phase, a stationary phase, and a period of involution, and may also be followed expectantly unless they impinge on vital structures, interfere with functions such as vision or feeding, cause grotesque

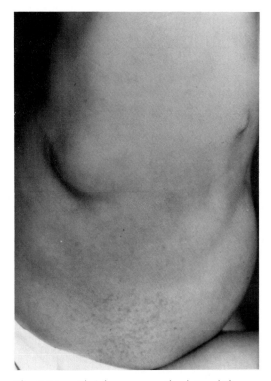

Fig. 3.11. Bluish mass on the lateral thorax representing a cavernous hemangioma.

disfigurement, or are associated with life-threatening complications such as thrombocytopenia and hemorrhage. Under these circumstances, it is appropriate to intervene promptly choosing the most effective and least damaging mode of therapy. As an alternative to surgery, prednisone in a dosage of 2–4 mg/kg/day has been efficacious in some instances. Cessation of growth and gradual decrease in size of the mass may be evident after 2–4 weeks of therapy. When a definite response has been obtained, prednisone should be tapered gradually or given in an alternate-day dosage regimen. Multiple courses of therapy may be required if growth resumes following discontinuation of the prednisone. Systemically administered corticosteroid should only be considered for selected patients and requires careful monitoring to prevent serious side effects.

Kasabach-Merritt Syndrome

The combination of a rapidly enlarging hemangioma and thrombocytopenia is known as Kasabach-Merritt syndrome. The hemangiomas are usually present at birth and typically are solitary and large, often involving an entire limb (Fig. 3.12); occasionally, however, Kasabach-Merritt syndrome has also been observed in patients with multiple small cutaneous and visceral hemangiomas. This complication seems to occur during the rapid growth phase of the hemangioma so that thrombocytopenia will occur most predictably early in infancy. The decrease in platelets may result in precipitous hemorrhage manifested by ecchymoses, petechiae, frank bleeding, and rapid enlargement of the hemangioma. Severe anemia is a consequence of this event, as is disseminated intravascular coagulation with consumption of fibrinogen and clotting factors. Normal numbers of megakaryocytes are present in the bone marrow, nevertheless, platelets are reduced due to sequestration and increased destruction within the hemangioma. The spectrum of severity ranges from mild depression of the platelet count to marked thrombocytopenia, hypofibrinogenemia and elevated levels of fibrin degradation products. Platelet and factor concentrates, fresh frozen plasma, and whole

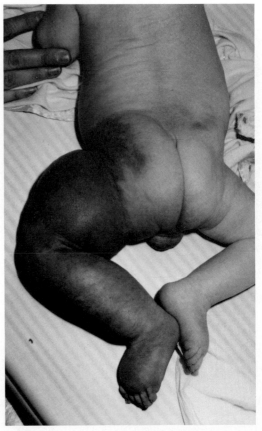

Fig. 3.12. Cavernous hemangioma involving the thigh of an infant with Kasabach-Merritt syndrome. Note bruising and edema of lower leg and foot.

blood or packed red cell transfusions may temporarily alleviate the problem but, in instances of active bleeding, heparin therapy may be required. Ultimately, the only effective means of controlling the hematological disorder is to reduce the size of the hemangioma. Oral corticosteroid therapy is often effective and may be given in combination with heparin and/or antiplatelet drugs such as aspirin and dipyridamole. Since none of these agents has been universally effective, surgical extirpation may be considered as an alternative choice of management. Frequently, however, the risk of bleeding is too great to hazard an operation. Irradiation also has been used in some patients but serious long-term sequelae are a deterrant to this mode of therapy.

Disseminated Hemangiomatosis (Diffuse Neonatal Hemangiomatosis)

This condition, like Kasabach-Merritt syndrome, is relatively rare but may also constitute another pediatric emergency. The cutaneous lesions may be few in number but are often profuse and are, typically, small, red, papular capillary hemangiomas (Fig. 3.13). Visceral hemangiomas most often involve the gastrointestinal tract, liver, central nervous system, and lung but may occur in other organs. The condition may be rapidly fatal due to onset of high output cardiac failure, respiratory tract obstruction, and compression of central neural tissue. When the patient presents with the triad of hepatomegaly, multiple cutaneous lesions, and high output cardiac failure the term hemangiomatosis of the liver is often used. A bruit may be present over the liver. An abdominal aortagram or celiac angiography will accurately delineate the size, location, and configuration of the lesions or, alternatively, a liver-spleen scan is a helpful noninvasive study.

Infants with multiple cutaneous and visceral hemangiomas may have a totally benign course or, conversely, may require intervention with life-saving measures. Digitalization is indicated for those patients in cardiac failure; the administration of prednisone in a dosage of 2–4 mg/kg/day has resulted in regression of the hemangiomas in some instances. Partial resection of the liver has also proved successful in situations where the hemangiomas are localized and amenable to a surgical approach. If the lesions are extensive, ligation of the hepatic artery has been performed but carries a serious risk.

Pigmented (Nevocytic) Nevi

Ordinary pigmented nevi or moles are also called nevus cell nevi to distinguish them from lesions formed by collections of mature mel-

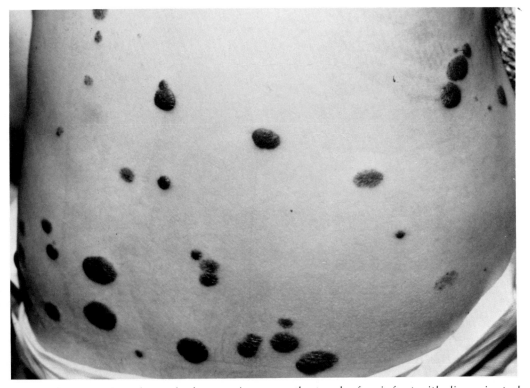

Fig. 3.13. Multiple red papular hemangiomas on the trunk of an infant with disseminated hemangiomatosis.

anocytes. Nevus cells are closely related to melanocytes, and one theory of origin proposes that they are derived from a common stem cell referred to as a nevoblast. An alternative theory suggests that nevus cells are of dual origin with the superficial cells arising from melanocytes and those in the deeper dermal layers arising from Schwann cells.

Acquired nevi have a definable life history. Early lesions are called junctional nevi because the melanized nevus cells are localized in nests on the epidermal side of the basement membrane. These nevi are discrete, flat, relatively small lesions of varying shades of brown. Although some nevi remain junctional in type indefinitely, most of them develop into compound or intradermal nevi, gradually changing morphologically as well as histologically. With maturation, the junctional nevus becomes elevated and dome shaped as the nevus cells move from epidermis into the dermis (compound nevus) and, finally, become localized only in the dermis (intradermal nevus).

It is important for the physician to be familiar with the natural history of acquired nevi so that these basically harmless lesions are not managed inappropriately. Parents often express anxiety when multiple nevi appear suddenly in a preschool child. One can comfortably reassure parents that the eruption of nevi is expected during early childhood. Likewise, the appearance of new nevi and darkening and growth of old nevi during adolescence are physiologic changes that should not be cause for alarm.

Acquired pigmented nevi are benign and need only be removed for cosmetic reasons or if the nevus is situated in an annoying site where it is subjected to repeated trauma causing chronic irritation and infection. A very small percentage of pigmented nevi undergo malignant transformation, but there is no means of determining which lesions are potentially dangerous, and random excision of nevi is neither feasible nor rational. Suspicious changes such as very rapid growth, development of satellite lesions, itching, pain, and bleeding are indications for excision and histologic evaluation. Most of these changes will be the result of irritation or maturation; however, if the patient or his parents continue to express anxiety, excision of the worrisome ne-

vus is a simple outpatient surgical procedure easily accomplished under local anesthesia.

Congenital Giant Pigmented Nevus (Giant Hairy Nevus)

The giant pigmented nevus which is always evident at birth, is considered to be a sporadic developmental anomaly although a few instances of multiple cases within families have been recorded. These nevi vary tremendously in size and may occupy large segments of the trunk or limbs (Fig. 3.14). Sites of predilection are the lower trunk, upper back and shoulders, scalp, and proximal limbs; the anatomic site is often indicated by certain designations such as bathing trunk, cape, or coatsleeve nevus.

The surface of the giant pigmented nevus can vary considerably in texture from flat to elevated, verrucous or nodular; a spectrum of hues of brown, blue, and black is also usual. Typical lesions develop a luxurious growth of coarse hairs but, occasionally, the giant pigmented nevus remains hairless and has a leathery surface texture. As the child ages, the nevus tends to become more variegated in

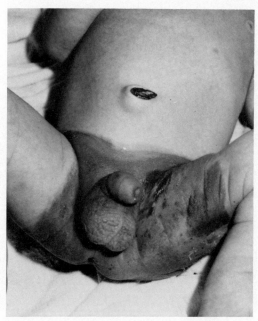

Fig. 3.14.   Giant congenital pigmented nevus in the bathing trunk area of an infant.

color and more nodular in texture. Most affected infants have numerous small satellite nevi scattered over the body surface, many of which may appear gradually during the first 2 years of life (Fig. 3.15).

On biopsy, the histologic features are usually those of an ordinary junctional, compound, or intradermal nevus and the pattern may differ in specimens obtained from multiple sites. The characteristic features of neural nevus, blue nevus, and spindle and epithelioid nevus may also be found interspersed. Characteristically, congenital nevi can be distinguished from acquired nevi because the nevus cells often extend deep into the lower dermis and even into the subcutaneous tissue. Sometimes, the cells are arranged in a band-like pattern or scattered in rows between the collagen bundles.

Giant pigmented nevi are of special significance for two reasons: 1) the association of leptomeningeal melanosis, and 2) the known predisposition for the development of malignant melanoma either within the nevus or in

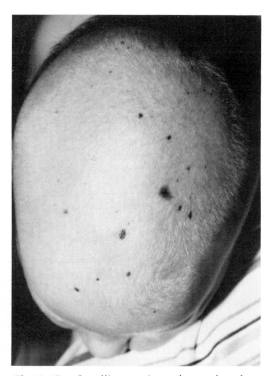

Fig. 3.15. Satellite nevi on the scalp of an infant with a giant congenital pigmented nevus.

the leptomeninges. Leptomeningeal involvement may be reflected clinically by developmental retardation, seizures, hydrocephalus, and motor deficits and may eventuate in malignant melanoma. This complication can be diagnosed by careful cytologic evaluation of the cerebrospinal fluid for cells containing melanin. The prognosis is guarded since most of these patients succumb despite palliative measures.

The reported incidence of malignant melanoma arising in giant hairy nevi ranges from 1–30% but is believed to be in the range of 10–15%. Unfortunately, reported series probably reflect bias in patient selection since those patients who experience complications are usually referred to large medical centers. Despite the lack of definitive data, the risk of developing a melanoma within a giant hairy nevus is considered high enough to make surgical excision and grafting the treatment of choice. Data on age of occurrence of malignancy indicate that this dreaded complication is as likely to arise in infancy as later, therefore, surgery should not be deferred. The task is formidable because of the large areas of skin that must be removed and because extensive involvement of the remaining skin with satellite lesions often limits its usefulness for grafting. If excision is delayed, frequent careful examination and biopsy of any enlarging nodules or suspicious areas is mandatory. These lesions can be extremely disfiguring and the cosmetic deformity may cause severe emotional problems.

Small Congenital Pigmented Nevi

The small congenital pigmented nevus (Fig. 3.16) poses a particular problem in that the true malignant potential of these lesions is simply not known. Those who advise routine removal of these lesions argue that histologically they represent the same entity as the large congenital pigmented nevus, therefore, they should be managed in a similar fashion. Conversely, it could be argued that data are lacking to support the view that small and medium-sized congenital pigmented nevi have significant malignant potential. Unfortunately, this controversy is not likely to be resolved until substantial long-

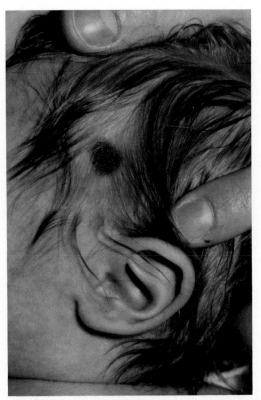

Fig. 3.16. Small congenital pigmented nevi on the scalp of an infant.

term statistical data are gathered from which risk for development of malignant melanoma can be predicted. At the moment, the onus is on the physician to discuss this problem honestly with parents and to help the family arrive at the most comfortable decision in the best interests of the child. If the lesion is not excised, periodic examination is indicated.

DIAPER AREA ERUPTIONS

Eruptions in the diaper area are mainly a problem of infants and young children but also occur in older children under special circumstances. Numerous disease entities can be included under this nonspecific heading, therefore, it is critical to define the etiologic factors as clearly as possible so that a diagnosis can be reached and appropriate management instituted. Often the morphology of the eruption is so characteristic that a diagnosis can be made on physical examination alone; in

addition, certain simple procedures such as a potassium hydroxide preparation of scales and a Gram stain of material from vesicular or pustular lesions may provide evidence to confirm the clinical impression.

Disorders that may present as a localized diaper area eruption are listed in Table 3.1. Some of these conditions such as epidermolysis bullosa, histiocytosis X and chronic bullous dermatosis of childhood are relatively rare, nevertheless, they must be considered in the differential diagnosis, particularly in instances of recalcitrant dermatitis when therapeutic failure cannot be attributed to noncompliance.

Noninfectious Eruptions

IRRITANT CONTACT DERMATITIS

The vast majority of infants with a diaper area eruption will have a simple irritant contact dermatitis. Although this eruption may be complicated by a secondary problem such as candidiasis, in the simple acute state, it is usually recognizable by certain clinical features (Table 3.2). Bright erythema resembling a scald and a parchment-like dryness occur in a patchy or confluent distribution over the entire lower trunk, but the sites in most pro-

Table 3.1
Diaper Area Eruptions

Noninfectious
  Irritant contact dermatitis
  Allergic contact dermatitis
  Seborrheic dermatitis
  Psoriasis
  Miliaria
  Atopic dermatitis
  Acrodermatitis enteropathica
  Epidermolysis bullosa
  Chronic bullous dermatosis of childhood
    (linear IgA dermatosis)
  Histiocytosis X
  Granuloma gluteale infantum

Infectious
  Candidiasis
  Pyoderma
  Herpes simplex
  Condylomata acuminata
  Syphilis
  Scabies

Table 3.2
Noninfectious Diaper Area Eruptions

Eruption	Clinical Description	Diagnostic Aids
Irritant contact dermatitis	Erythema, scaling, nodules, vesicles, erosions; folds relatively spared; accentuation at edges of diaper.	None
Allergic contact dermatitis	Erythema, scaling, vesicles, erosions; distribution dependent on allergen.	History of contactants applied. Patch tests occasionally.
Seborrheic dermatitis	Sharply demarcated erythematous dry scaly plaques; folds involved; scalp, face, axillae, neck, retroauricular skin usually involved; pruritus absent.	None
Psoriasis	Sharply demarcated erythematous dry scaly plaques; Köbner response, nail pitting common.	Skin biopsy. Family history positive for psoriasis.
Atopic dermatitis	Erythematous weeping acute eczema or dry, lichenified plaques; pruritus intense; lesions elsewhere on skin.	Family history positive for atopic diseases.
Histiocytosis X	Papules, vesicles, pustules, ulcerations, particularly in inguinal folds and axille; seborrhea-like generalized eruption; may be hemorrhagic; may have evidence of visceral involvement.	Skin biopsy; histiocytic infiltrate. Tzank smear of pustules; numerous histiocytes. EM: Langerhans granules in histiocytes.
Miliaria	Vesicles; erythematous papulopustules; pruritus usual.	None

longed contact with the diaper, usually the convex surfaces, are most severely involved. As the dermatitis becomes more chronic the brilliant erythema fades and the skin becomes scaly, often with superimposed papulovesicular or bullous lesions, fissures, and erosions (Fig. 3.17). Chronic hypertrophic, flat-topped papules and infiltrative nodules may develop simulating syphilitic condylomata. Erosion of the perimeatal skin is common in male infants. Frequently, the dermatitis is accentuated at the margins of the diapers on the thighs and abdomen. This phenomenon has been referred to as "tide-mark dermatitis" and is due to friction and the alternating states of wetness and dryness at the edges of the diaper.

Irritant contact dermatitis in the diaper area is usually attributed to prolonged contact with urine, feces, retained soaps, and topical preparations. The assumption that ammonia plays a major role in the initiation of this type of dermatitis has recently been challenged. In a clinical study of infants with and without diaper rash there was no difference in free

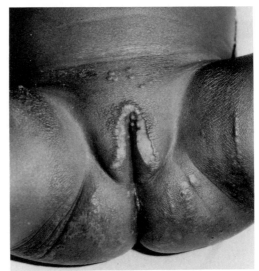

Fig. 3.17. Irritant diaper dermatitis showing hypertrophic papules and labial erosions.

ammonia in urine from children with irritant diaper dermatitis compared to urine from a group without dermatitis, and the incidence of organisms capable of splitting ammonia from urea was the same in both groups. In addition, experimental application of ammoniacal urine to intact skin of infants and adults failed to produce a dermatitis; however, experimental findings suggested a secondary role for ammonia as aggravating already damaged skin. Probably a number of other nonidentified odoriferous breakdown products of food present in urine and feces are also contributory factors to irritant diaper dermatitis.

ALLERGIC CONTACT DERMATITIS

True allergic contact dermatitis, in contrast to irritant contact dermatitis, occurs infrequently and is often misdiagnosed. The morphology is similar to allergic contact dermatitis elsewhere on the body. The rash is pruritic, edematous, erythematous, and often vesicular initially, becoming lichenified when chronic. The distribution varies depending on the particular sites of contact with the allergen. The most common offenders are ingredients in medications such as neomycin in topical antibiotic preparations, Paraben preservatives in creams and ethylenediamine in Mycolog Cream. Chemicals in diaper or clothing, laundry products, and other topical medications used in the diaper area may also be responsible for initiating a contact dermatitis.

SEBORRHEIC DERMATITIS

Seborrheic dermatitis of infancy often appears during the first month of life and may be intermittently troublesome for the first year. Diffuse or focal scaling and crusting of the scalp, sometimes called cradle cap, may be the initial or only manifestation. More often, there is generalized flexural involvement with the diaper area as a site of predilection as well as the axillae, retroauricular areas, face, and neck. The eruption is nonpruritic, erythematous, dry and patchy, or plaquelike with a yellow or white surface scale (Fig. 3.18). Postinflammation pigmentary changes are common, particularly in black infants.

When scaling is pronounced, the eruption

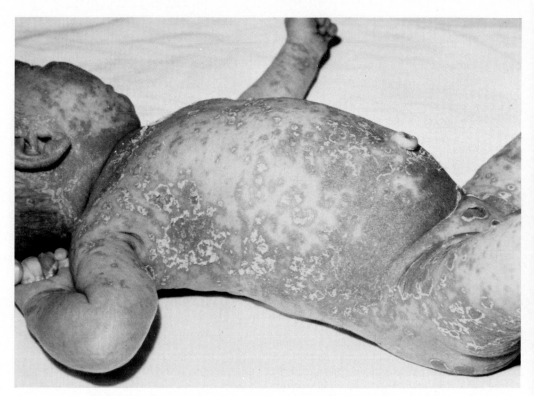

Fig. 3.18.   Widespread seborrheic dermatitis in a young infant.

may resemble psoriasis which can be distinguished only with difficulty. A complicating candidal eruption can also be recognized in some infants. The possibility of coexistant atopic dermatitis must be considered in infants who exhibit pruritus or who have a more exudative type of dermatitis. More often than not, a simple question about who is more bothered by the dermatitis, parent or child, will separate the patients with seborrheic dermatitis and atopic eczema.

PSORIASIS

When psoriasis presents in the young infant it is most frequently found initially in the diaper area. This phenomenon can probably be accounted for by the Köbner (isomorphic) response which reflects the tendency for psoriatic lesions to appear in areas of traumatized skin (Fig. 3.19). Differentiation from other scaly red diaper-area eruptions is difficult, however, characteristic plaques elsewhere on the integument and nail pitting are helpful diagnostic clues. Although thick silvery scales are typical, often the scales are absent due to

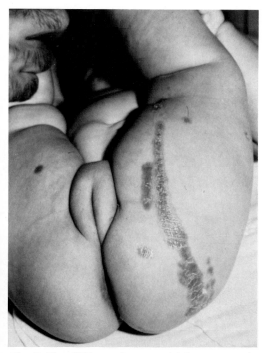

Fig. 3.19. Köbner (isomorphic) response in an infant with psoriasis due to a brace for congenital dislocation of the hip.

the constant moisture and maceration in the diaper area. Linear lesions resulting from friction do not occur in seborrheic dermatitis or candidiasis and are indicative of psoriasis, if present.

Biopsy may be diagnostic in some instances; however, if the histopathologic changes are not entirely typical, it can only provide supportive but not absolute evidence for the disease. A family history of psoriasis should be sought but, again, may only be considered circumstantial evidence if present. Often long-term observation provides the most reliable information as to the nature of the eruption.

MILIARIA

Two forms of miliaria occur in the diaper area: miliaria crystallina, which is more common in the neonate (see Transient Lesions of the Neonate), and miliaria rubra or "prickly heat," an ubiquitous rash of infants and toddlers. The latter eruption consists of groups of small, sterile papulopustules with an erythematous base. The lesions are usually randomly scattered over the lower abdomen and thighs as well as elsewhere on the integument, particularly in the flexural areas. Differentiation from staphylococcal pustules and candidiasis is easily accomplished if Gram-stained smears and KOH of intralesional material are examined and if bacterial fungal cultures are performed.

HISTIOCYTOSIS X

This sometimes fatal, rare infiltrative disease often initially presents as a diaper area eruption. Although the usual textbook description is that of a hemorrhagic seborrhea-like rash, in fact, a variety of lesions are characteristic of this condition. Vesicles, pustules, erythematous papules (often with an umbilication and a tiny central crust), and an eczematous plaque-like eruption are all typical. Purpura is found only if the bone marrow is involved and there is accompanying thrombocytopenia; frequently this is a relatively late manifestation.

The initial sites of involvement are usually the inguinal folds, axillae, and retroauricular areas. Erosion of lesions in the inguinal folds is extremely suggestive of histiocytosis X since ulceration is the result of invasion of epidermis by the infiltrating histiocytes (Fig. 3.20). Any persistent diaper area eruption, particularly if associated with typical lesions in other flexural areas, if accompanied by hematologic disturbances or organomegaly, or if progressive and erosive, should be biopsied to exclude this diagnostic possibility. Infants with histiocytosis X should be referred to a hematologist-oncologist for evaluation and further management.

GRANULOMA GLUTEALE INFANTUM

This relatively newly described entity consists of well circumscribed, angioma-like painless nodules that may be found on the buttocks, thighs, and lower abdomen. The nodules may become quite large and have been compared to cherries or plums since they may become deep red or purple in color. Affected infants are otherwise well, and the nodules resolve spontaneously without therapy. All of the reported infants with this condition had a history of prolonged repetitive applications of topical fluorinated corticosteroids to the affected skin, and the nodules are believed to

be an adverse reaction to those agents. Topical corticosteroids should be immediately discontinued in any infant with this problem.

MISCELLANEOUS ERUPTIONS

Three rare vesiculobullous eruptions that may affect the diaper area are chronic bullous dermatosis of childhood (linear IgA dermatosis), epidermolysis bullosa and acrodermatitis enteropathica. Chronic bullous dermatosis of childhood can be distinguished by the morphology and distribution of the bullae, the histologic finding of a subepidermal blister, and the direct immunofluorescence finding of linear IgA distributed along the basement membrane. The severe forms of epidermolysis bullosa are characterized by blisters induced by heat or trauma to the skin and mucous membranes. Once again, light and electron microscopy to determine the exact site of cleavage in the skin is often helpful diagnostically. Acrodermatitis enteropathica, an autosomal recessive disease of zinc deficiency, causes lesions in the perioral area, hands, feet, knees, elbows, and diaper area. The lesions are initially vesicobullous, then psoriasiform and eczematous (Fig. 3.21). Associated features such as hair loss, change in hair color, photophobia, apathy, diarrhea, and nail dystrophy are usually present. Diagnosis is made by determination of the plasma zinc as well as levels of zinc-dependent enzymes, such as alkaline phosphatase, which are also low.

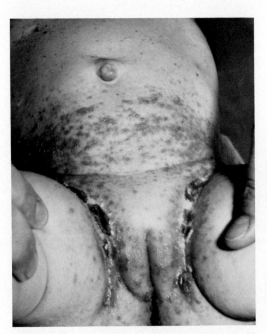

Fig. 3.20. Multiple erythematous infiltrated papules and inguinal ulcerations of histiocytosis X.

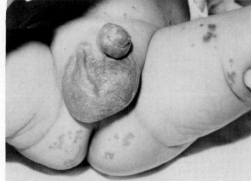

Fig. 3.21. Eczematous dermatitis in the inguinal area in an infant with acrodermatitis enteropathica.

Infectious Eruptions

CANDIDIASIS

Candidiasis of the diaper region is an extremely common problem during the early months of life. The relatively high incidence of localized cutaneous lesions can be attributed to acquisition of *Candida albicans* as normal flora in the gastrointestinal tract. The usual source of the yeast, in most instances, is the mother who may be a vaginal or intestinal carrier of the organism and who may have had overt vaginitis during her pregnancy. *C. albicans* is not a normal skin saprophyte but is deposited onto the skin of the diaper area via the feces.

Typical candidiasis of the diaper area is a bright red scaly plaque often with a scalloped edge bordered by a fringe of epithelium (Table 3.3). Multiple tiny vesicopustules, so called satellite lesions, develop beyond the margins of the plaque and represent one of the characteristic features of this condition. The plaque often involves the entire lower abdomen, perineum, vulva or scrotum, inguinal flexures, and inner aspects of the thighs (Fig.

3.22). Since the eruption results from contamination of the perineal skin with feces containing *C. albicans*, it is usual to have involvement of the perirectal skin as well. The moisture and maceration of the diaper and flexural areas encourages proliferation of the yeast; pruritus and burning associated with the dermatitis may cause extreme discomfort. Diagnosis is made by identification of budding yeasts and pseudomycelia on KOH preparation of scales obtained from the border of the lesion. Alternatively, a Gram stain of material from a vesicopustule may also demonstrate the organism. The organism can be grown on blood agar or on Mycosel agar for confirmation of diagnosis. Stool culture is usually also positive for *C. albicans* in these infants.

Some infants with long-standing candidal diaper dermatitis may develop a widespread candidal eruption over much of the trunk, proximal limbs, and face. Others who also develop generalized dermatitis appear to have an "id" reaction in that lesions outside of the diaper area are KOH- and culture-negative for *C. albicans*. The term "psoriasiform napkin dermatitis" has been used in the British literature to describe this phenomenon, causing

Table 3.3
Infectious Diaper Area Eruptions

Eruption	Clinical Description	Diagnostic Studies
Bullous impetigo	Variable-sized superficial blisters with clear or turbid fluid, red base	Gram stain: Gram-positive cocci Culture: *Staphylococcus aureus*
Pustular pyoderma	Small → large pustules; may be crusted or necrotic	Gram stain: positive for infecting organism Culture: causative organism
Candidiasis	Sharp-edged, red, scaly plaques with satellite vesicopustules; folds involved, also perirectal skin	KOH prep: positive for budding spores and mycelia Gram stain: positive for spores Culture: *Candida albicans*
Herpes simplex infection	Grouped small vesicopustules on erythematous base	Tzank smear: multinucleated giant cells, balloon cells Viral culture: Herpes simplex
Condylomata acuminata	Multiple papillomatous lesions on genitalia, perineum, perirectal	None
Scabies	Papules, vesicles, eczematous plaques, burrows; lesions elsewhere including palms and soles	Scraping with oil: positive for mites, eggs, feces
Syphilis	Maculopapular scaly rash, annular lesions, moist papules	VDRL-positive FTA-positive

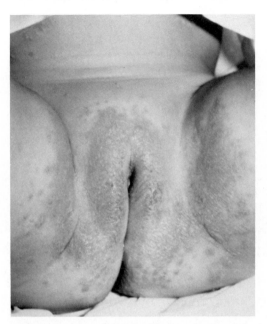

Fig. 3.22. Candidiasis of the diaper area with satellite vesicopustules. In this infant, the folds are relatively spared.

considerable confusion since the eruption is often mistakenly diagnosed as psoriasis. In fact, many of these infants have seborrheic dermatitis complicated by secondary infection with *C. albicans* and, unfortunately all three conditions (seborrhea, candidiasis, psoriasis) can mimic each other clinically.

PYODERMA

Several bacterial organisms may be responsible for infection in the diaper area, but the most common organism is *Staphylococcus aureus* which may variably cause a superficial pustular eruption resembling folliculitis (Fig. 3.23), bullous impetigo, localized cutaneous abcesses, and flaccid bullae, and denudation as part of a more generalized staphylococcal infection, scalded skin syndrome. The superficial pustular eruption mimics candidiasis and miliaria and requires Gram stain and culture of intralesional material for definitive diagnosis. The infant is not ill, is usually afebrile, and may be treated in a conservative fashion. In contrast, deeper lesions require a more aggressive approach particularly since the infants are usually systemically ill.

Bullous impetigo is probably the most com-

mon of the superficial infections in the diaper area. It may appear during the first week of life and may involve a number of infants in the newborn nursery simultaneously or sequentially. In the hospitalized newborn, it is particularly worrisome not only because of the risk of sepsis, but also because of the possibility of epidemic spread.

The lesions of bullous impetigo most frequently arise in the diaper area and periumbilical skin but may spread to contiguous areas and become widespread. The blisters vary considerably in size often forming arcs or circles as they spread, but less often they form the grape-like clusters characteristic of Herpes simplex infection. Since the cleavage plane is high in the epidermis, the blisters are thin-roofed and, therefore, flaccid, filled with straw-colored or turbid fluid, and rupture readily leaving a moist, red, raw base that acquires a thin varnish-like covering as it dries (Fig. 3.24). These lesions reepithelialize easily and do not leave scars. Unlike the fluid from the flaccid bullae of staphylococcal scalded skin syndrome, the blister fluid of bullous impetigo always contains the infectious organism which can be demonstrated by a Gram stain and/or bacterial culture.

Other organisms that less commonly cause

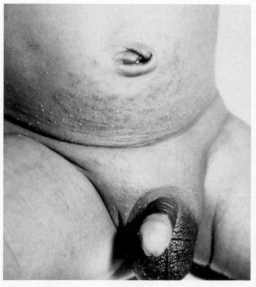

Fig. 3.23. Multiple tiny pustules over the lower abdomen and groin. Culture grew *Staphylococcus aureus*.

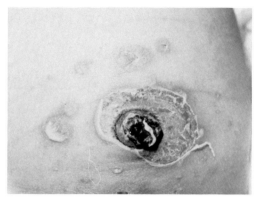

Fig. 3.24. Multiple flaccid and eroded bullae in the periumbilical area representing staphylococcal bullous impetigo.

diaper area pyoderma include group B streptococci (a bullous eruption) group A β-hemolytic streptococci (pustules and erythematous eroded lesions with amber-colored sticky crusts) and the Gram-negative rods (necrotic pustules).

HERPES SIMPLEX INFECTION

Herpetic infection in the diaper area is uncommon but may occur as part of a generalized cutaneous infection in the newborn or as a primary infection in the toddler, either as an isolated focus or concurrent with the primary episode of gingivostomatitis. The lesions are always grouped, small, vesicles that evolve into pustules and finally become crusted as they mature. Affected infants are usually systemically ill with significant fever and neonates are often desperately ill with involvement of viscera and the central nervous system. A Tzank smear is a rapid preliminary procedure that can be used to confirm the diagnosis. In addition, newer techniques permit rapid identification of the organism both by immunofluorescence and by viral culture.

MISCELLANEOUS INFECTIOUS CONDITIONS

Other nonbacterial infectious conditions in the diaper area include viral exanthems, syphilitic lesions (maculopapular, annular, condylomata lata), scabies, and condylomata acuminata (mucous membrane warts). The lat-

ter are not uncommon in the toddler age group and, although the question of sexual abuse must be considered, it should not be assumed without substantial evidence.

Treatment

Critical to successful management of diaper dermatitis is defining the specific cause. Once the etiology is known, the proper therapeutic program can be instituted. Any weeping or bullous condition will benefit from open compressing with Burow's solution (available as Domeboro Powder Packets or Effervescent Tablets) or saline at least four times daily for 10–20 minutes. Following compressing, the topical agent may be applied. If the skin is dry rather than moist, and particularly if there is generalized dryness, daily bathing with a bath oil (Alpha Keri, Domol Bath and Shower Oil, Lubath) and a soap substitute (Aveeno Bar, Lowila Cake) or superfatted soap (Dove, Lubriderm Soap, Alpha Keri, Basis) followed immediately by total body inunction with a bland emollient (Eucerin, Lubriderm Cream or Lotion, Nutraderm, Neutragena Lotion for Hand and Skin, Shepard's Cream Lotion) is indicated. If miliaria is the primary problem, or has complicated an underlying dermatitis, then, avoidance of humid conditions and occlusive topical preparations is particularly important.

Primary irritant diaper dermatitis will often respond to simple preventative measures, although some infants seem predisposed to this problem. The damaging effects of prolonged contact with urine and feces can be obviated by frequent changing and meticulous washing of the genitalia with plain water. The additional deleterious effects of maceration of an already inflamed skin from contact with a urine-soaked diaper can be avoided to some degree if modern disposable paper diapers are substituted for cloth diapers and plastic pants. Frequent application of a bland protective ointment with a petrolatum or zinc oxide base following thorough gentle cleansing may suffice to prevent dermatitis. Care should be taken to avoid abrasive coarse-milled powders and creams containing sensitizing, irritating, or toxic ingredients such as boric aicd, balsam of Peru, menthol, and topical anesthetics. Cornstarch powder facilitates the growth of yeast and should never be used in the diaper area. If true allergic contact dermatitis is suspected, all previously applied medications as well as any suspected contactants should be discontinued.

If the skin is very inflamed, a corticosteroid may be required. Hydrocortisone in a concentration of 0.5 or 1% may be applied at each diaper change (or four to six times/day). If the dermatitis is erosive, a cream base may burn or sting causing the infant considerable distress. Substitution of an ointment base will usually alleviate discomfort. Gels are drying and should not be used in the diaper area, but lotions provide another alternative base, if necessary. If the dermatitis does not heal with these measures, a brief course of a dilute fluorinated corticosteroid may be given, but it should be remembered that these products can cause local skin changes including striae. Additional protection of the skin by zinc oxide paste applied as a thick covering over the steroid may be helpful.

Seborrheic dermatitis, atopic dermatitis, and psoriasis will also respond to applications of a topical corticosteroid. Psoriasis is the most recalcitrant of these eruptions, and the physician is cautioned against succumbing to the temptation to prescribe a strong corticosteroid. Very often, parents must settle for partial resolution in the best interests of the child. Liquor carbonis detergens, 5–10% in a water washable base, may also be effective for psoriatic lesions, and regular use of emollients is usually helpful.

Infectious lesions must be treated with specific antiinfectious agents. Candidal dermatitis responds to typical nystatin, amphotericin B, miconazole, clotrimazole, and haloprogin in cream or lotion bases. It is not unreasonable to combine antifungal therapy with a topical steroid if the skin is very inflamed; however, it is preferable to avoid multiple agent "shotgun" type preparations. Pyoderma may respond to compresses and a topical nonsensitizing preparation antibiotic such as Polysporin Ointment or Bacitracin Ointment, however, in some instances, depending on the age of the child and the extent of the infection, systemic therapy may be indicated. Ultimately, the sensitivities of the organism cultured should determine the choice of systemic and topical antibiotics.

References

General

1. Jacobs, A.H.: Symposium on pediatric dermatology. Pediatr. Clin. N. Am. *25:* 2, 1978.
2. Solomon, L.M., and Esterly, N.B.: *Neonate Dermatology*, W.B. Saunders, Philadelphia, 1973.
3. Weinberg, S., and Hoekelman, R.A.: *Pediatric Dermatology for the Primary Care Practitioner*, McGraw-Hill, New York, 1978.

Transient Lesions of the Neonate

1. Bhaskar, S.N.: Oral lesions in infants and newborn. Dent. Clin. N. Am., July, 421, 1966.
2. Carr, J.A., Hodgeman, J.E., Freedman, R.J., and Levan, N.E.: Relationship between toxic erythema and infant maturity. Am. J. Dis. Child., *112:* 129, 1966.
3. Cunliffe, W.J., Coterill, J.P.: *The Acnes, Clinical Features, Pathogenesis and Treatment*. W.B. Saunders, London, 1975.
4. Mortensen, O., and Stougard-Andresen, P.: Harlequin color change in the newborn. Acta Obstet. Gynecol. Scand., *38:* 352, 1959.
5. Ramamurthy, R.S., Reveri, M., Esterly, N.B., Fretzin, D.F., and Pildes, R.S.: Transient neonatal pustular melanosis. J. Pediatr. *88:* 831, 1976.
6. Smith, M.A., Manfield, P.A.: Salmon patches in the first year of life. Br. J. Dermatol., *74:* 31, 1962.
7. Weary, P.E., Graham, G.F., Selden, and R.F., Jr.: Subcutaneous fat necrosis of the newborn. South. Med. J., *59:* 960, 1966.

Nevoid Lesions (Birthmarks)

1. Braun, P., Ducharme, J.C., Riopelle, J.L., and Davignon, A.: Hemangiomatosis of the liver in infants. J. Pediatr. Surg., *10:* 121, 1975.
2. Brown, S.H., Jr., Neerhout, R.C., and Fonkalsrud, E.W.: Prednisone therapy in the management of large hemangiomas in infants and children. Surgery *71:* 168, 1972.
3. Burman, D., Mansell, P.W.A., and Warin, R.P.: Miliary haemangiomata in the newborn. Arch. Dis. Child., *42:* 193, 1967.
4. Corrigan, J.J.: Disseminated intravascular coagulopathy. Pediatr. Rev. *1:* 37, 1979.
5. Didisheim, P., and Fuster, V.: Actions and clinical status of platelet-suppressive agents. Semin. Hematol., *15:* 55, 1978.
6. Evans, J., Batchelor, A.D.R., Stark, G, and Uttley, W.S.: Haemangioma with coagulopathy: sustained response to prednisone. Arch. Dis. Child., *50:* 809, 1975.
7. Fost, N.C., and Esterly, N.B.: Successful treatment of juvenile hemangiomas with prednisone. J. Pediatr., *72:* 351, 1968.
8. Hagerman, L.J., Czapek, E.E., Donnellan, W.L., and Schwartz, A.D.: Giant hemangioma with consumption coagulopathy. J. Pediatr. *87:* 766, 1975.
9. Hoffman, H.J., and Freeman, A.: Primary leptomeningeal melanoma in association with giant hairy nevi.

Report of two cases. J. Neurosurg., *26:* 62, 1967.

10. Kaplan, E.N.: The risk of malignancy in large congenital nevi. Plast. Reconstr. Surg., *53:* 421, 1974.

11. Kopf, A.W., Bart, R.S., and Hennessey, P.: Congenital nevocytic nevi and malignant melanomas. J. Am. Acad. Dermatol., *1:* 123, 1979.

12. Lampe, I., and Latourette, H.B.: Management of cavernous hemangiomas in infants. Pediatr. Clin. N. Am., *6:* 511, 1959.

13. Lanier, V.C., Pickrell, K.L., and Georgiade, N.G.: Congenital giant nevi: clinical and pathological considerations. Plast. Reconstr. Surg., *58:* 48, 1976.

14. Mark, G.J., Mihm, M.C., Liteplo, M.G., Reed, R.J., and Clark, W.H.: Congenital melanocytic nevi of the small and garment type. Clinical, histologic and ultrastructural studies. Hum. Pathol., *4:* 395, 1973.

15. Reed, W.B., Becker, S.W., Sr., Becker, S.W., Jr., and Nickel W.R.: Giant pigmented nevi, melanomas and leptomeningeal melanocytosis. Arch. Dermatol., *91:* 100, 1965.

16. Schiliro, G., Guarneri, B., and Russo, A.: A case of multiple neonatal haemangiomatosis with favorable outcome following steroid therapy. Acta Paediatr. Scand., *65:* 267, 1976.

17. Stevenson, R.F., and Morin, J.D.: Ocular findings in nevus flammeus. Can. J. Ophthalmol., *10:* 136, 1975.

18. Stigmar, G., Crawford, J.S., Ward, C.M., and Thomson, H.G.: Ophthalmic sequelae of infantile hemangiomas of the eyelids and orbit. Am. J. Ophthalmol., *85:* 806, 1978.

Diaper Area Eruptions

1. Andersen, S.L.C., and Thomsen, K.: Psoriasiform napkin dermatitis. Br. J. Dermatol., *84:* 316, 1971.

2. Farber, E.M., and Jacobs, A.H.: Infantile psoriasis. Am. J. Dis. Child., *131:* 1266, 1977.

3. Fergusson, A.G., Fraser, N.G., and Grant, P.W.: Napkin dermatitis with psoriasiform "ide." Br. J. Dermatol., *78:* 289, 1966.

4. Koblenzer, P.J.: Diaper dermatitis—an overview. Clin. Pediatr., *12:* 386, 1973.

5. Kozinn, P.J., Taschjian, C.L., and Burchall, J.J.: Diaper rash, a diagnostic anachronism. J. Pediatr., *59:* 75, 1961.

6. Leyden, J.J., Katz, S., Stewart, R., and Kligman, A.M.: Urinary ammonia and ammonia-producing microorganisms in infants with and without diaper dermatitis. Arch. Dermatol., *113:* 1678, 1977.

7. Neville, E.P., and Finn, O.A.: Psoriasiform napkin dermatitis—a followup study. Br. J. Dermatol., *92:* 279, 1975.

8. Robertson, A.F., and Sotos, J.: Treatment of acrodermatitis enteropathica with zinc sulfate. Pediatrics, *55:* 738, 1975.

9. Uyeda, K., Nakayasu, K., and Takaiski, Y., et al.: Kaposi sarcoma-like granuloma on diaper dermatitis. Arch. Dermatol., *107:* 605, 1973.

CHAPTER 4

ATOPIC DERMATITIS

C. RAYMOND ZEISS

HISTORY AND DEFINITION

Atopic dermatitis is a special form of eczema which emerged as a clinical entity in the 1800s and had the designation neurodermatitis. Eczema is a general term for a cutaneous response to various stimuli which is characterized in acute stages by vesciculation and erythema and in the chronic stages by scaling and thickening of the skin. Atopic dermatitis, then, comes under the general heading of eczema and the terms atopic dermatitis and atopic eczema can be used interchangeably. Atopic dermatitis is set apart from the other forms of eczema by its association with a personal or family history of allergic rhinitis or asthma. This association was noted by Besnier in the late 1800s and its hereditary nature was firmly established by Cooke and VanderVeer in 1916. The name, atopic dermatitis, was suggested by Wise and Sulzberger in 1933. In a recent review, atopic dermatitis was defined as a chronic, itching, superficial inflammation of the skin often occurring in association with a personal or family history of allergic rhinitis or asthma. Manifestations can be as severe as a generalized exfoliative erythroderma or as mild as a small round patch of chronic dermatitis. Erythema, edema, excoriations, and oozing characterize the acute condition while scaling, lichenification, hyperpigmentation, and fissuring denote the chronic state.

NATURAL HISTORY AND INCIDENCE

Atopic dermatitis is a very common disease which has its major impact on the young. In a large perspective study of infants by Halpern et al. in the United States, there was a 4.3% incidence of the disease. In Great Britain, Walker and Warin have reported a 3.1% incidence of infantile eczema. In a comprehensive study of the prevalence of dermatologic diseases in the United States population from the National Center for Health Statistics, an incidence of 6.9/1000 was found.

The natural history of the disease has been remarkably well described and three phases have been delineated. Each phase is characterized by a distinctive distribution of the dermatitis. The *infantile phase* begins during the fourth to sixth month of life. Dermatitis is found on the face, the extensor surfaces of the extremities, and the scalp. Sixty per cent of the individuals who will develop this disease develop it in the first year of life. Dermatitis tends to improve and may disappear between the third and fifth years of life. The *childhood phase* has its onset between the ages of 2 and 4 with predilection for the flexural areas, the hands, feet, and perioral areas. The childhood phase by definition terminates at 10 years of age. In this stage, lichenification is common. The *adult form* of atopic dermatitis is characterized by layers of highly pruritic dermatitis involving the flexural areas, face, neck, upper trunk, and feet. In individual patients, all of these stages may appear in sequence or may occur only as a single phase in a particular patient.

Although the course of atopic dermatitis is highly variable, some observations have been made. Atopic dermatitis of early onset usually resolves (60% of the patients) within the first

49

6 years of life. Dermatitis may persist into the 20s and 30s with only 2% of the patients continuing beyond the age of 45 years. It has been noted that if the dermatitis is severe initially, only 30% will clear in a 20-year period. Additionally, 50% of the patients will develop allergic rhinitis and 20–30% will develop asthma.

DIAGNOSTIC FEATURES

To be included in a diagnosis of atopic dermatitis, the patient should have prominent pruritus, the typical pathology and distribution of the lesions (see Fig. 4.1 on color Plate I, and Fig. 4.2) consistent with the age of the patient, the tendency for chronic relapsing dermatitis, and a background of a personal or family history of atopic disease. Other markers have been associated with the disease. Intense pruritus, xerosis (dry skin), lichenification (Fig. 4.3), palmar markings, elevated immunoglobulin E (IgE) serum levels, depressed cell mediated immunity, increased susceptibility to bacterial and viral infections of the skin, and abnormal vascular abnormalities have all been considered to be prominent markers of this disease. Less common features include anterior subcapsular cataracts, facial pallor, infraorbital darkening, the Dennie-Morgan infraorbital fold, and keratoconus. At present, there is no fully consistent genetic marker for the disease such as a specific histocompatibility antigen (HLA) type. Most authorities agree that there is a polygenic inheritance with environmental factors needed to have the gene express itself. Monozygotic twins have a 10-fold greater concordance for the disease than do dizygotic twins.

PATHOLOGY

Pathologic changes in atopic dermatitis depend upon the stage of the disease; that is, acute, subacute, or chronic. The *acute stage* is characterized by epidermal microvesicles containing a mixed inflammatory exudate of lymphocytes, eosinophils, and neutrophils. There is spongiosis (intracellular edema) accompanied by an infiltration in the epidermis

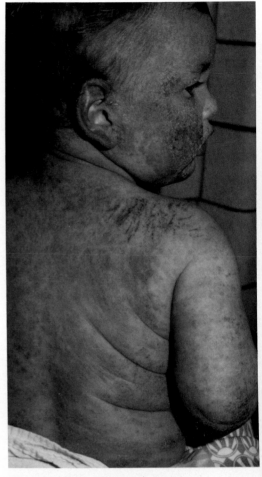

Fig. 4.2. Generalized eczematous atopic dermatitis demonstrating crusting exudative lesions on the face and elbows as well as excoriations on the shoulders.

with lymphocytes and neutrophils. The upper dermis shows vascular dilatation and edema with a perivascular infiltrate composed of eosinophils, neutrophils, and lymphocytes. In the *subacute stages*, there is less spongiosis and smaller microvesicles within the epidermis. The dermal inflammatory infiltrate is more pronounced than seen in the acute phase with lymphocytes predominating. In the *chronic* stage of atopic dermatitis, pathologic changes switch from spongiosis and microvesiculation seen in the acute stages to acanthosis with elongation of the rete ridges and a hyperkeratotic stratum corneum. There continues to be a prominent perivascular infiltrate in the

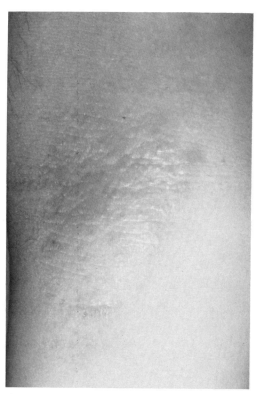

Fig. 4.3. Lichenified and eczematous patch on flexure surface of arm—*atopic eczema.* (Reproduced with permission from E. E. Johnson et al., *The Journal of Allergy and Clinical Immunology, 54:* 54, 1974.)

dermis with an infiltrate composed primarily of lymphocytes, eosinophils, and macrophages. A recent study of lichenified plaques with special attention to the absolute number of mast cells found that there was almost twice the number of mast cells seen in lichenified areas compared to clinically uninvolved skin or in skin biopsied during an acute eruption. This is consistent with the earlier findings of increased tissue histamine in lichenified areas.

PATHOPHYSIOLOGIC MECHANISMS

Pathophysiologic studies in this disease can be divided into physiologic studies and the more recent immunologic studies. There has been an explosion in immunologic observa-

tions made over the last 15 years and highlights of this work will be given.

The close association of atopic dermatitis with allergic rhinitis and extrinsic asthma led to several studies of the skin reactivity to common allergens. Positive immediate wheal and flare reactions to common allergens can be found in 70% of patients without rhinitis or asthma and in over 90% of the patients with concomitant respiratory disease. With the discovery of immunoglobulin E as the carrier of reaginic activity, it was natural to measure total serum IgE in these patients. In approximately 87% of patients with atopic dermatitis, elevated levels of serum IgE are evident averaging 4–10 times normal. There is a tendency for the IgE levels to be correlated with the severity of the dermatitis (Fig. 4.4). The IgE levels are highest in patients with associated allergic rhinitis and extrinsic asthma. The enthusiasm for IgE being a central marker of the disease has been tempered somewhat by more recent studies which show approximately 57% of patients with atopic dermatitis having normal levels and a carefully controlled study by Johansson demonstrating that the elevated IgE correlated better with the presence of allergic rhinitis and/or asthma. Significantly, elevated IgE has been found in other dermatoses such as contact dermatitis, psoriasis, and acral dermatitis. Specific IgE against given allergens can be measured by the radioallergosorbent test (RAST) and elevated specific IgE can be found in patients with atopic dermatitis related to a variety of common allergens such as pollens, molds, and foods. In these patients, the elevation of IgE to a specific allergen correlates poorly with immediate wheal and flare skin test reactivity in the same patients.

Another area of continued interest is the study of cell-mediated immunity in patients with atopic dermatitis. Clinical observations indicated that these patients have increased susceptibility to viral infections such as herpes simplex, vaccinia, and Coxsackie viruses. A relative inability to sensitize patients with atopic dermatitis to dinitrochlorobenzene (DNCB) was shown in 1966. In addition, a depression of the total number of circulating T lymphocytes and a depression of T cell response to mitogens has been reported. In many diseases with depressed cell-mediated

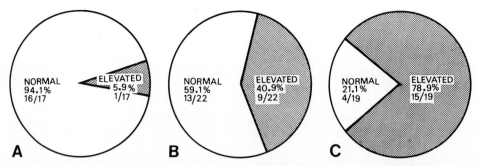

Fig. 4.4. Frequency of elevated serum IgE concentrations by combined disease classifications. *A*, Mild atopic dermatitis with atopic respiratory disease. *B*, Mild atopic dermatitis with atopic respiratory disease or severe atopic dermatitis without atopic respiratory disease. *C*, Severe atopic dermatitis with atopic respiratory disease. (Reproduced with permission from E. E. Johnson et al., *The Journal of Allergy and Clinical Immunology*, *54:* 94, 1974.)

immunity, there are abnormal elevations of IgE and dermatitis which resembles atopic dermatitis. Examples of these diseases include the extreme hypergammaglobulin E syndrome described by Buckley, these patients having undue susceptibility to cutaneous bacterial and fungal infections, and the Wiskott-Aldrich syndrome. In certain patients with the Wiskott-Aldrich syndrome, transfer factor has restored cell-mediated immunity and the eczema has cleared. In addition to cell-mediated immunity, depressed monocyte and neutrophil chemotactic responses have been found in small percentages of patients with atopic dermatitis.

There is, therefore, a general consensus that defects in T cells can lead to overproduction of IgE. Pioneering work by Tada and others presented evidence in animals that IgE responses were under regulation by thymus-derived T lymphocytes.

Many physiologic studies have been done in patients with this disease with abnormal vascular responses receiving a good deal of attention. It has been noted that stroking of the skin of patients with atopic dermatitis would result in a response which was termed "white dermographism." Stroking a normal skin usually produces an erythematous line along the tract within a few seconds. Approximately a minute later, an erythematous flare extends along the scratch mark. In patients with atopic dermatitis, this response is altered in that the initial erythematous response is quickly superseded by a white blanch extend-

ing outward from this line of trauma. In addition, intracutaneous injection of methacholine chloride in these patients produces blanching around the wheal instead of the normal red flare. These reactions were believed to be characteristic of the disease entity. Older studies by Reed, and a recent study by Uehara and Ofuji, have shown that this phenomenon is not specific for atopic dermatitis and can occur in patients with allergic contact dermatitis. In addition, normal uninvolved skin in both patients with atopic dermatitis and patients with contact dermatitis failed to show these vascular abnormalities. More recently, Kaliner has demonstrated significant increases in sweat response to concentrations of methacholine chloride in patients with atopic disease. Patients with allergic rhinitis and asthma without eczema showed increased sensitivity to cholinergic stimulation as measured by the eccrine sweat response. Abnormal vascular responses and responses to methacholine chloride, then, can be characteristic of inflamed skin and/or the result of the underlying atopic state and may not be at all specific for atopic dermatitis.

In summary, a variety of interesting immunologic and physiologic observations have been made in patients with atopic dermatitis. The areas of most intense investigation center upon the relationship of IgE and depressed cellular immunity in these patients and the connection of these observations to the final explanation for the disease state. A summary of this recent information into a unified hypothesis of the pathogenesis of this disease has been given by Blaylock.

TREATMENT

There is at the present time no curative therapeutic strategy in the treatment of patients with this hereditary dermatitis. The therapeutic strategy to control the eruption divides itself into several areas.

The strategy of avoidance has centered around two specific areas. In a family with both parents having atopic disease, certain foods have been withdrawn from the newborn in an attempt to prevent the development of atopic dermatitis. Early studies, either retrospective or nonblinded, tended to demonstrate the lower incidence of rhinitis, asthma, and/or atopic dermatitis when milk, eggs, wheat, and beef were avoided for the first 9 months. Halpern, in a large scale prospective study, demonstrated that substitution of soy or breast milk for cow's milk formula in the first 6 months of life did not effect the incidence of childhood allergy or atopic dermatitis. However, another study of neonates at high risk of developing allergic disease showed that substituting soy or breast milk and excluding cow's milk, eggs, and fish led to a decrease in incidence of atopic dermatitis. This area remains controversial and withholding of cow's milk in these high risk families may not be efficacious.

Once the atopic dermatitis has established itself, one should avoid those foods which the parents are strongly convinced cause a flare-up of the disease. Fully 50% of infants and children with atopic dermatitis will have no reaction on scratch tests to milk or other common foods. When the food is strongly suspected historically, challenge with that food usually results in hives and not flaring of the eczema. The use of a battery of skin tests to common foods and/or the use of the RAST test have not been found to be a benefit in determining which foods to eliminate from the diet. At the present time, the clinical history appears to be the best guide to food elimination and highly restricted diets are to be avoided.

Thorough allergy investigation with skin testing and possible institution of allergy injection therapy (immunotherapy) is indicated when there is the presence of severe seasonal or perennial allergic rhinitis and/or asthma. There is no evidence that immunotherapy will improve atopic dermatitis and, in the face of eczema and other inhalant disease, immunotherapy should be instituted by a well trained allergist.

There is probably no other skin disease which is so characterized by chronic intense pruritus. The antipruritic action of antihistamines can afford benefit by suppressing the itch, thereby reducing trauma to the skin. Hydroxyzine is a potent, long-acting antihistamine which also has an antianxiety effect. It is usually well tolerated by both adults and pediatric patients but drowsiness does occur.

Local corticosteroids applied to the skin are the most effective form of topical therapy. Widespread use of chronic, potent, corticosteroid preparations under occlusion can produce adrenal suppression and skin atrophy with the formation of striae. Use of the lower potency corticosteroids (hydrocortisone 1% or the quarter-strength fluorinated corticosteroids) are effective and rarely produce adrenal suppression or side effects. There are now many topical fluorinated steroids on the market and some attention should be given to the wide variation in cost of these materials especially as compared to the 1% hydrocortisone cream (see Chapter 22).

When extreme dryness of the skin is a problem, especially in the chronic stages, several emollients may be applied to prevent loss of moisture from the skin. These may include Cetaphil Lotion, Eucerin cream, and 10% urea-containing preparations. Infrequent bathing with the addition of mineral oil and moisturizers such as Alpha Keri may be helpful.

Antibiotics may be used judiciously for the treatment of infected lesions. Studies of the microbial flora of patients with this disease demonstrate a carriage rate of *Staphylococcus aureus* in over 90%. Erythromycin is a good choice since many of these strains of *S. aureus* have been found to be resistant to penicillin.

Systemic corticosteroids may be used in those few extremely difficult cases, or patients with the explosive onset or reexacerbation of the skin lesions which make thorough topical application impossible. Prednisone in a single morning dose of 0.5 mg/kg for a week is appropriate therapy with a switch to alternate day therapy with cautious tapering and eventual discontinuation of the steroids when the disease process is controlled.

References

1. Holta, A: Conference on infantile eczema. J. Pediatr., *66:* 158, 1965.
2. Rajka, G: Atopic dermatitis. In W. Rooks (Ed.) *Major Problems in Dermatology*, Vol. 3. W. B. Saunders, Philadelphia, 1975.
3. Blaylock, W. K.: Atopic dermatitis. Diagnosis and pathobiology. J. Allergy Clin. Immunol. *57:* 62, 1976.
4. Rasmusen J. E., and Provost T. T.: Atopic dermatitis. E. Middleton, C. E. Reed, and E. F. Ellis, (Eds.) In *Allergy Principles and Practice*, p. 1039. C. V. Mosby, St. Louis, 1978.
5. Katz S: Atopic dermatitis. *Task Force on Asthma and Other Allergic Diseases.* NIH publication No. 79-387, p. 373. United States Department of Health, Education, and Welfare, Washington, D. C., 1979.

CHAPTER 5

OTHER ECZEMATOUS DISEASE

PAUL LAZAR

KINDS OF ECZEMA

Diaper Dermatitis

Diaper dermatitis is a common problem that occurs primarily due to friction and moisture. The presence of microorganisms may contribute to the changes. Disease that is resistant to therapy may be atopic dermatitis in diaper area with secondary factors aggravating the situation. In the obese infant, often the inguinal creases are spared when friction and urine are the most important etiologic factors. Associated or primary *Candida* infections usually have outlying superficial pustules beyond the main seat of the disease. Any primary disease (atopic dermatitis, psoriasis, etc.) may occur in the diaper area.

Dyshidrotic Eczema

Dyshidrotic eczema (pompholyx) is a recurrent blistering disease of the palms and soles. Usually, the lesions are pin head size but may be larger. Eccrine glands are involved only secondarily and involvement of the sides of the fingers and palms is more common than involvement of the feet. The high incident of familial atopy and other areas of atopic dermatitis suggest that this is atopic disease in a particular location. Recurrences are frequent and the problem is to be differentiated from contact dermatitis, dermatophytid, pustular psoriasis, and food allergies.

Nummular Eczema

Nummular eczema (orbicular eczema) (Fig. 5.1) is an eruption that consists of roughly round patches or plaques with crusted vesicles located on the dorsum of the extremities and elsewhere. The dermatitis tends to be recurrent and resistant to clearing although it is responsive to topical and systemic treatment. The condition frequently follows prolonged exposure to, or explosive reactions to, primary irritants and contact allergens, particularly on xerotic skin. As always, the question of underlying atopic disease arises whenever eczematous disease is present and persistent. Unfortunately, recurrences are frequent, new patches commonly arise, and resistance to absolute cure is frustrating. Once established, the dermatitis can continue for months and years. Associated staphylococcal colonization may respond to appropriate systemic antibiotic therapy.

Hand Eczema

This common dermatitis represents a number of different entities. Defatting of the skin which is dry and low humidity are commonly associated with these changes. The problem is a major one for the housewife and all those

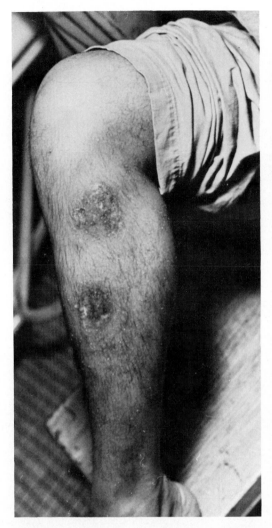

Fig. 5.1. Nummular eczema involving the legs.

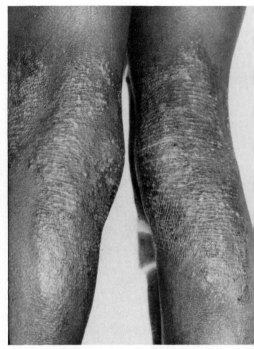

Fig. 5.2. Typical lichenification in popliteal area of localized neurodermatitis.

working with water, solvents, cleansers, and other irritant chemicals. True allergic contact dermatitis is a less frequent cause of eczematous hand changes.

Heat and humidity support fungal and bacterial involvement expressed as eczematous changes. Frequently, the dermatitic features have a primary cause but they are perpetuated and complicated by many factors such as allergic, photoallergic, and physical reactions, ingestants, inhalants, and xerosis.

Foot Eczema

This has many of the same elements as hand eczema with the added dimension of occlusion and allergic reaction to footwear. Shoe materials including dyes, preservatives, rubber, adhesives, and many other components have contributed to the frequent occurrence of dermatitis of the feet. In addition, the warmth, moisture, and friction accompanying the use of footwear contribute to the eczematous changes. Microorganisms add another factor to skin problems affecting the feet as primary and secondary etiologic agents.

Eczema Hiemalis

Eczema hiemalis (winter eczema, erythema craquelé) is an erythematous eruption with superficial crack-like lesions in the skin. The skin is xerotic with the changes usually evident during the winter and primarily in the elderly. Itching and dry skin warn of the imminent appearance of the gross changes. Adequate lubrication will ordinarily prevent or reverse the process; however, if the physiologic capability of the skin is extended beyond its natural ability to recover, eczematous changes appear. The process rests on a balnce between adequate lubrication of the skin and loss of the cutaneous integrity.

Localized Neurodermatitis

Localized neurodermatitis (lichen Vidal, lichen simplex chronicus, lichenification with pruritus). This lichenified dermatitis is usually confined to one area. It is unrelated to atopy and more common in women and orientals. This must be differentiated from stasis dermatitis, lichen planus and psoriasis. The essential elements are friction, excoriations, pruritus, and lichenification (Fig. 5.2). The margin of the typical patch fades imperceptibly into normal skin.

Disseminated Neurodermatitis

Disseminated neurodermatitis is synonymous with atopic dermatitis (Fig. 5.3). This label seems too restrictive and overemphasizes the psychiatric aspects of the condition. Initially, the term was started because it was thought the changes were related to neurological rather than psychiatric changes. It is unrelated to urticaria and other skin changes related to emotional upsets.

Infectious Eczematoid Dermatitis

Infectious eczematoid dermatitis, in the classic sense, is the well known dermatitis which occurs in the area bathed by drainage from an infected area (see Fig. 5.4 on color Plate I). Sources leading to such changes are infected ears (Fig. 5.5), noses, and draining sinuses. The dermatitis is usually subacute in appearance with pustules present within and around the affected area. Similar clinical disease may be associated with draining varicose ulcers and osteomyelitis.

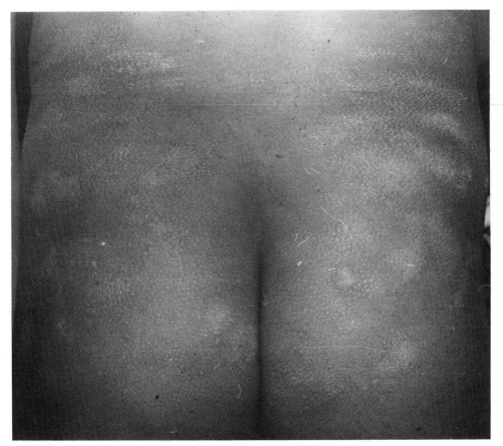

Fig. 5.3. Atopic dermatitis manifested as hypopigmented pityriasis alba.

The basic approach to treatment of these other eczemas is similar to that for atopic dermatitis. Specific treatment and recommendations for special situations must be selected as for all medical problems. Infectious components are treated best with systemic antibiotic therapy.

LOCAL THERAPY

Topical therapy is the cornerstone and often the only treatment necessary to control eczematous dermatitis. Steroid preparations (Table 5.1) are easily the most effective remedies with selection of the appropriate vehicle for maximum effectiveness and patient acceptability critical for getting the best results. Nonfluorinated steroid preparations are desirable for prolonged use on the face, genital, and intertriginous areas. Other preparations may give relief more rapidly and are designated more appropriately for use on other body surfaces. Systemic absorption of topically applied steroid preparations must always be kept in mind, especially in infants and children. Cost may be a consideration in using topical steroid preparations so other remedies may aid in controlling that factor and the patient's problem.

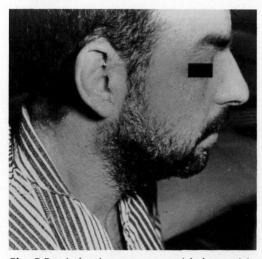

Fig. 5.5. Infectious eczematoid dermatitis involving the bearded area, cheeks, and eyelids. Source of the disease was drainage from the ear.

Table 5.1
Topical Corticosteroids

Alphaderm Cream (1% hydrocortisone cream), Norwich-Eaton
Aristocort Topical Products (triamcinolone acetonide), Lederle
Cetacort Lotion (hydrocortisone), Texas Pharmacal
Cordran SP Cream (flurandrenolide), Dista
Cordran Tape (flurandrenolide tape) Dista
Decaderm 1% Topical in Estergel (dexamethasone), Merck Sharp & Dohme
Diprosone Cream 0.05% (betamethasone dipropionate), Schering
Florone Cream (diflorasone diacetate), Upjohn
Halog Cream/Ointment/Solution (halcinonide), Squibb
Hydrocortisone creams—many companies alone or in combination with urea, vioform
Hytone Cream (hydrocortisone), Dermik
Kenalog Cream/Protein/Ointment/Spray (triamcinolone acetonide), Squibb
Lidex Cream 0.05% (fluocinonide), Syntex
Synalar Cream 0.025% (fluocinolone acetonide), Syntex
Synemol (fluocinolone acetonide), Syntex
Topicort Emollient Cream 0.25% (desoximetasone), Hoechst-Roussel
Topsyn Gel 0.05% (fluocinonide) same as Lidex, Syntex
Tridesilon Creme 0.05% (desonide), Dome
Uticort Gel (betamethasone benzoate gel), Parke-Davis
Valisone Cream 0.1% (betamethasone valerate), Schering
Westcort Cream 0.2% (hydrocortisone valerate), Westwood

Baths to hydrate the keratin and alleviate itching and inflammation may be invaluable. The water temperature should be comfortable for the patient. Other uses of water, such as wet dressings to combat infection and weeping, should be employed. Lubrication of the wet skin by use of bath additives (Table 5.2) or direct applications of emulsions (Table 5.3) do much for the patient's comfort. Cool compresses usually provide significant and immediate relief from itching.

Individual remedies may be improved by the addition of menthol, phenol, and camphor to help control pruritus (Table 5.3). Enhanced response to topical steroids may follow occlu-

Table 5.2
Systemic Antipruritics[a]

Atarax Tablets and Syrup (hydroxyzine hydrochloride), Roerig
Benadryl (diphenhydramine hydrochloride USP), Parke-Davis
Chlor-Trimeton (chlorpheniramine maleate USP), Schering
Co-Pyronil (pyrrobutamine compound), Dista
Dimetane (brompheniramine maleate NF), Robins
Drammamine (dimenhydrinate), Searle
Forhistal Maleate Lontabs (dimethindene maleate NF), Ciba
Histady (methapyrilene hydrochloride), Lilly
Periactin (cyproheptadine HCl), Merck Sharp & Dohme
Pyribenzamine (tripelennamine HCl), Ciba
Tacaryl Tablets and Syrup (methadilazine HCl), Westwood
Teldrin Spansule Capsules (chlorpheniramine) maleate, Smith Kline & French
Temaril (trimeprazine tartrate), Smith Kline & French
Vistaril Capsules and Oral Suspension (hydroxyzine pamoate), Pfizer

[a] Tranquilizers, soporifics, and antiinflammatory drugs (including aspirin) may be helpful, as may systemic antibiotics.
  Please note that this is only a partial list of available drugs and is just a guide for treatment of eczematous disease.

Table 5.3
Antipruritic Products

Bath Oils and Additives
  Almay-Tar Bath
  Alpha Keri
  Aquasol Bath Oil
  Balnetar, and Balneol
  Derma Lab Bath and Body Oil
  Domol Bath and Shower Oil
  Lubath
  Neutrogena Sesame Seed Body Oil
  Zetar Emulsion

Lotions and Emollients
  Aquacare Dry Skin Cream & Lotion
  Carmol HC Cream
  Derma Lab Lotion and Cream
  Formula 405 Cream
  Keri Lotion, and Creme
  Lubriderm Cream, and Lotion
  Neutrogena Hand Cream, and Lotion for Hand and Skin
  Shepherd's Cream Lotion, and Dry Skin Cream
  Wondra Lotion

Soaps, Shampoos, and Cleansers
  Almay-Tar Shampoo
  Aquasol Body Lotion
  Aveeno Bar
  Basis Soap
  Cetaphil Lotion
  Danex Shampoo
  Derma Lab Soap
  DHS Tar, and regular, Shampoo
  Exsel Shampoo
  Head and Shoulders Shampoo
  Lubriderm Soap
  Neutrogena Dry-Skin Soap
  Neutrogena Solid Soap Shampoo
  Oilatum Soap
  Purpose Brand Soap, and Shampoo
  Regular Selsun Shampoo
  T & C Shampoo
  Vanseb-T Tar Shampoo
  Zetar Shampoo
  Zincon Dandruff Shampoo

Local Anesthetics
  Benzocaine ointment
  Xylocaine 5% Ointment

Powders
  Baby powders
  ZeaSorb Medicated Powder

sion by plastic film and other occlusive dressings. However, one must always consider the problems of sweating, associated infection, and patient acceptability.

Tar preparations give relief, still, and are less expensive to use over large surfaces. A water washable and nonstaining preparation such as liquor carbonis detergens may be incorporated in a variety of vehicles. Topical antibiotics can be useful as well as oxyquinoline compounds and antifungal remedies alone or in combination with topical steroids.

Vehicle selections for all topical treatment must be considered very carefully. The choice will depend on the clinical features of the disease, its location, the weather, patient activities, and age, cost, and patient willingness to use the preparations. Cleansers and shampoos should be selected carefully. (Table 5.3). Mechanical occlusions or restraints ranging from cotton gloves or socks to splints or ace bandages aid in controlling itching and scratching. Unna's zinc paste gelatin type dressing has been used with great success.

Ultraviolet exposure has helped many, although some atopics are sun-sensitive. In addition, temporary removal to a new climate or even a hospital bed will result in clearing or a diminution of the severity of the process. Every attempt to keep the dermatitis from exacerbations should be tried.

SYSTEMIC THERAPY

For serious problems and acute exacerbations, the administration of oral or injectable steroids (Table 5.4) usually will control the dermatitis rapidly. One should attempt to limit the total dose and length of administration time whenever possible. Injectable steroids give the physician control of the situation and allows one to keep the dose at a level lower than with oral preparations. However, the hypothalamic-pituitary-adrenal axis is more apt to be suppressed by intramuscular long-acting steroids. A short course of oral prednisone given every morning in a single dose need not be tapered (1). Longer courses should be given every other day and in the mornings. If such a course controls the disease, it is usually free of most side effects and suppresses the internal endocrine balance very little.

Systemic antibiotics frequently aid in the management of recalcitrant atopic dermatitis. Although not grossly infected, apparently the organisms on the eczematized skin keep it from responding completely to topical and systemic medications.

To combat sleeplessness and help alleviate itching, oral sleeping remedies, antihistamines, and mild tranquilizers may be very helpful (Table 5.2). A drowsy patient may have difficulty performing day-to-day activities so a work and activities history should be evaluated when one prescribes remedies which may make the patient tired or drowsy.

Finally, the patients should be educated to understand the problems of management and the disease. Frequently, the patients are able to relate important information about their own dermatitis. The physician and family

Table 5.4
Oral and Injectable Preparations

Celestone Phosphate Injection (betamethasone sodium phosphate NF), Schering
Aristocort Intralesional (triamcinolone diacetate), Lederle
Meticortelone Acetate Aqueous Suspension (prednisolone acetate USP), Schering
Prednisone (many suppliers)
Solu-Medrol (methylprednisolone sodium succinate for injection USP), IV and IM, Upjohn
Kenalog-40 Injection (sterile triamcinolone acetonide suspension), Squibb
Medrol Tablets (methylprednisolone tablets NF), Upjohn
Hydrocortisone Tablets and Cortisone Acetate Tablets, Purepac
Decadron Phosphate Injection (dexamethasone sodium phosphate MSD), Merck Sharp & Dohme

should do everything reasonable to support and encourage the patient afflicted with atopic dermatitis. One should always encourage them to believe they will be the fortunate ones whose dermatitis will clear eventually although no specific predictions can be made in that regard. However, it is essential that patients with active eczema lead as normal a life as possible.

REFERENCES

1. Storrs, F.J.: Use and abuse of systemic corticosteroid therapy. J. Am. Acad. Dermatol., *1*: 95, 1979.
2. Chendwith, B.R., and Lobitz, W.C., Jr.: Atopic dermatitis. *Clinical Dermatology*. Vol. 3., Unit 13-2, p.1. Harper & Row, New York, 1971.
   Demis, D.J.; Crounse, R.G.; Dobson, R.L.; and McGuire, J.
3. Frick, O.L.: The Atopic state—a particular kind of immune reaction, a review. Ann. Allergy, *24*: 95, 1966.
4. Baer, R.L.: *Atopic Dermatitis*. New York University Press, New York, 1955.
5. Roth, H.C., and Kierland, R.R.: The natural history of atopic dermatitis. Arch. Dermatol. *89*: 209, 1964.
6. Rostenberg, A., and Bogdonoff, D.R.: Atopic dermatitis and infantile eczema, In M. Samter (Ed.) *Immunological Diseases*, p. 635. Little, Brown, & Company, Boston, 1965.
7. Callen, J.P.: Eczema (dermatitis)—classification, diagnosis and treatment. J. Ky. Med. Assoc. *76*: 485, 1978.
8. Huff, J.C.: Eczematous dermatitis. Major Probl. Clin. Pediatr., *19*: 86, 1978.

CHAPTER 6

CONTACT DERMATITIS

CHARLES ZUGERMAN

Contact dermatitis is an inflammatory reaction caused by direct contact of the skin with an inciting agent. It may be either irritant or allergic in nature and may be caused by a confusing array of different materials.

BACKGROUND

An irritating substance is one which can cause a reaction in most individuals tested if it is applied for a significant length of time at a sufficient concentration (Table 6.1). Percutaneous penetration of the involved material occurs and a nonimmunologically mediated inflammatory reaction takes place. Irritation may occur through several mechanisms, including denaturation of the epidermal proteins, altering the capacity of the stratum corneum to hold water. Because this is not immunologically mediated, the concentration of an irritant must exceed a threshold before the reaction can take place and this threshold may be very high according to the irritancy of the compound. It is not necessary for the skin to be previously sensitized and, therefore, an irritant reaction may occur immediately following contact with the material. Eighty per cent of all cases of contact dermatitis are of the irritant variety. Examples of this process include contact dermatitis to soap, detergent, or strong acid.

Allergic contact dermatitis is a T cell-mediated immune response which requires the percutaneous penetration of a low molecular weight hapten. Unlike irritant contact dermatitis, an induction period of 5–7 days is required before the first appearance of hypersensitivity, and the peak reaction on the skin occurs 24–48 hours after being rechallenged with the same antigen. Allergic contact dermatitis occurs in only 20% of patients suffering from contact dermatitis and is typified by reactions to poison ivy, nickel, and potassium dichromate. It is very difficult to tell the difference, clinically, between irritant contact dermatitis and an allergic contact dermatitis. Indeed, many irritants may be allergenic and some allergens are irritating if the concentration is too high. In general, allergic contact dermatitis appears more polymorphic with erythema, edema, and vesiculation. Irritant contact dermatitis, on the other hand, looks more like a severe burn with large blisters or marked erythema and edema.

Occasionally, a contact dermatitis only occurs in the presence of sunlight. This type of eruption, mediated by the T cell system, is known as a photoallergic dermatosis. If, on the other hand, the problem is not immunologically mediated and sunlight is still required in order to initiate it, it is known as a phototoxic eruption. The following discussion will deal primarily with ordinary allergic contact dermatitis.

Natural Course

Acute contact dermatitis begins within hours or days of contact with the antigen. Initially the lesions are characterized by erythema limited to the precise area of contact.

This erythema may become markedly indurated and eventually edema, papules, vesicules, and blisters occur with subsequent exudation and erosion (Fig. 6.1). As the reaction becomes more severe, new sites distant from the original site of contact become inflammed with occasional total body involvement (Fig.

Table 6.1
Comparison of Allergic and Irritant Contact Dermatitis

	Allergic	Irritant
First appearance of hypersensitivity	5–7 days	Immediate
Peak reaction	24–48 hr	12–24 hr
Transferred with lymphocytes	+	No
Threshold	Low	High
Examples	Nickel	Soap
	Chrome	Detergents

6.2). Without further contact with the provocative material, the eruption will heal within a period of a few days to a few weeks. Because the skin is still recovering from a severe inflammatory reaction, the skin barrier is not normal and other antigens can easily be absorbed percutaneously. If the patient self-medicates himself with home remedies and over-the-counter products, he may develop a new allergy to the medication. Also, bacterial superinfection occurs more easily at this time.

Chronic dermatitis, on the other hand, results from persistent contact with the provocative antigen and is characterized by hyperkeratotic, lichenified, scaly, and pruritic lesions which can develop painful fissures (as shown in Fig. 6.3, see color Plate I). Often, the antigenic stimulus is inapparent and thus the eruption does not clear rapidly and may persist for many years. Usually, this problem

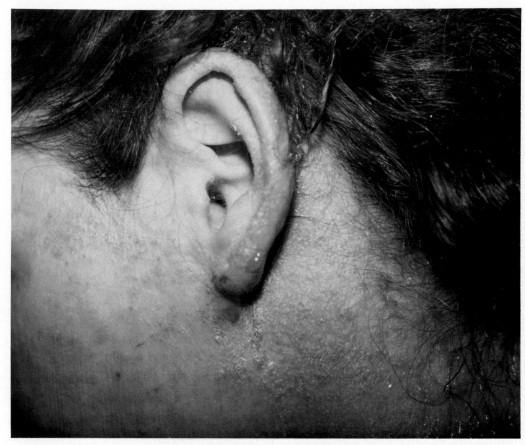

Fig. 6.1.   Acute allergic contact dermatitis to *p*-phenylenediamine in hair dye.

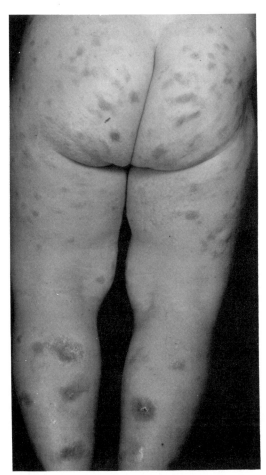

Fig. 6.2. A generalized allergic contact dermatitis.

is caused by less antigenic materials rather than potent antigens. Therefore, chronic dermatitis is difficult to diagnose and often it is impossible to treat adequately without determining the source of the antigenic stimulation.

Pathogenesis of Allergic Contact Dermatitis

Allergic contact dermatitis is a type IV cell-mediated hypersensitivity requiring an initial 5- to 7-day contact with the antigen. Upon reapplication of the antigen, the reaction will reoccur and reach its peak in 24–48 hours.

BASIC IMMUNOLOGY OF CONTACT DERMATITIS

The inductive phase (Table 6.2) of the immune response first begins at the time an antigen contacts the skin. During the preparatory segment of the inductive phase, a low molecular weight hapten comes in contact with the skin surface. It reacts with epidermal proteins, and when a hapten·protein complex occurs, a complete antigen is formed. Once a hapten·protein complex penetrates the epidermis, the reaction enters its second segment, the recognition phase.

In order for a reaction to occur, the complete antigen must be recognized by lymphocytes. Initially, however, all T lymphocytes are "antigen inexperienced" since they have never before been in contact with the antigen in question. A chance encounter with an antigen-inexperienced lymphocyte may occur within the dermis leading to the "turning on" of that lymphocyte to the antigen. More likely, however, the antigen is picked up by lymphocytes and is transported to the lymph node where sensitization of uncommitted T lymphocytes takes place.

The final phase of induction is that of proliferation of white blood cells. As a consequence of sensitization, committed T lymphocytes enter the draining lymph nodes through afferent lymphatics and induce the production of immunoblasts within the paracortical areas. These are probably precursors of the effector cells which induce the inflammatory reaction of allergic contact dermatitis.

Upon reapplication of the same hapten to the skin surface, a similar sequence of events occurs. The antigen is absorbed percutaneously and, in the process, complexes to an epidermal protein. This time, however, antigen-experienced cells, created from antigen-inexperienced lymphocytes as a consequence of the initial sensitizing episode, are present. The experienced T lymphocytes produce lymphokines (products of activated lymphocytes) and, as a consequence, recruit numerous other

Table 6.2
Phases of Development of Allergic Contact Dermatitis

Inductive phase
Preparatory phase
Recognition phase
Proliferative phase
Elicitation phase

cells very rapidly in order to produce the inflammatory reaction. The lymphokines attract other mononuclear cells, cause tissue damage, cause damage to other cell types, retain other cells in the immediate vicinity, and increase vascular permeability. The end result is a rapid, severe inflammatory response.

Table 6.3
Molecular Weights of Some Allergenic Haptens

Hapten	Molecular Weight
Formaldehyde	30
p-Phenylenediamine	108
Benzocaine	165
Tetramethylthiuram disulfide	240
Mercaptochlorobenzene	167
Dinitrochlorobenzene	202

Factors Influencing Development of Allergic Contact Dermatitis

ANTIGENIC FACTORS

Not all haptens are equally capable of producing allergic contact dermatitis. Poison ivy

Table 6.4
Risk of Developing Contact Dermatitis According to the Area of the Body

High Risk	Low Risk
Face	Palms
Scalp	Soles
Vulva	Back of forearms
Penis	
Groin	
Dorsum of hands	
Scrotum	
Perianal area	

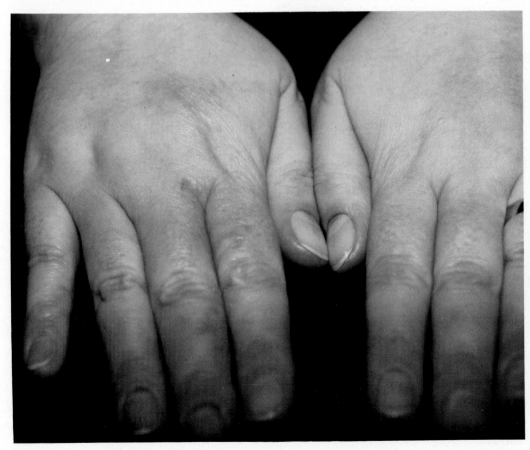

Fig. 6.4.   Irritant contact dermatitis to soap and water.

(*Rhus toxicodendron*) dermatitis may occur in a large percentage of those exposed to the antigen while nickel dermatitis occurs in 4% of exposed males and in 14% of exposed females. Most individuals never develop allergy to antigens such as erythromycin ointment. This variability is explained, in part, by specific features of the antigen.

First, the size of the antigen is an important consideration (Table 6.3). Most allergic haptens have molecular weights of less than 400 while those with progressively large molecular weights are increasingly less sensitizing. For example, epoxy resin oligomers with a molecular weight of 340 sensitized 100% of guinea pigs tested while the oligomer with a molecular weight of 908 sensitized none.

In addition to having a small molecular weight, the hapten must be fat soluble in order to facilitate percutaneous penetration

through the skin. It must also be capable of binding to epidermal proteins in order to form a complete antigen, and it must not be easily carried away by the circulation once it arrives at its destination. Finally, and most importantly, it must be easily recognized by inexperienced T lymphocytes during the process of sensitization

HOST FACTORS

Host susceptibility varies from individual to individual, and is, in part, dependent upon the degree of contact the patient has with the offending antigen. Women wear jewelry more than men and would therefore be expected to have a proportionately higher incidence of allergic contact dermatitis to nickel. Chromate, on the other hand, is used extensively in industry and an allergy to this compound

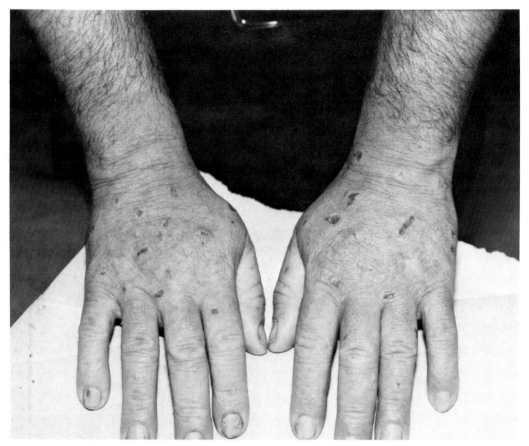

Fig. 6.5.   Chronic allergic contact dermatitis secondary to wood stain used at work.

is more commonly among men than among women.

Inflamed or infected skin allows for greater percutaneous penetration of an antigen and is, therefore, an important consideration in the host's ability to develop contact dermatitis. Neomycin applied topically to uninflamed skin is relatively nonallergenic. When used on a stasis ulcer, however, over one-third of the patients treated will eventually develop an allergic contact dermatitis.

The area of contact is important in two respects (Table 6.4). Thin macerated tissue allows for greater percutaneous penetration. In addition, areas which are especially exposed to antigens (for example hands (Fig. 6.3) and face) more frequently develop allergic contact dermatitis.

Etiology

Any material in the patient's environment is capable of evoking an irritant or allergic contact dermatitis depending upon the compound's concentration, molecular weight, and formulation as well as upon the host factors discussed above. Irritating compounds include mechanical irritants such as fiberglass; chemical irritants such as soap, (Fig. 6.4)

acids, water, alkali, and detergents as well as biological irritants including bacteria, fungi, and viruses. These materials are abundant in our environment and are related in their ability to cause dermatitis without setting off the T lymphocyte-mediated immune response.

Allergic reactions comprise only 20% of contact dermatitis cases but are important because of the economic and physical hardship they cause and because they are potentially preventable. One can compromise a virtually endless list of possible sensitizers depending upon a patient's occupation, hobbies, place of residence, state of health, hygiene, and age (Figs. 6.1, 6.5, and 6.6). Common allergens in North America include nickel, potassium dichromate, *p*-phenylenediamine, lanolin, mercaptobenzothiazole, and balsum Peru (Table 6.5) which are found in a bewildering array of diverse products, cosmetics, occupations, and environments (Table 6.6).

Occupational exposure is quite common and can sometimes be predicted by the astute physician (Table 6.6). Finally, the area of the body which is involved may give the investigating physician an idea as to the etiologic agent. If the patient's eruption is confined to the face, one should consider perfume, emollients, or preservatives in cosmetics as a possible cause. Periorbital lesions might be

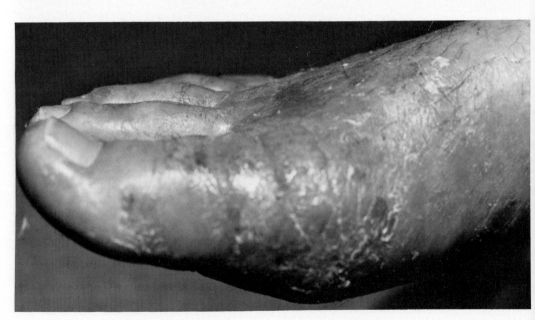

Fig. 6.6. Allergic contact dermatitis to a rubber accelerator in the patient's shoe.

caused by the materials brought to the eyes on the patient's fingers, eye medications, shampoo, and eye liners (Table 6.7).

Differential Diagnosis

Contact dermatitis occurs more commonly in situations where the skin barrier is disrupted and percutaneous penetration is more rapid and complete. Therefore, contact dermatitis may complicate other inflammatory diseases of the skin. For instance, allergic shoe dermatitis occurs more commonly in patients with severe dyshidrotic eczema of the feet. Keeping this in mind, the following are sometimes confused with contact dermatitis.

Atopic dermatitis occurs in individuals with a family history of atopy. It is chronic, occurs first in early childhood, and is localized to anticubital spaces, neck, posterior popliteal spaces, and the face. It is frequently complicated by a superimposed allergic contact dermatitis.

Lichen simplex chronicus is an idiopathic disease consisting of multiple chronic lichenified plaques localized to the legs, arms, intergluteal cleft, and hands. It is worsened by repeated local trauma.

Dyshidrotic eczema occurs occasionally in individuals who demonstrate hyperhidrosis of the palms and soles. It is characterized by fine vesicles which erode leaving behind crusted scaly lesions.

Seborrheic dermatitis is a chronic idiopathic eczema confined to the scalp, nasolabial folds, ears, axillae, and groin. It is characterized by greasy, yellow, scaling patches. *Psoriasis* is often difficult to distinguish from seborrheic dermatitis and should be considered in the differential diagnosis of contact dermatitis.

Fungus infections, particularly of the hands and feet, can be confused with contact dermatitis. Scrapings from the involved areas when prepared with potassium hydroxide and

Table 6.6
Common Occupational Exposures

Occupation	Exposure
Barber	Depilatories, dyes, perfumes, soaps, metals
Carpenter	Adhesives, cement, fiberglass insulation wood, metals, varnish
Cement worker	Cement, epoxy, oils
Florist	Fungicides, herbicides, antibiotics, insecticides, plants
Painter	Cleansers, dyes, metals, paint, paint removers, putty, solvents
Roofer	Asphalt, dichromate, formaldehyde
Shoemaker	adhesives (mercaptobenzothiazole, resin), dyes, tanning compounds (chromates), soaps, cleaners

Table 6.5
Common Sensitizers in North America

Sensitizer	(Concentration)	Incidence (Female/Male)	Present In
Nickel	2.5%	14.9/5.5	Coins, metal objects, ceramics, jewelry
Dichromate	0.5%	5.9/9.8	Cement, dyes, leather, preservatives, photo materials, matches
Formalin	2.0%	3.4	Textile finishes, fixatives, and preservatives
Mercaptobenzo-thiazole	1.0%	3.0	Rubber
p-Phenylenedi-amine	0.6%	6.1	Dyes
Balsum Peru	25.0%	7.2	Perfumes, cosmetics
Thiuram	1.0%	5.0	Rubber

Table 6.7
Regional Diagnosis of Contact Dermatitis

Location	Material
Hands	Irritants (soaps, water, detergents, solvents)
	Food additives
	Medications and cosmetics (anesthetics, lanolin, preservatives, perfumes)
	Metals (nickel, dichromate) in coins, jewelry, metal pots and pans
	Nail polish
Feet	Medications and cosmetics
	Shoes (metals, rubber, dyes)
Mouth	Food preservatives
	Tooth pastes
	Mouth wash
	Dentures
	Yeast infections
Scalp	Hair dyes
	Shampoos
	Conditioners
Eyes	Eye shadow
	Shampoos
	Metal eyelash curlers
	Eyeliner
	Medications

viewed under the microscope will allow a physician to make the correct diagnosis.

Stasis dermatitis occurs on the lower extremities as a result of chronic venous insufficiency. It is characterized by brown eczematous areas which frequently ulcerate and are sometimes complicated by allergic contact dermatitis due to applied medications. Signs of venous insufficiency such as varicosities may also be present.

Diagnosis

Careful history and physical examination are critical to the correct diagnosis of contact dermatitis. In addition, patch testing, which entails the application of a standard concentration of a pure material to the patient's upper back in an attempt to reproduce the contact dermatitis, may also be useful in the diagnosis of allergic contact dermatitis and is described more completely in Chapter 2, Procedures and Techniques in Dermatology.

Therapy

Treatment of contact dermatitis is most effective if the cause can be determined through patch testing and through a careful history and physical examination. If etiology cannot be determined, then treatment must be symptomatic.

Acute contact dermatitis is treated with frequent soaks using tap water, saline, Burow's solution (aluminum subacetate) or potassium permanganate. Burow's solution is readily available in the form of tablets or powder and can be used in 1:20, 1:40, or 1:80 dilution concentrations in treating this disease. Between soaks, the area is allowed to air dry and a topical steroid lotion is applied. Once the blisters have broken and begun to crust over, soaking may be discontinued and a topical steroid cream may be used. In cases of severe acute contact dermatitis where the cause is known (such as poison ivy), a short course of systemic cortisone in intermediate doses can be employed. Prednisone in doses of 40–60 mg tapered over a 7–10 day period is effective.

Chronic contact dermatitis is a much more difficult therapeutic problem. Often, tar or steroid ointments must be used over long periods of time with only partial effect. Ultraviolet light as well as avoidance of nonspecific irritants such as soap, water, and detergents may be partially helpful. Patch testing with "standard" antigens is indicated and may occasionally yield the etiologic agent. In the long run, however, chronic contact dermatitis responds poorly and often leads to significant morbidity.

References

1. Fregert, S., et al.: Epidemiology of contact dermatitis. St. John's Medical Journal, *55:* 17,1969.
2. Shelley, W.B., and Juhlin, L.: The Langerhans' cell: its origin, nature and function. Acta Derm. Venereol. 1., *79:* (Suppl)7, 1978.
3. Rudner, E.J., Clendennning, W.E., Epstein, E., et al.: Epidemiology of contact dermatitis in North America, 1972. Arch. Dermatol., *108:* 537, 1973.
4. Adams, A.A.: *Occupational Contact Dermatitis*, Ed. 1. J.B. Lippincott, Philadelphia, 1969.
5. Marzulli, F.N., and Maibach, H.I.: *Advances in Modern Toxicology—Dermatotoxicology and Pharmacology*, Ed. 1, Vol. 4. John Wiley & Sons, New York, 1977.
6. Fisher, A.A.: *Contact Dermatitis*, Ed. 2. Lea & Febiger, Philadelphia, 1973.
7. Baer, R.L., and Gigli, I.: Allergic eczematous contact dermatitis. In T.B. Fitzpatrick et al. (Eds.) Dermatology in General Medicine, Ed. 2, McGraw-Hill, New York, 1979.

CHAPTER **7**

ACNE, ROSACEA, AND SEBORRHEIC DERMATITIS

RUTH K. FREINKEL

These three disorders are grouped together despite the fact that they are clinically very different and distinct from each other, have differing pathological findings, and follow different courses. They are related, however, in that all three have the tendency to affect the same individual and all three are primarily expressed in areas of the skin rich in sebaceous secretions and resident microbial flora. Whether or not similar pathogenic factors are operative and how these relate to sebum and/or the microbial flora is as yet unknown. Although all three are primarily inflammatory disorders, corticosteroids are more useful in rosacea and seborrheic dermatitis than in acne where they may exacerbate the lesions. On the other hand, broad spectrum antibiotics are effective in both acne and rosacea but relatively ineffective in seborrheic dermatitis, suggesting that the bacterial flora plays a primary role in the first two but not in the last.

Despite these uncertainties regarding pathogenesis, these three extremely common disorders, which cause significant cosmetic and symptomatic distress, are for the most part controllable by relatively simple medical treatment readily administered by any physician.

ACNE

Acne is one of the most common skin diseases and it has been estimated that 20–25%

of individuals in the age group at risk have clincally significant disease. A much larger group, which includes the milder cases, buys over-the-counter medication in an amount estimated at 18–24 million dollars annually. The devastating effects of the facial disfigurement in psychosocially vulnerable teenagers and young adults cannot be overemphasized. Although acne is self-limited, the psychic trauma is often not, and significant residual scarring from even rather moderate acne remains as a life-long burden. Thus, acne requires active treatment to control the lesions until the disease resolves spontaneously. Treatment should never be discouraged by physicians, school health personnel, or parents on the grounds that the disorder is temporary or common.

The clinical manifestations of acne are familiar to physician and layman, alike, and comprise three types of lesions, all of which involve the common follicle of the hair and the extremely large sebaceous glands of the face, neck, and upper trunk. The comedo presents either as a patulous follicle filled with debris (keratin, sebum, microorganisms) which turns black due to oxidation (blackhead) or as a small flesh-colored papule (closed comedo) which is equivalent to the blackhead except that the follicular orifice has not been dilated. Normal drainage of the follicle is blocked in these comedones, allowing the content to increase and bacterial products to accumulate. Microcomedones, not visible also are present. Red papules and pustules represent the inflammatory stage of the disease and may arise from closed comedones or clinically normal follicles, but rarely develop around open comedones unless these are traumatized by picking and squeezing. The third stage of the disease is represented by deep nodules and pseudocysts. Scarring is the final stage and is most frequently present as deep triangular pits; it may, however, be hypertrophic especially as the result of nodular and cystic lesions.

Comedones are more common early in the course of most acne while nodulocystic lesions are present as a late state. However, all three may coexist in severe acne. Most acne becomes clinically important when puberty is well established and resolves in the late teens. However, acne may begin in prepubescent children usually coinciding with adrenarche. The incidence is equal between the sexes. However, very severe acne is more common in males, while in females the disease tends to persist more frequently into adult life. It is not uncommon for women to have acne into the mid-thirties and this is often more disturbing for the patient than adolescent acne since she believes it to be "abnormal" and since it may impose occupational problems.

Etiology and Pathogenesis

The pathogenesis of acne is understood to a significant degree. The process is initiated when androgenic hormones (gonadal and adrenal) are produced in sufficient amounts to activate the dormant and potentially very large sebaceous glands of the face, neck, and upper trunk. The increased production of sebum permits heavy colonization of the follicle by anaerobic diptheroids (*Proprionibacterium acnes*). It appears likely that excessive and abnormal keratinization of the follicle, which can block its patency, is due in part to androgenic stimulation but is probably also due to irritant effects of bacterial products. Some of these products include lipases that generate free fatty acids from sebum triglycerides. Free fatty acids are known to be comedogenic and may also act as inflammatory agents. The products include other lytic enzymes and have chemoattractant effects of leukocytes. In the

blocked follicles of the blind comedo or its micro counterpart, the accumulation of bacterial products provides the stimulus for inflammation and ultimately rupture of the follicle. Papules and pustules result (Fig. 7.1). Pathogenic organisms play no role in most acne and the resident microorganisms do not invade the skin around the damaged follicle. In repeatedly damaged follicles, granulomatous inflammation may occur in response to the extruded follicular contents giving rise to persistent and recurrent nodules and "sterile" abscesses (cysts). Scarring is a result of the destructive process that involves the follicle.

Exacerbating Factors

Many myths are propagated by physician and layman about acne. It is not true that exogeneous dirt contributes to acne; however, oily cosmetics have a comedogenic effect. Very few foods, including carbohydrates, have been shown to really exacerbate the disease, although chocolate and nuts seem to worsen the disease in a small number of individuals. Exacerbations related to the second-half of the menstrual cycle and probably caused by androgenic ovarian hormones occur in a large proportion of women (but not all),

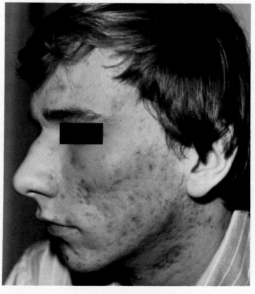

Fig. 7.1. Acne vulgaris with multiple papules, pustules, and comedos over the face.

but the effect of pregnancy is unpredictable. In most women with persistent postadolescent acne, there is no detectable endocrine disturbance. However, postadolescent acne, in conjunction with menstrual irregularities and/or hirsutism, may be due to excessive androgen production and warrant an endocrine evaluation. Some oral contraceptive agents contain androgenic progestins which worsen acne.

Acne is often exacerbated by heat, humidity, and excessive sweating. On the contrary, ultraviolet light tends to improve the disease. Whether patients are better or worse in the summer depends in good measure on the balance between these conflicting effects.

Exposure to halogens and halogenated industrial products may actually initiate an acnelike eruption or worsen preexisting acne. Glucocorticoids given for a protracted time also cause and exacerbate acne (so-called steroid acne).

Genetic factors play a role and severe acne tends to be familial.

Treatment

Treatment should be guided by the extent and severity of the disease. There is little evidence that intensive therapy, early, alters the duration of the disease. However, efforts should be directed towards suppression of inflammatory lesions to prevent scarring and nodulocystic acne. It is important to involve the patient in the treatment since success depends on continued therapy until the disease resolves spontaneously.

Mild or early acne usually responds to topical applications, once or twice a day, of drying lotions containing precipitated sulfur, sodium thiosulfate, salicylic acid, resorcinol in various combinations with alcohol or lotions, and gels containing 5–10% benzoyl peroxide (Table 7.1). A number of such preparations are available over the counter and may suffice for the treatment of mild acne. Benzoyl peroxide is a potent irritant and, initially, patients experience redness and scaliness. If this is too distressing, administration can be decreased until the skin becomes tolerant and irritation disappears. Since benzoyl peroxide, unlike other drying agents, actually prevents new lesions, it should be used on the entire acne area and continued even when lesions are suppressed. True irritant, and even allergic, contact dermatitis occurs occasionally due to benzoyl peroxide.

Table 7.1
Topical Medications for Acne, Seborrheic Dermatitis and Rosacea

Acne
Mild drying lotions: Komed Mild Acne Lotion, Sulforcin Lotion, Sulfacet-R Lotion, and Rezamid Acne Lotion, Klaronacne Lotion
Benzoyl peroxide—mild lotions: 2.5–10% lotions
Benzoyl peroxide—stronger gels, available as 5% or 10%
Retinoic acid: Retin A Brand tretinoin Cream (0.05% or 0.1%), and Retin A Brand tretinoin Lotion (0.05%)
Antibiotic lotions: erythromycin, tetracycline, and clindamycin lotions

Seborrheic Dermatitis
Shampoos containing sulfur and salicylic acid: Ionil, Sebulex, and Venseb Dandruff Shampoo
Shampoos containing tar: Sebutone, Ionil T, and Vanseb T Tar Shampoo
Scalp lotion: Sebucare
Scalp lotions for thick crusts: P & S Liquid
Corticosteroid lotions: Synalar Solution (0.01%), Valisone Lotion 0.1%, and Kenalog Lotion (0.1%)
For skin lesions: hydrocortisone cream 0.5–1% (Hytone Ointment), sulfacetamide lotion (Sulfacet-R Lotion), sulfacetamide with 0.5% hydrocortisone (Sulfacet R-HC), and a sulfur, salicylic and tar ointment (Pragmatar)

Rosacea
Hydrocortisone cream 0.5–1%
Benzoyl peroxide lotions or gels
Sulfur lotions (Sulforcin Base or Lotion, and Sulfacet R)

Little is to be gained by using hydrocortisone which is often incorporated in commercial preparations.

Excessively harsh soaps, abrasive lotions or soaps, and abrasive cosmetic aids do little good and are too irritating to use in conjunction with benzoyl peroxide. Topical vitamin A acid in creams or lotions is a useful adjuvant especially in comedonal acne since it has a comedolytic effect; it is, however, extremely irritating and may meet patient resistance. Appropriate combinations of drying lotions and vitamin A acid may produce a satisfactory effect. Recent data suggests that Retin A Brand Tretinoin may potentiate the carcinogenic effect of ultraviolet light. Caution should, therefore, be exercised in its use until the findings have been studied further. Cosmetics should be limited to those formulated without oil (oil free) which are commercially available. Face washing, by hand only, should be encouraged two or three times a day with care to remove all cosmetics at night. Moisturizers and cold creams are contraindicated. Dietary restrictions are usually useless, except when the patient recognizes adverse effects, and they should not be stressed.

The physician should be aware that acne often occurs in patients with dry skin (this is especially common in patients of Celtic descent). Such patients do not tolerate the irritating effects of benzoyl peroxide or vitamin A acid well. To avoid the need for moisturizing creams, very mild soaps (e.g. Neutrogena or Basis soap) should be used and tolerance to medication gradually built up by restricted use.

When such simple methods are insufficient, or in the face of significant inflammatory acne, antibiotics are usually indicated. The rationale for their use involves suppression of *Corynebacterium acnes* and possibly of inflammation by inhibition of chemotaxis. Oral administration of 500–1000 mg of tetracycline or erythromycin is effective in most cases. If tetracycline is used, it must be taken on an empty stomach usually 2 hours after and 2 hours before meals. In many cases, 500 mg taken at bedtime provides an adequate dose and there is no merit in divided doses. Once the lesions are adequately suppressed for 2 or 3 months, it may be possible to drop to a maintenance dose of 250 mg/day. Intermit-

tent treatment tailored to exacerbation is not advisable; however, some patients can discontinue antibiotics during the summer months. This therapy is remarkably free of side effects and may be continued for months and years if the dose is kept to 500 mg or less.

The major adverse effects are 1) gastrointestinal intolerance, and 2) vaginal candidiasis. In patients who experience such effects, the antibiotic usually has to be discontinued. Although very few well documented instances of hepatic, renal, or hematological complications have been recorded, most have occurred after prolonged administration of large doses. For this reason, blood counts and urinalysis should be performed at regular intervals if the patient has been on antibiotics for more than 2 years. Antibiotics should not be used in pregnant women and tetracycline must be discontinued immediately if pregnancy occurs to avoid deposition in bones and teeth of the fetus. Tetracycline can cause phototoxic effects. Other broad spectrum antibiotics have not been proven safe and should be used cautiously. Clindamycin, which is an effective drug, should be used only in exceptional cases and for short periods because of its role in causing pseudomembranous colitis.

Topical antibiotics are currently used by many dermatologists and are becoming commercially available. Formulations include clindamycin, erythromycin or tetracycline in lotion type vehicles. If the reported efficacy of these preparations is confirmed by more extensive and chronic use, they may largely replace oral antibiotics in all but the most severe cases.

Hormone therapy (e.g. contraceptive pills) is not used as widely as formerly for several reasons. Although those containing high estrogen and low progestin are effective in many women, there are serious questions about their long-term safety and their use is contraindicated in women under the age of 18. However, there are occasional patients with severe postadolescent acne who will benefit from hormonal treatment when more routine measures are not successful.

Estrogens exert their effect by suppressing the activity of sebaceous glands and hence sebum production. In many patients, this can be accomplished with oral contraceptives containing relatively little estrogen and is probably due primarily to suppression of ovarian androgens. However, estrogens probably also act directly on sebaceous glands by inhibiting androgen effects. This effect would interfere with activities of androgens of adrenal origin, as well, and may account for the greater effectiveness of those oral contraceptives containing high levels of estrogens. It should be remembered, moreover, that certain oral contraceptives contain progestins which have androgenic effects and which actually exacerbate the disease (e.g. Ovral, Norlestrin, Ortho-Novum).

Although low doses of glucocorticoids reduce adrenal androgen production, their use in common acne is not recommended. In those cases where there is a significant abnormality of adrenal function and excessive production of androgenic hormones, however, low doses of glucocorticoids have been used to good effect.

A number of other treatments have been advocated in the past but have not withstood the test of time. Of these, some mention of the use of systemic vitamin A is indicated. There is no evidence that a deficiency of vitamin A or any other vitamin or trace metal plays a role in acne. Nonetheless, chronic administration of large doses of vitamin A continues to be used. This treatment is not only not effective but is hazardous, since it may cause severe toxic effects. In this connection, it is worth noting that the retinoids, which are vitamin A analogs, hold some promise for the future if their toxic effects can be overcome. Certain of these drugs have been shown to be remarkably effective in suppressing sebum production and early studies suggest that they are clinically effective in severe acne. Bacterial vaccines and oral zinc have not been proven effective.

Acne surgery is an important adjunct to treatment. This includes opening and draining blind comedones and cystic lesions. The nodules and cysts frequently fail to respond to topical and antibiotics therapy but will resolve when injected with 0.1–0.3 ml of a suspension of 3–5 mg/ml triamcinolone acetonide. In severe cystic acne, an effective treatment may be warm compresses of Vleminckx's solution (sulfurated lime solution) (available as Vlem-dome); patients, however, frequently object to the pungent odor. Light freezing with liquid nitrogen or carbon dioxide slush is sometimes helpful in nodulocystic acne. Similarly, ultraviolet light (sun lamp) treatment may be a useful adjunct if administered frequently. It should not be used with vitamin A acid and patients should be cautioned about excessive exposure and the use of protective eye goggles.

Scarring, especially of the pitted type can be helped in selective patients by dermabrasion. (See Chapter 33, Dermabrasion).

ROSACEA

This disorder occurs primarily in middle-aged and elderly individuals but can develop in young adults. Women are more frequently affected than men but the disease is often more disfiguring in the latter.

Although its location and certain clinical features resemble those of acne, it is a clinically distinct entity and probably is mediated by a different pathogenetic mechanism.

Rosacea is characterized by persistent erythema of the central portion of the face (as shown in Fig. 7.2 on color Plate I). Telangiectasia are usually present even early in the course and tend to be most prominent on the nose and cheeks. Papules, often surmounted by tiny superficial pustules, are the second component of the disease (Fig. 7.3). Although they tend to come and go, they may be quite persistent and in some severe cases eventuate as recalcitrant nodular lesions. In general, the papulopustular lesions are also confined to the central portion of the face (Fig. 7.4). As the disease progresses, the soft tissues of the nose become hyperplastic leading to a disfiguring enlargement known as rhinophyma. This complication is more common in males. Comedones and cystic lesions are not a feature of rosacea.

The onset of the disorder is insidious, usually between the ages of 30 and 50. If the disease begins early, it may concur with post-adolescent acne and present difficulties in differential diagnosis. A history of easy facial flushing from anxiety, embarrassment, or alcohol intake is frequently present suggesting an excessive lability of the facial vasculature as an underlying feature.

Exogenous factors which exacerbate the

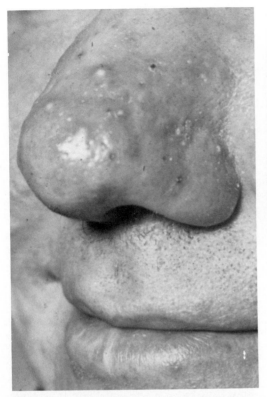

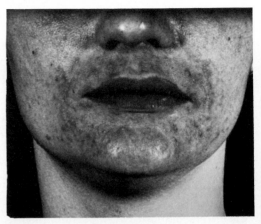

Fig. 7.4. Perioral dermatitis with erythema, papules, and some pustules. Related to rosacea.

acterized by chronic granulomatous nodules and was formerly considered to be a tuberculid because of the presence of epitheloid and giant cells. The reaction, however, is probably a response to the extrusion of follicular contents following a destructive inflammatory process.

Fig. 7.3. Rosacea—papules surmounted by tiny superficial pustules on the nose.

disease frequently are those which cause dilatation of facial blood vessels. These include alcoholic beverages, coffee, excessive heat and humidity, ingestion of very hot or spicy foods, and exposure to sunlight. The role of the latter is not well appreciated. However, in some cases, sun exposure is a triggering factor and in its initial phase the lesions may occur only after exposure to sunlight.

Varient Forms

So-called perioral dermatitis is considered by some to be a varient of rosacea. This disorder, which is not uncommon, is characterized by papulopustular lesions and erythema in the lower portion of the face, particularly around the mouth. It is most commonly seen as a consequence of the administration of topical fluorinated corticosteroids but can occur spontaneously.

An especially severe form of rosacea is char-

Associated Findings

The most common other physical findings involve the eyes. Blepharitis and conjunctivitis are frequently present. Keratitis is a more serious associated disorder which may progress to ulceration and visual impairment.

Etiology and Pathogenesis

The etiology of rosacea remains unknown. A role was formerly attributed to a resident mite, *Demodex folliculorum*, in the follicles; although the numbers of these parasites may be increased, no evidence for their role in the pathogenesis has been advanced. Pathologic studies have demonstrated only vascular dilation and a nonspecific inflammatory reaction in the dermis and, unlike acne, the disease is not primarily a folliculitis. Although the disease occurs in an area richly supplied with sebaceous glands, sebum, per se, does not seem to be an etiological factor. This is supported by the fact that rosacea is most common in

women at a time of declining sebum production. A possible role of the cutaneous flora cannot be ruled out, however. The recent demonstration that a toxin elaborated by *Staphylococcus epidermidis* may produce recurrent blepharoconjunctivitis, suggests that exploration of the role of the products of the bacterial flora in producing inflammation may be fruitful.

Treatment

Unlike acne, rosacea is not self-limited. Treatment is required for remission of the disease. Most cases of rosacea respond to the chronic administration of broad spectrum antibiotics (e.g. tetracycline and erythromycin) in moderate doses (250–500 mg/day). This usually produces the resolution of the papulopustular component and may in time reduce the erythema. Intermittent use of hydrocortisone creams (0.5–1%) is also helpful especially for the erythema. Fluorinated corticosteroids are detrimental and chronic usage of any corticosteroid is to be avoided since these may be acnegenic and cause telangiectasia. Other topical agents used for acne may be useful especially those containing sulfur. Benzoyl peroxide creams and lotions are sometimes of help but may also cause irritation and worsening of the underlying erythema. A necessary part of therapy includes the avoidance of excessive heat, humidity, alcohol ingestions, and excessive exposure to sunlight.

Rhinophyma tends to be progressive and does not resolve with medical treatment although its progress may be arrested. Removal of the excess tissue by shaving it off, dermabrasion, or electrosurgery produces good cosmetic results. Recurrence in time, is unfortunately common.

SEBORRHEIC DERMATITIS

This common skin disorder has a wide age distribution, affects both sexes, often overlaps with acne and rosacea, and appears to be associated with a constitutional diathesis with chronic, intermittent signs and symptoms.

The disease is characterized by poorly de-lineated erythema with scales that are often waxy and yellowish. Although the lesions may resemble psoriasis, they lack the characteristic sharp borders and the fluffy white scales of the latter. Seborrheic dermatitis almost invariably involves the scalp in a diffuse manner. The presence of dandruff in the absence of redness is not diagnostic of seborrheic dermatitis. Shedding of visible scales from the scalp is not necessarily abnormal and may be due only to a greater than usual rate of shedding of the stratum corneum together with excessive oiliness.

Redness and scaling of the eyebrows, nasolabial folds, retroauricular folds, and bearded area are commonly present (Fig. 7.5). Blepharitis and conjunctivitis are often present. In obese individuals, especially, the eruption often involves axillary and inframammary folds (in women) and the perineum. From time to time patients will also note scaly patches on the anterior chest and around the umbilicus. Seborrheic dermatitis is one of the cutaneous disorders that can progress from localized and patchy lesions to a universal cutaneous involvement with a chronic and intractable exfoliative dermatitis. Itching, es-

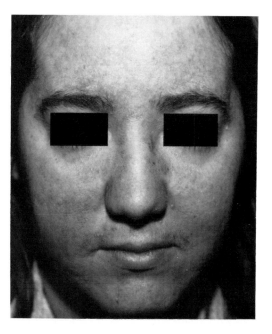

Fig. 7.5. Seborrheic dermatitis with erythema and scaling of face.

pecially on the scalp, is troublesome to the patient. Whether or not the disease produces loss of scalp hair is a matter of dispute, although in severe cases this seems to be the case.

The disease is common in infants where it begins on the scalp as cradle cap and in the perineal area as a recalcitrant diaper rash. Especially in infants, but also in adults, involvement of skin folds is often complicated by superimposed infection with *Candida albicans*; this is accompanied by typical small pustules at the edges or beyond the boundaries of the involved areas. Bacterial superinfection of the dermatitic areas occurs in severe, neglected cases especially on the scalp and behind the ears leading to a moist exudative and sometimes purulent appearance.

Differential diagnosis may be difficult. With involvement of the scalp and skin folds, it may closely mimic psoriasis. However, absence of well defined plaques, lesions of extensor surfaces such as elbows and knees, and of dystrophic nail changes help to differentiate the two disorders. Patches of the disease on the trunk may mimic tinea versicolor; a positive potassium hydroxide (KOH) preparation will confirm the diagnosis. In its more severe forms, the disease also may resemble atopic eczema; however, the characteristic involvement of the anticubital and popliteal fossae and a personal or family history of atopy will be absent.

Etiology and Pathogenesis

The pathologic features of the lesions are not very specific showing an inflammatory reaction in the dermis and sometimes psoriasis-like changes in the epidermis (without the characteristic features of psoriasis). Etiology of the disease remains obscure. It occurs in areas rich with sebaceous glands but also shows a preference for less oily areas in the skin folds. Sebum, thus, does not seem to play a determining role. On the other hand, it is very common in certain central nervous system disorders in which the skin also becomes oily (e.g. strokes, and Parkinson's disease). It frequently exacerbates during severe chronic debilitating diseases of diverse sorts. Although bacteria flourish in the scaly lesions and pyod-

ermas are common, suppression of bacteria does not cure the dermatitis.

Treatment

Treatment of the disease is usually satisfactory in the short run but patients quickly learn that the disease is recurrent and requires chronic attention. Mild scalp involvement can usually be controlled with "anti-dandruff" shampoos containing antiseptics, sulfur, salicylic acids, and tars which are readily available over the counter. Similarly, scalp lotions containing the same types of agents are helpful. Selenium sulfide lotions and shampoos are also widely used; reports of hair loss due to this compound have not been confirmed.

The use of scalp lotions and sprays containing hydrocortisone or fluorinated steroids may be required to control erythema and itching. Corticosteroid creams are the most effective topical medication for the lesions elsewhere. Fluorinated steroids should be avoided, however, since their use on the face and skin folds and on infant skin is likely to lead to adverse effects. Lotions and ointments containing 1–3% precipitated sulfur and 3% salicylic acid or sulfacetamide are often useful adjuncts and reduce the exposure to corticosteroids. Dietary manipulations, and vitamins have demonstrated little usefulness in the therapy of seborrheic dermatitis. Secondarily infected lesions may require compresses and systemic antibiotics. Topical antibiotics have little value except in otitis externa which may be due to seborrheic dermatitis. When a candidal infection is present as well, it requires the topical use of effective anticandidal agents such as Mycostatin, miconazole, or clotrimazole.

References

Acne

1. Akers, W.A., et al.: Systemic antibiotics for treatment of acne vulgaris. Arch. Dermatol., *111:* 1630, 1975.
2. Esterly, N.B., Furey, N.L., and Flanagan, L.E.: Effect of antimicrobial agents on leukocyte chemotaxis. J. Invest. Dermatol., *70:* 51, 1978.
3. Kligman, A.M., and Mills, O.H., Jr.: Acne cosmetica. Arch. Dermatol., *106:* 843, 1972.
4. Peck, G. et al.: Prolonged remissions of cystic and conglobata acne with 13-*cis* retinoic acid. N. Engl. J. Med. *300:* 329, 1979.
5. Plewig, G., and Kligman, A.M.: *Acne: Morphogenesis and Treatment.* Springer-Verlag, Berlin, 1975.

6. Sebaceous glands and acne vulgaris: *Proceedings of the 22nd Annual Symposium on Biology of Skin.* W. Montagna, M. Bell, and J.S. Strauss, (Eds.) J. Invest. Dermatol., *62:* Part 3, 1974.

Rosacea

1. Bovrie, P.: Rosacea with special reference to its ocular manifestations. Br. J. Dermatol. *65:* 458, 1953.
2. Marks, R., and Harcourt-Webster, J.N.: Histopathology of rosacea. Arch. Dermatol., *100:* 683, 1969.
3. Sneddin, I.B.: Adverse effects of topical fluorinated corticosteroids in rosacea. Br. Med. J., *1:* 671, 1969.
4. Sneddin, I.B.: Peri-oral dermatitis. Br. J. Dermatol., *87:* 430, 1972.
5. Wereide, K.: Long term treatment of rosacea with oral tetracycline. Acta Derm. Venereol., *49:* 176, 1969.

Seborrheic Dermatitis

1. Krestin, D.: Seborrheic facies as a manifestation of post encephalitic parkinsonism and allied disorders. Q. J. Med., *21:* 177, 1927.
2. McGinley, K. J., et al.: Quantitative microbiology of the scalp in nondandruff, dandruff and seborrheic dermatitis. J. Invest. Dermatol., *64:* 401, 1975.

CHAPTER **8**

PSORIASIS

HENRY H. ROENIGK, JR.

Psoriasis is a common scaly erythematous disease of unknown etiology showing wide variation in severity and distribution of skin lesions. It usually follows an irregular chronic course which is marked by remissions and exacerbations of unpredictable onset and duration.

Approximately six million people in the United States have psoriasis. Psoriasis vulgaris produces stigmatizing, chronic, recurrent lesions that often become emotionally and physically debilitating to the patient. Moreover, it is an expensive disease and frequently requires lifelong treatment.

ETIOLOGY AND PATHOGENESIS

The cause of psoriasis is not known. There is a genetic predisposition to the disease, but the exact modes of inheritance also are unknown. Recent studies have found common HL-A antigens in psoriatic patients. Kinetic studies have shown that in psoriasis the epidermal cells proliferate rapidly, completing a germinatic cell cycle every 37.5 hours compared with 19 days for normal skin. This is important in understanding some of the proposed mechanisms for systemic therapies.

Structural changes in dermal capillary loops and enzyme abnormalities having an effect on neutrophils may play a part in development of psoriasis. Chemical regulators of cyclic-AMP are reduced in psoriasis and may affect skin changes in psoriasis.

CLINICAL FEATURES

Most commonly, the characteristic cutaneous lesions of psoriasis are round, erythematous dry patches of various sizes covered by abundant, grayish white imbricated scales (see Fig. 8.1 on color Plate I; Figs. 8.2–8.4; and see Fig. 8.5 on color Plate II). They may occur as small or large plaques or small guttate, generalized lesions. Although they have a predilection for the scalp, (Fig. 8.4), nails, and extensor surfaces of the limbs, the lesions may cover the entire body, producing an erythroderma (Fig. 8.5).

Another, rarer form, pustular psoriasis, can produce generalized sterile cutaneous pustules (Fig. 8.6) and severe systemic involvement that can be fatal. Another form of pustulation may be localized to palms and soles and not associated with systemic symptoms. Psoriatic arthritis (Fig. 8.7), which simulates rheumatoid arthritis, appears in approximately 10% of psoriatic patients. HL-A B-27 histocompatible antigen is strongly associated with psoriatic arthritis, ankylosing spondylitis and Reiter's disease. This form of the disease primarily affects the distal joints and may become deforming as it progresses. Nail dystrophies and pitting of the nail plates (Fig. 8.8) occur frequently and are often mistaken for onychomycosis (fungal infection of the nails).

The Köbner phenomenon occurs in psoriasis by new lesion of active disease appearing on skin at sites of irritation, physical injury, wounds, sunburn, etc.

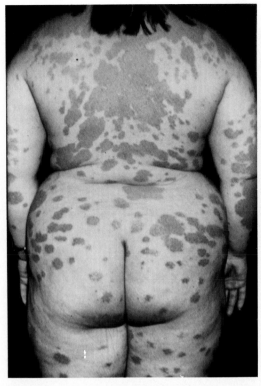

Fig. 8.2. Generalized plaques of psoriasis over trunk and extremities.

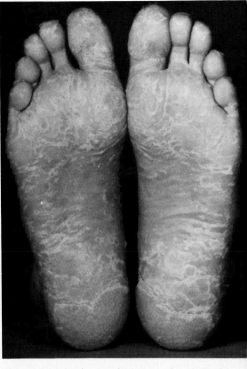

Fig. 8.3. Scaling plaques of psoriasis on soles of feet.

TREATMENT

General Factors

The nature of psoriasis and the lack of a single specific cure can be discouraging to both the patient and the physician, who often adopts a nothing-can-be-done attitude. This is unwarranted; instead, the patient should be assured at the first visit that, although there is no cure for psoriasis, it can always be controlled by one or more treatment modalities.

Initially, the patient should be cautioned about factors that exacerbate psoriasis (Table 8.1). In addition, the lesions of psoriasis may disappear spontaneously or as a result of therapy, but recurrences are almost certain to occur in a week, a month, a year, or perhaps several years. Many forms of therapy have been tried. For example, the Goeckerman tar and light therapy is still used today, while others—the turkey diet, arsenic, and x-ray—have been discontinued because they were either ineffective or too dangerous.

Proper attention should be given to such things as sound nutrition and avoiding stress and fatigue, because these factors affect the patient's response to therapy. The literature contains numerous reports of certain foods having a beneficial or deleterious effect on psoriasis. No specific dietary component seems to play a role in the disease, although the obese psoriatic patient will likely benefit in several respects from losing weight.

Whatever specific regimen is chosen for treatment of psoriasis, the psychologic approach must be stressed. Many psoriatic patients, even those with disease of long duration, do not understand the natural course of psoriasis and the many factors that seem to precipitate it. By spending some time instructing patients in the basic pathophysiology of the disease, the physician can obtain a high degree of cooperation. This is essential for successful management of psoriasis.

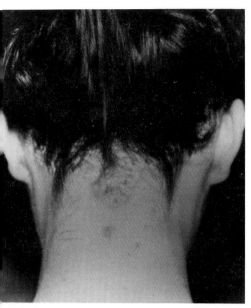

Fig. 8.4. Plaques and scales of psoriasis of scalp.

Outpatient Therapy

Most psoriatic patients can be managed as outpatients using the following guidelines to treatment.

Topical therapy is always the first approach. Even when systemic treatment becomes necessary, topical treatment should continue to avoid overusing systemic drugs.

TOPICAL CORTICOSTEROIDS

Patients with limited areas of psoriatic plaques respond well to therapy aimed at removing the scales and lubricating the lesions. Thus, topical corticosteroids are among the most useful agents (Table 8.2), and adding 3–6% salicylic acid, 5% liquor carbonis detergens or other tar bases to the topical steroids may enhance their efficacy.

Occlusive, pliable, plastic dressings increase the effectiveness of topical steroids, although such dressings are usually used only during

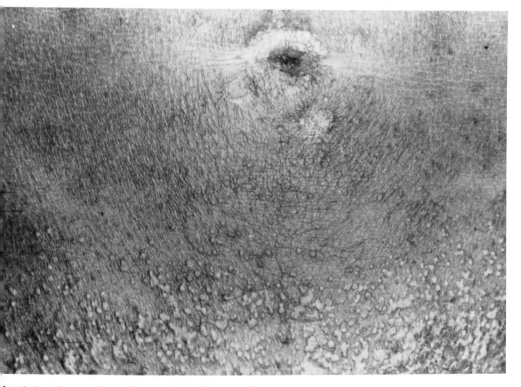

Fig. 8.6. Generalized flare of sterile pustules associated with high fever and systemic symptoms. von Zumbusch type of pustular psoriasis.

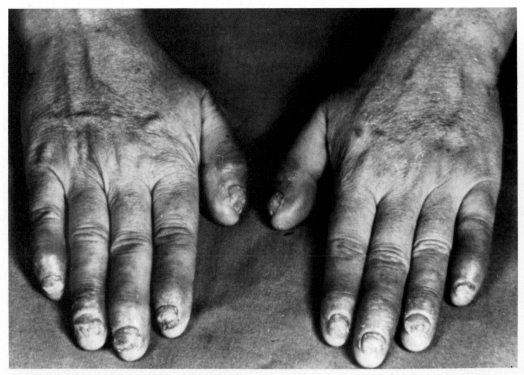

Fig. 8.7. Psoriatic arthritis with swelling and erythema of distal interpharangeal joints. Often associated with nail changes.

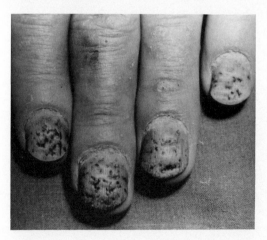

Fig. 8.8. Nail abnormalities from psoriasis consists of pitting, dystrophic changes, onycholysis, and discoloration of the nail plate.

sleeping hours (6–8 hours). Plastic wrap is used on the extremities, dry cleaning bags on the trunk, plastic food bags on the feet, and disposable plastic gloves on the hands. Whole-

Table 8.1
Factors that Exacerbate Psoriasis

Excessive intake of alcohol
Excessive weight gain
Emotional disturbances
Infection
Trauma to skin
Excessive dryness of skin
Drugs (lithium carbonate, antimalarials)

body reusable plastic suits usually can be purchased at department or sporting goods stores. Flurandrenolide-impregnated tape (Cordran tape) is satisfactory for occluding small areas of the body.

Topical corticosteroids are available in several different bases. Generally, the gel is superior to the ointment base, which is superior to the cream base (Table 8.2). Remember, however, that prolonged use of topical corticosteroids, especially fluorinated agents, can lead to complications, such as atrophy of the skin, telangiectasia, striae, and overgrowth of bacterial and fungal infections of skin.

Table 8.2
Topical Corticosteroids in Order of Potency[a]

Corticosteroid	%
Group I	
Diprosone Ointment	0.05
Halog Cream	0.1
Lidex Cream	0.05
Topicort Ointment	0.05
Topsyn Gel	0.05
Group II	
Aristocort A Cream	0.05
Diprosone Cream	0.05
Flurobate Gel	0.025
(Benisone Gel)	0.25
Topicorte Emollient Cream	0.01
Valisone Lotion	0.01
Valisone Ointment	
Group III	
Aristocort A Ointment	0.01
Cordran Ointment	0.05
Kenalog Ointment	0.1
Synalar-HP	0.2
Synalar Ointment	0.025
Group IV	
Cordran SP Cream	0.05
Kanalog Cream	0.1
Kenalog Lotion	0.025
Synalar Cream	0.025
Valisone Cream	0.1
Group V	
Tridesilon Creme	0.05
Locorten Cream	0.03
Group VI	
Topicals with hydrocortisone, dexamethasone, flumethasone, prednisolone, and methyl prednisolone	

[a] Group I is the most potent and potency descends with each group to group VI, which is least potent. There are no significant differences among agents within any given group.

Systemic absorption can cause temporary suppression of adrenal steroid production. This usually can be reversed in a few days by discontinuing topical steroids.

Tachyphylaxis is a phenomenon in which high potency topical steroids lose their effectiveness after about 1 week of intensive applications. Sometimes, switching to a lower strength topical steroid may be useful for maintenance but changing therapy to a pure tar preparation may be better at this point.

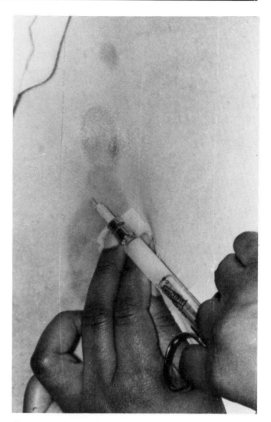

Fig. 8.9. Intralesional steroids with a 30-gauge needle into plaque of psoriasis.

INTRALESIONAL STEROIDS

Intralesional therapy with corticosteroids is effective for localized resistant plaques of psoriasis. Suspensions of triamcinolone acetonide (Kenalog) given parenterally, 10 mg/ml, are often used. Diluting 1 ml of triamcinolone acetonide with 1 ml of saline or water makes a final dilution of 5 mg/ml that helps prevent the occasional atrophy of subcutaneous tissue. The suspension is injected with a 26- or 30-gauge (Fig. 8.9) disposable needle until blanching occurs. About one injection per square centimeter is sufficient.

TAR PREPARATIONS

Tars, either crude or refined, are effective topical agents used alone in psoriasis or in combination with ultraviolet light therapy. The color, smell, and staining qualities of tar make it unaesthetic.

A bath containing two capfuls of Zetar

Emulsion (30% coal tar) or Balnetar (2.5% coal tar) will leave a barely visible coating of tar on the skin. Additional tar should be applied to the skin at bedtime, preferably in the form of a cream or ointment. The traditional preparation of 5% coal tar in petrolatum is effective but extremely messy. It may not be practical for home use, since greasy tar will stick to everything the patient touches. A similar problem arises with the use of a coal tar derivative, anthralin (dithranol 0.1, 0.2, or 0.4%) in paste form, which crumbles and falls off the skin, staining bedclothes and carpets. Anthralin paste has an irritant potential for normal skin, so that it must be applied to psoriatic plaques, which is very time-consuming. The advantages of anthralin paste are that it causes rapid flattening of thick psoriatic plaques.

A more cosmetically acceptable tar-derived preparation is liquor carbonis detergens (LCD), commonly applied in 5–10% concentrations in cold cream. If the patient's skin tends to dry out with daily bathing, a bath oil such as Alpha Keri may be added to the water.

Cosmetically acceptable tar preparations are available for baths or as shampoo, and some tars have been placed in a gel base (Estar, Psoragel) that makes them effective, safe, and more acceptable to patients.

SCALP PREPARATIONS

The scalp is difficult to treat, especially in patients with thick hair. The scalp may be treated with Baker's P&S Liquid for several hours before shampooing to loosen the scales. Thick scalp plaques may respond to oil of cade, 20%; sulfur, 10%; salicylic acid, 5%; and about 90 g of unibase. Most patients require at least one shampoo daily with either an antiseborrheic or a tar shampoo. This may be done by hand or with an automatic hair shampooer that has an automated, 3-minute wash and rinse cycle. Topical corticosteroid lotions or gels may be applied to the scalp between washings.

ULTRAVIOLET LIGHT THERAPY

Natural sunlight is an effective adjunctive therapy for psoriasis if it is readily available.

If natural sunlight is unreliable, a substitute source of ultraviolet light should be found. Small portable sunlamps promoted for home use are not suitable because only a small area of skin can be exposed at any one time. It is too impractical, unreliable, time-consuming, and dangerous to keep shifting a small light from place to place in order to irradiate all involved areas.

Artificial sunlight exposure can be provided best in a walk-in ultraviolet light booth containing eight or more four-foot-long UVB (290–320 nm) sunlamp bulbs. A "light box" allows an initial safe exposure time of 1 minute in Caucasians, 2 minutes in Orientals and Latins, and 3 minutes in blacks. The treatment time can then be increased by 1-minute increments with each successive treatment until the desired point of minimal erythema is reached. Treatment may be given every day or two or three times a week. The maximum exposure tolerated without burning is usually 10–15 minutes for Caucasians and 15–25 minutes for blacks.

UVB light sources are also available in many health clubs. UVB light booths are available commercially and may be purchased for home use, although these booths are not standardized. Plans are available for constructing a home light box, using an empty closet lined with aluminum foil and containing eight bulbs (Fig. 8.10).

During any ultraviolet light therapy, special sunglasses or goggles must be worn to prevent eye damage.

Hospitalization

When topical outpatient therapy fails or when psoriasis becomes more extensive and complications develop, hospitalization is necessary. It is helpful, of course, if the hospital has an area where the nurses are specially trained to care for the many problems of psoriatic patients.

In acute, spreading psoriasis, local applications should be soothing and aggressive therapy should be avoided. Cool baths and petrolatum or other lubricants are safe to use.

The Goeckerman regimen and its variations have been a standard inpatient treatment for psoriasis for more than 50 years. The

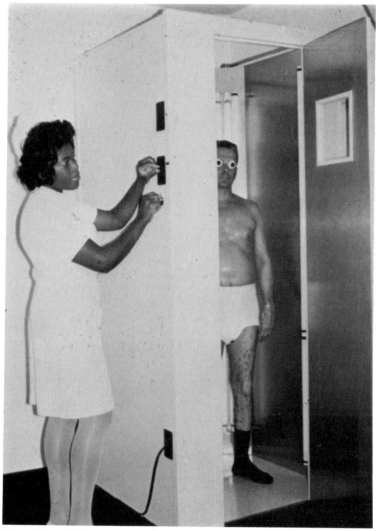

Fig. 8.10.   Ultraviolet light box with UVB bulbs (Westinghouse FS-40) and aluminum siding.

average hospitalization period is 2–3 weeks. Clinical improvement results in remission in almost all patients for 6–8 months after discharge.

The Goeckerman procedure starts with the application of 5% crude coal tar ointment to the entire body at bedtime.

In the morning, excess tar is removed with mineral oil. The patient is then given total body ultraviolet light using a light box equipped with ordinary fluorescent light bulbs (UVB) (290–320 nm) or blacklight (UVA) (320–400 nm) and aluminum reflecting sides. It is important to test the patient for the minimal erythema dose before starting ultraviolet light therapy, because a small percentage of psoriatics are "light sensitive," and the therapy will exacerbate the psoriasis rather than improve it. The amount of ultraviolet light (UVB) should be increased by 1 minute each day to a suberythema dose. Two doses of UVB per day may be given if tolerated by the patient. The patient then bathes to remove the remaining tar. Rest and relaxation during the remainder of the day are part of treatment.

A modified version of the Goeckerman routine can be used to shorten the hospital stay. Instead of applying crude coal tar at night, the patient applies topical corticosteroids under a plastic occlusive suit. In the morning, the remaining topical steroids are removed and a tar bath is given before ultraviolet light therapy.

Hospitalization also may be necessary to treat psoriatic arthritis, do a liver biopsy, or perform other tests in preparation for systemic therapy.

Psoriasis Day Care Centers

These centers are an outgrowth of the successful treatment of patients during hospitalization. The same type of treatments used for hospital patients may be used in the day care centers, where the patient stays only from 8 AM to 5 PM. This reduces costs and provides the same effective therapy as that given to inpatients.

The same combination of tar, tar gel, or anthralin plus ultraviolet light is used during daytime hours. The patient goes home or to the job in the evenings and returns to the psoriasis day care center the next morning.

Remissions from day care centers are similar to inpatient Goeckerman therapy.

Systemic Therapy

Antihistamines often help relieve pruritus associated with acute flare-ups of psoriasis. Sedatives and tranquilizers may help alleviate some of the anxiety that accompanies the disease. Antibiotics, such as penicillin or erythromycin, are indicated if there is an acute guttate, a type of psoriasis characterized by teardrop-shaped lesions and often accompanied by infection, after streptococcal infection. Vitamins, especially vitamin B_{12}, have been advocated for patients with psoriasis, but there is no evidence to support vitamin deficiency as a cause.

SYSTEMIC CORTICOSTEROIDS

Systemic treatment of psoriasis with corticosteroids was enthusiastically recommended 20 years ago, but it quickly became obvious that steroids were only controlling psoriasis and that long-term therapy caused many complications that are well known today. When steroids were withdrawn, the patients experienced a "rebound"—often the disease is worse than it had been before therapy. However, small doses of systemic corticosteroids may be indicated for severe disabling arthritis associated with psoriasis.

ANTIMETABOLITES

Since kinetic cell studies have shown that part of the pathogenesis of psoriasis involves rapid turnover of epidermal cells, it was reasonable to turn to antimitotic agents for treatment. *Methotrexate* (MTX) is among the oldest of these and has been used for 20 years in treating psoriatic patients. However, the agent carries a number of serious risks and should be administered only by, or under the supervision of, a physician experienced with antimetabolite therapy. MTX is the only antimetabolite currently approved by the FDA for psoriasis therapy.

The indications for starting MTX therapy or any form of systemic therapy must be individualized.

Because of the high risks attending its use, MTX is indicated in the symptomatic control of recalcitrant psoriasis that is not responsive to other forms of therapy and only when the diagnosis and need for MTX therapy have been established after dermatologic consultation. Each patient should be evaluated for severity of the disease, amount of discomfort, and degree of incapacity, as well as general physical condition. Generally, psoriasis should be so severe that it cannot be adequately controlled by standard topical antipsoriatic therapy.

Some patients with the following may be candidates for MTX: psoriatic erythroderma or arthritis, acute pustular psoriasis (von Zumbusch type), localized pustular psoriasis, psoriasis that prevents employment, extensive psoriasis, and a need to withdraw from systemic corticosteroids.

Contraindications. The relative contraindications to MTX therapy include significant abnormalities of renal or liver function, pregnancy, active or recent hepatitis, fibrosis or cirrhosis of liver, severe leukopenia or thrombocytopenia, active peptic ulcer, excessive alcohol consumption, active infectious disease such as tuberculosis or pyelonephritis, unreliable patient, and anemia.

Consultation with physicians familiar with antimetabolite therapy is advisable before starting MTX. It is necessary for many pre-MTX laboratory studies and a liver biopsy. Close follow-up is also essential.

PHOTOCHEMOTHERAPY

Photochemotherapy (PUVA) is a new form of systemic therapy combining the use of 8-methoxypsoralen and ultraviolet light (UVA range) given in special ultraviolet boxes (Fig. 8.11). It has proven highly effective in treating severe psoriasis (Fig. 8.12 and 8.13). Special artificial lights that have a peak irradiation on the skin about 350 mm irradiate the skin with increasing doses (Joules/cm^2 of light) 2 hours after taking oral 8-methoxypsoralen. Two large cooperative studies (1, 2) have shown that complete clearing of psoriasis can be achieved in over 90% of patients treated with an average of 20 PUVA treatments. Some patients will go into a prolonged remission, and require no further treatment, but most patients need maintenance doses of PUVA at 1- to 2-week intervals to remain clear. Guidelines to correct use of PUVA therapy including indication, complications and precautions are available. Long-term side effects could include skin cancer, aging of skin, and cataracts.

PUVA is primarily an outpatient therapy. It obviates the use of topical steroids, tars, anthralin and other agents that often are unacceptable to patients. It also avoids the use of methotrexate and other cytotoxic drugs that require constant monitoring for hematologic, hepatic, and other potential long-term side effects.

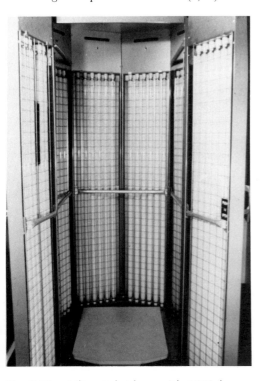

Fig. 8.11. Ultraviolet box with UVA lamps (General Electric) for use in photochemotherapy (PUVA).

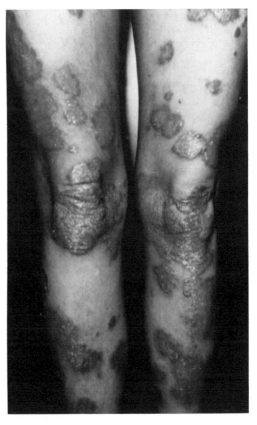

Fig. 8.12. Psoriasis before treatment with photochemotherapy (psoralen + UVA).

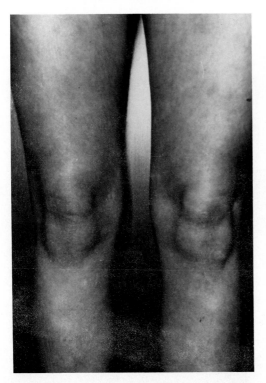

Fig. 8.13. Complete remission of psoriasis after 20 treatments with photochemotherapy.

RETENOIDS

Retenoids are a group of compounds related to vitamin A. They have specific effects on the skin which in early experiments make them a valuable oral treatment for psoriasis which lacks the hematologic and hepatic problems of methotrexate and the potential long term side effects of PUVA. Retenoids can be used to reduce the number of PUVA treatments to clear psoriasis or used alone or combined with UVB light therapy to clear psoriasis. Side effects include dry mouth and irritation of the eye.

References

1. Melski, J.W., et al.: Oral methoxsalen photochemotherapy for treatment of psoriasis: a cooperative clinical trial. J. Invest. Dermatol., *68:*1 328, 1977.
2. Roenigk, Jr., H.H., et al.: Photochemotherapy for psoriasis—a clinical cooperative study of PUVA-48 and PUVA-64. Arch. Dermatol., *115:*576, 1979.
3. Farber, E.M., and Cox, A.J.: Psoriasis—*Proceedings of the Second International Symposium.* Yorke Medical Books, New York, 1977.
4. Bailin, P.L., Roenigk, Jr., H.H., and Steck, W.D.: Hospital management of psoriasis. Cutis, *14:*201, 207, 1974.
5. Roenigk, Jr., H.H.: Don't give up on the patient with psoriasis. Mod. Med., 59, 1977.
6. Epstein, J.A., Farber, E.M., et al.: Current status of oral PUVA therapy for psoriasis. J. Am. Acad. Dermatol., *1:*106, 1979.

CHAPTER 9

"OTHER" PAPULO-SQUAMOUS DISEASES

HENRY H. ROENIGK, JR.

The list of skin diseases usually grouped together because of their morphological similarities of developing macules, papules, and a scaling surface are:

Psoriasis vulgaris
Seborrheic dermatitis
Parapsoriasis
Lichen planus
Lichen nitidus
Lichen striatus
Pityriasis rosea
Pityriasis rubra pilaris
Fungus diseases
Syphilis

Because of their major importance, certain of these diseases have been discussed in separate chapters: psoriasis (Chapter 8), seborrheic dermatitis (Chapter 7), fungus diseases (Chapter 11). Because all of the papulosquamous diseases should be considered in a differential diagnosis, it is often necessary to obtain a serology (to rule out syphilis) or a potassium hydroxide (KOH) (to rule out fungus). Skin biopsy may help differentiate some of these disorders, but frequently the biopsy of the papulosquamous diseases will be nonspecific and then clinical patterns of disease may help establish the diagnosis (Chapter 1).

PARAPSORIASIS

The term parapsoriasis is confusing since

the disease is not psoriasis and does not result from psoriasis. It is a confusing group of diseases which are superficial, scaling plaques of various sizes, usually nonpruritic and resistant to therapy. Some of the diseases are chronic and result in no serious problems, but one form of the disease can eventuate into mycosis fungoides lymphoma. The initial lesion is usually a macule or maculopapule covered with a fine scale which tends to spread peripherally. Initial lesions are usually on the trunk or extremities. There are four main types.

Parapsoriasis Guttata

The lesions are fine maculopapular lesions like guttate psoriasis, with the fine silvery scale of psoriasis but failing to respond to antipsoriatic therapy. The lesions are mainly on the trunk. Secondary syphilis lesions are chronic and remain from months to years.

No specific therapy is indicated although the lesions may improve with natural sunlight. Topical corticosteroids occasionally induce remissions.

Parapsoriasis Lichenoides

This form of parapsoriasis (retiform) presents with elevated, dull, red and scaly, lichenoid papules which are mainly over the trunk. They tend to coalesce giving a retiform (netlike) appearance. The eruption is more generalized affecting the neck, trunk, and limbs. There is no pruritus and general health is excellent. The disease is chronic and no specific therapy is effective.

Parapsoriasis en Plaque

These lesions present as larger plaques than the guttate and lichenoid types of parapsoriasis. They are yellowish red to brownish in color with a fine definite scale and occurring mainly on the trunk, buttock, and thigh (Fig. 9.1). These lesions, in contrast to the previous two types of parapsoriasis, may be associated with itching. Skin biopsies and careful clinical observation of these patients are essential since many of these cases will eventuate into mycosis fungoides lymphoma.

Natural sunlight may cause some temporary improvement, but photochemotherapy with psoralens and UVA will cause complete clearing of lesions similar to the clearing in the plaques stage of mycosis fungoides.

Parapsoriasis Varioliformis Acuta

This disease (also known as acute parapsoriasis, pityriasis lichenoids et varioliformis acuta, and Mucha-Habermann syndrome) should probably no longer be classified with the parapsoriasis group since clinically and histologically it is quite different from the other forms of parapsoriasis.

The onset is acute with a clinical picture similar to chickenpox showing papules, vesicles, and pustular or crusted lesions. The le-

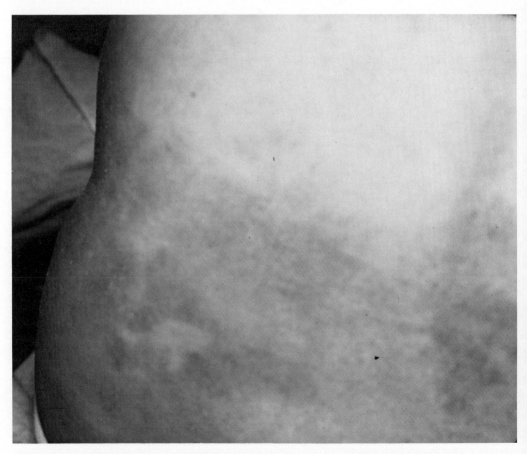

Fig. 9.1.   Parapsoriasis in plaque with erythematous plaque-like lesions on trunk.

sions go through stages of evolution from papule to pustule to necrosis and, finally, leaving varioliformis scars (Fig. 9.2). The lesions occur primarily in the second and third decades and appear to have two phases. The condition may last a few weeks or months and then heal spontaneously, or the condition may persist for 10 or more years.

The basic lesion is a vasculitis, and skin biopsy of an early lesion will show features of the vasculitis along with destruction of the epidermis by hemorrhage and invasions with lymphocytes.

Treatment with large doses of antibiotics (either tetracycline (1.5 gm/day), penicillin, or erythromycin) have been reported effective, but fail in the cases with a longer course. Small doses of methotrexate (5.0–7.5 mg) will control the disease, but discontinuation of the drug results in return of lesions. Close monitoring of blood counts and liver function studies are necessary.

LICHEN PLANUS

The characteristic lesions of lichen planus is polygonal, flat-topped papule with a violaceous hue which tends to be symmetrical, bilateral, and very pruritic (as shown in Fig. 9.3 in color Plate II). There is a fine, cloudy, whitish network over the surface (Wickham's striae) and the lesions may coalesce to form groups or larger patches. Scratching of the lesion frequently results in a linear pattern (Köbner's phenomenon). Annular lesions are common on the trunk, mucous membranes, or penis. The distribution pattern of lichen planus favors the development of lesions on the anterior surface of the wrist and ankle, inner thigh, sacral region, under the breasts, and on the buccal mucosa (Figs. 9.4 and 9.5). Lesions on the dorsum of the tongue are usually annular. Lichen planus may involve only the mucous membranes of the vagina, mouth, or rectal areas and differentia-

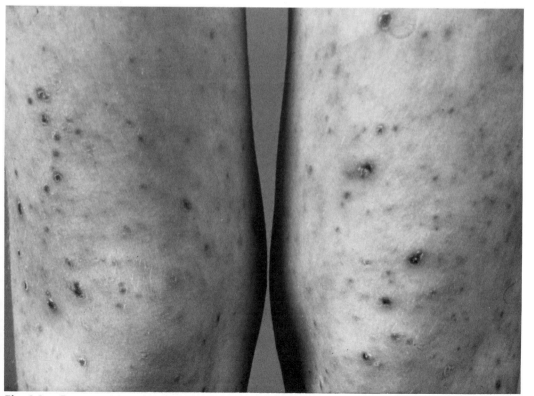

Fig. 9.2. Parapsoriosis varioliformis acuta (Mucha-Habermann syndrome) Chronic chickenpox-like eruption with vesicles, papules, crusts, and scars.

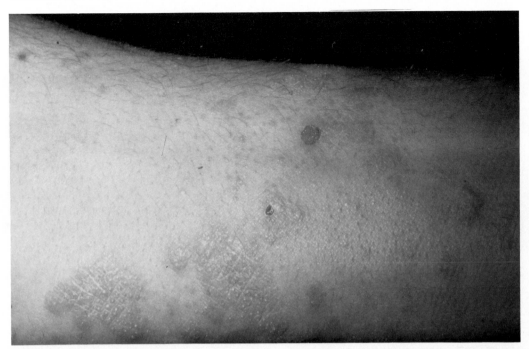

Fig. 9.4.   Lichen planus. Papular lesions and erythematous plaques.

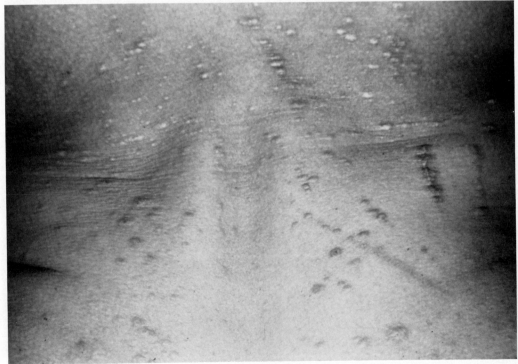

Fig. 9.5.   Lichen planus of back with erythematous papular lesions. Köebnerized lesions on right side of back.

tion of the lacy white patches from leukoplakia and other whitish plaques of these areas are necessary. Hypertrophic lichen planus develops, usually, on the anterior aspects of lower legs, but also on back of the hands or, rarely generalized.

Differentiation from neurodermatitis is often difficult. The lesions which are much thicker than other forms of lichen planus may persist for years. The scalp may be involved with lichen planopilaris in which follicular, spiny papules appear which result in atrophy and scarring alopecia. Nails may be associated with acute or chronic lichen planus showing pitting, linear lines, or subungual keratosis. Occasionally, only the nails present with disease (twenty-nail syndrome) and differentiation from psoriasis may be impossible.

The histopathology of lichen planus, especially in the acute phase with small papular lesions, is charactistic. Therefore, a skin biopsy should be done to confirm the diagnosis. Direct immunofluorescences of the lesions show deposition of immunoglobulin below the basement membrane which may represent Civatte bodies. This technique may be helpful if the histopathology is not diagnostic.

Treatment of lichen planus depends on the extent of the lesions and symptoms. Topical or intralesional corticosteroids are effective in resolving lesions. Intralesional steroids are especially effective for hypertrophic lichen planus. For acute, spreading, generalized, intensely pruritic lichen planus, systemic corticosteroids are indicated. Prednisone 40-60 mg/day until clear (1–2 weeks) may then be rapidly tapered and stopped in 2–3 weeks. Occasionally, the disease will recur after stopping steroids but there is no rebound flare as seen with psoriasis. Griseofulvin has been reported effective in double-blind studies, but the reasons for this antifungal drug being effective are not clear.

Oral or vaginal lesions of lichen planus respond to vitamin A acid topically or topical corticostoids in Orabase. Oral psoralens followed by long wave UVL (PUVA, see Chapter 8) is effective for resistant lichen planus.

LICHEN NITIDUS

Lichen nitidus presents as skin-colored or pinkish, shiny, circinate flat-topped papules which develop in groups or remain pinhead size. They tend to develop on the genital, abdomen, and on the flexor surface of the forearms. Lichen nitidus is more common in blacks than Caucasions. There is usually no itching and mucus membranes are seldom involved. The lesions occasionally resemble lichen planus. Skin biopsy will help make the diagnosis since the biopsy of lichen nitidus shows a localized papule of inflammatory cells in upper dermis with epithelioid cells, lymphocytes, and histiocytes. The epidermis is flattened by the inflammation.

The etiology is unknown and, since the lesions eventually disappear spontaneously,

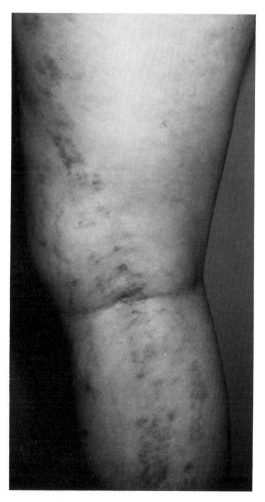

Fig. 9.6. Lichen striatus with linear distribution down the leg.

no treatment is necessary. Lubrication of the skin may be helpful.

LICHEN STRIATUS

The development of lichenoid papules re-

sembling planus in a linear distribution down an extremity of a child is characteristic of lichen striatus (Fig. 9.6). The lesion is asymptomatic and usually involutes spontaneously

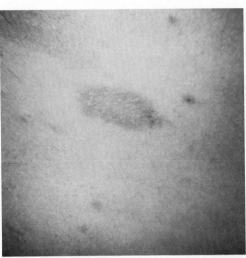

Fig. 9.7. "Herald patch" of pityriasis rosea.

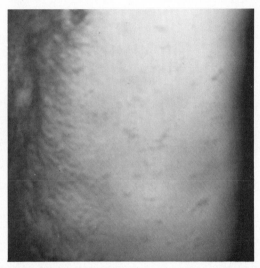

Fig. 9.8. Pityriasis rosea. Fawn-colored oval lesions on the trunk.

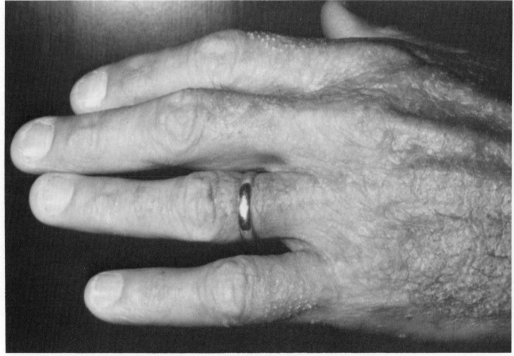

Fig. 9.10. Follicular papules on the dorsum of phalanges in pityriasis rubra pilaris.

in a few months without residua. No therapy is needed.

PITYRIASIS ROSEA

Pityriasis rosea is a self-limited disorder which develops abruptly usually in the spring and fall of the year. It presents a typical pattern over the trunk and proximal upper and lower extremities which is symmetric but is preceded by a "herald patch" (Fig. 9.7) which resembles a tinea infection of the skin. Several days later multiple lesions appear, usually first on the trunk. The lesions tend to be oval with the long axis following lines of cleavage ("Christmas tree pattern") (Fig. 9.8). They tend to be fawn-colored at the center with a reddish edge with a fine peripheral scale. The eruption may be extensive (as shown in Fig. 9.9, see color Plate II) and itching may be severe or absent completely. Differential diagnosis should include tinea corporis which can be excluded by KOH exams, secondary syphilis (always do a serology), and drug eruptions. Guttate parapsoriasis should be suspected if lesions persist longer than the usual 6–8 weeks.

Spontaneous cure regularly occurs in 6–8 weeks, therefore active treatment is not necessary. Symptomatic antiprusitic lotions and systemic antihistimine help the generalized puritus. Ultraviolet radiation (UVB) given daily often hastens involution of the disease if given in suberythema doses. Systemic corticosteroid are only rarely necessary in a short course for extensive lesions and severe itching.

PITYRIASIS RUBRA PILARIS

Pityriasis rubra pilaris is a rare disease with characteristic lesions and distribution. The lesions are firm, reddish brown papules which are follicular. They tend to coalesce to form patches and groups to eventually cover the entire body surface. Diffuse scaling of scalp and typical conical papules pierced by hair occur on dorsal surfaces of phalanges (Fig. 9.10). When the lesions become generalized,

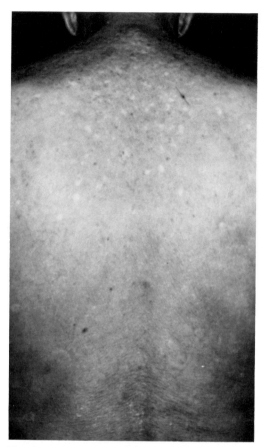

Fig. 9.11. Pityriasis rubra pilaris with erythroderma. Note the small areas of clear skin on back.

producing an erythroderma (Fig. 9.11), there are typically a few small clear areas of normal skin on the trunk. The palms and soles often show diffuse hyperkeratosis (Fig. 9.12).

The skin biopsy is not diagnostic and the course is usually chronic, lasting several years. There is a congenital form which persists a lifetime and is often confused with psoriasis, and an acquired type which may resolve in a few years.

Therapy has generally been ineffective, but high doses of vitamin A (200,000–600,000 units) may produce remission. Retenoids, a derivative of vitamin A, may be effective. Topical agents are generally ineffective. Methotrexate has been reported effective in a few cases.

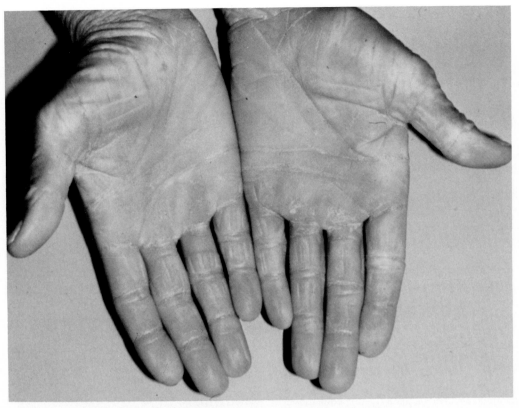

Fig. 9.12. Hyperkeratosis of palms in pityriasis rubra pilaris.

References

1. Lepine, E.M.: Parapsoriasis; a re-evaluation. Cutis, *14:* 729, 1974.
2. Samman, P.D.: The natural history of parapsoriasis in plaque—chronic superficial dermatitis—and prereticulotic poikiloderma. Br. J. Dermatol., *87:* 405, 1972.
3. Solberg, K., Hersle, K., Mobachen, H., and Thelander, H.: Topical tretenoin therapy and oral lichen planus. Arch. Dermatol., *115:* 716, 1979.
4. Wilkinson, J.P., Dawber, R.P.R., Bowers, R.P., and Fleming, K.: Twenty-nail diptrophy of childhood: case report and histopathological finding. Br. J. Dermatol., *100:* 217, 1979.
5. Ortonne, J.P., Thioolet, J., and Sannwald, C.: Oral photochemotherapy in the treatment of lichen planus. Br. J. Dermatol., *99:* 77, 1978.
6. Black, M.M.: The pathogenesis of lichen planus. Br. J. Dermatol., *86:* 302, 1972.
7. Schgal, V.N., Abraham, G.J., and Molik, G.B.: Griseofulvin therapy in lichen planus—a double-blind controlled trial. Br. J. Dermatol., *87:* 383, 1972.
8. Stewart, W.M.: Pathology of lichen planus. Br. J. Dermatol., *95:* Supp 14, 18, 1976.
9. Burch, P.R., and Rowell, N.R.: Pityriosis rosea—an autoaggressive disease—statistical studies in relation to aetiology and pathogenesis. Br. J. Dermatol., *82:* 548, 1974.
10. Beamer, J.E., Newman, S.B., Reed, W.B., and Cram D.: Pityriosis rubra pilaris. Cutis, *10:* 419, 1972.
11. Griffiths, W.A.: Pityriosis rubra pilaris: clinical features and natural history in a study of 93 patients. Br. J. Dermatol., *96:* (Sup 15), 18, 1977.

CHAPTER 10

PYODERMAS

SUSAN CHAPPE

Pyoderma is a bacterial infection of the skin, usually caused by streptococci or staphylococci. Primary infections are produced by invasion of normal skin by pathogenic bacteria. Secondary infections develop in areas of damaged skin and often show a mixture of organisms. Normal skin is highly resistant to invasion by bacteria. The following factors may play a role in resistance to infection:

Relative dryness of normal skin
Natural antibacterial substances in sebum
   (polyunsaturated fatty acids)
Low pH (5.5) of skin
Suppressive effect of one bacterial strain on another
   (bacterial interference)
Circulating immunoglobulins and delayed
   hypersensitivity

NORMAL SKIN FLORA

Organisms that survive and multiply on the skin constitute the normal "resident" flora. The "transient" bacteria are merely present on the skin and may temporarily colonize. The composition of the normal flora varies over the body surface. The exposed areas, such as face, neck, and hands, have a higher bacterial density than the skin on the trunk and legs.

Staphylococcus epidermidis is uniformly present on the skin surface. *Staphylococcus aureus* is carried in the nose in about 50% of the population, in the perineum in about 20%, and on normal exposed skin in about 20% of the population. *Streptococcus viridans* (α-hemolytic)

is frequently present in the mouth and may spread to the hands and other areas. *Streptococcus pyogenes* (β-hemolytic) is not ordinarily present on the skin surface except in epidemics. *Propionibacterium acnes* is present in the sebaceous follicles. Aerobic diphtheroids (*Corynebacterium*) are present primarily in the axillae and interdigital skin. Moist intertriginous areas are frequently colonized by Gram-negative bacilli such as *Escherichia coli*, *Proteus*, *Enterobacter*, and *Pseudomonas*.

GENERAL GUIDELINES TO TREATMENT

Pyodermas are caused primarily by *S. aureus* or *S. pyogenes*. Common types of infections include impetigo, cellulitis, and folliculitis. A rapidly developing lymphangitis is typical of streptococcal involvement. Mild-to-moderate cutaneous infections can be treated with local compresses, topical drugs, oral antibiotics, or a combination of these. Severe infections should be treated with parenteral antibiotics. The selection of the antibiotic should be based on the clinical appearance of the skin lesion, the presence of systemic signs, Gram stain, and bacterial culture and sensitivity results.

Numerous topical antibacterial cleansers are available. Povidone-iodine (Betadine Skin Cleanser) is a broad range microbicidal substance available in several vehicles. Betadine is active against Gram-positive and Gram-negative bacteria, viruses, fungi, protozoa, and yeast. Hexachlorophene (pHisoHex) is a

bacteriostatic agent active against staphylococci and other Gram-positive bacteria. With
repeated use, an antibacterial residue remains
on the skin. Chlorhexidine gluconate (Hibiclens Antimicrobial Skin Cleanser) is a topical
bactericidal agent producing a persistant
antimicrobial effect against both Gram-positive and Gram-negative bacteria.

Topical antibiotics can be used to suppress
bacterial growth. Bacitracin is a polypeptide
antibiotic that is bactericidal against many
Gram-positive organisms, including β-hemolytic streptococci. It is inactive against most
Gram-negative organisms except *Pseudomonas*.
Neomycin is an aminoglycoside antibiotic effective against most Gram-negative organisms
except *Pseudomonas*. Neomycin is also active
against many Gram-positive organisms, including staphylococci, but β-hemolytic streptococci may be resistant. In the hospital, a
large proportion of staphylococci are resistant
to neomycin, and gentamicin is the preferred
aminoglycoside. Gentamicin (Garamycin
Cream) has a spectrum similar to neomycin,
and is also active against *Pseudomonas*. Widespread use of topical gentamicin may increase
the background of gentamicin-resistant organisms. Polymyxin B is a cyclic polypeptide
antibiotic active against Gram-negative bacilli, including *Pseudomonas*, but is not effective
against *Proteus*. A combination of two or three
antibiotics (Neosporin Ointment, Polysporin
Ointment) may be necessary to cover the
spectrum of bacteria. These agents are capable of producing a contact dermatitis in a
small number of patients. Excessive application of ointments can lead to tissue maceration and the propagation of infection. Topical
antibiotics may help control the bacteria in
superficial wounds, but systemic antibiotics
are often necessary.

Penicillin is the drug of choice for systemic
treatment of infections due to group A streptococci and sensitive staphylococci. For oral
administration, penicillin V (phenoxymethyl
penicillin) is the preferred penicillin, and for
parenteral therapy of severe infections, penicillin G is the drug of choice. Infections caused
by penicillinase-producing *S. aureus* should be
treated with a penicillinase-resistant penicillin, such as parenteral nafcillin or oxacillin.
Oxacillin is similar to nafcillin but is less
active against other Gram-positive cocci and

is not as efficiently excreted by the liver.
Cloxacillin and dicloxacillin are penicillinase-
resistant penicillins which are reliably absorbed from the gut and can be used orally.
Ampicillin, amoxicillin, and carbenicillin are
not effective against penicillinase-producing
staphylococci. When a staphylococcal infection is suspected, nafcillin may be used to
initiate therapy, pending bacterial culture
and sensitivity results. If the organism is sensitive to penicillin G, the antibiotic can then
be changed. Patients allergic to one penicillin
should be considered allergic to all penicillins.
Erythromycin is a broad spectrum antibiotic
effective against group A streptococci, staphylococci, *Corynebacterium*, and many other organisms. Erythromycin is useful in treating
the penicillin-allergic patient and in treating
patients in whom streptococci and staphylococci may coexist. It is not recommended in
the treatment of severe staphylococcal infections, because of the rapid development of
resistance. Cephalosporins are active against
most Gram-positive cocci, including penicillinase-producing staphylococci, and many
strains of Gram-negative bacilli. Patients allergic to penicillin may develop allergic reactions to cephalosporins. Clindamycin and
vancomycin are also effective in the treatment
of staphylococcal infections. Clindamycin,
ampicillin, and many other antibiotics can
cause severe diarrhea and pseudomembranous colitis. Vancomycin is potentially oto-
toxic and nephrotoxic.

IMPETIGO CONTAGIOSA

Impetigo contagiosa is a common superficial bacterial infection, caused by group A
β-hemolytic streptococci. A mixture of streptococci and *S. aureus* is isolated in about one-
half the patients. *S. aureus* appears to be a
secondary invader, and is not of the group II
phage type associated with bullous impetigo.
S. aureus, alone, is isolated from less than 10%
of cases of nonbullous impetigo. Group B
streptococci have been cultured from newborn skin.

Impetigo contagiosa is more common in the
summer and early fall. The disease is usually
found in children and is highly contagious.

Predisposing factors include crowded living conditions, poor health and hygiene, malnutrition, and a warm, humid climate. Impetigo contagiosa may complicate antecedent scabies, varicella, atopic eczema, and other skin disorders.

The earliest clinical lesion is a small vesicle which becomes pustular and crusts. The surrounding skin may be slightly inflamed. As the lesion enlarges, a thick golden yellow "stuck on" crust is produced (Fig. 10.1). With removal of the crust, a red weeping surface can be seen and another crust soon forms. Lesions often develop on the face, arms, and legs. Occasionally, lesions spread peripherally with central healing giving the appearance of a superficial fungal infection. Patients may notice pruritus and burning. Regional lymphadenopathy is frequently present, but systemic symptoms are uncommon.

Studies of impetigo in children show that group A streptococci appear on normal skin about 10 days prior to developing lesions. The organisms probably invade the skin through areas of microscopic trauma. Organisms later spread to the respiratory tract. Acute nephritis may follow streptococcal pyoderma or pharyngitis. More cases of poststreptococcal nephritis are caused by impetigo than by pharyngitis. The nephritogenic serotypes causing pharyngitis, M-types 1, 4, 12, 25, and 49, generally differ from the strains causing pyoderma, M-types 2, 49, 55, 57, and 60. The latent period for nephritis following pyoderma is 3 weeks, whereas nephritis follows pharyngitis by 10 days. Asymptomatic microscopic hematuria occurs in a few patients during the acute episode of pyoderma. In tropical climates, nephritogenic strains commonly cause impetigo. The frequency of acute glomerulonephritis following infection with a nephritogenic strain is 10–15%. The overall incidence of postpyoderma nephritis is probably about 2%. Rheumatic fever does not follow streptococcal pyoderma. The antistreptolysin O (ASO) titre following a streptococ-

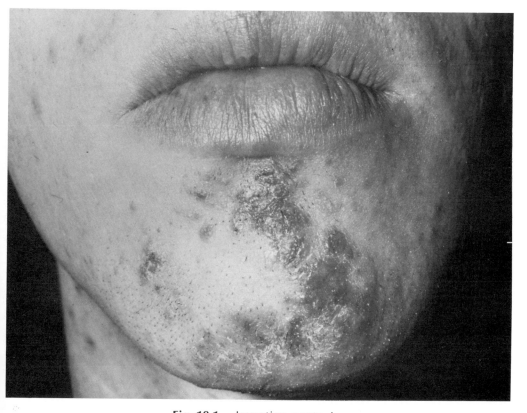

Fig. 10.1. Impetigo contagiosa

cal pyoderma is not consistently elevated. The antideoxyribonuclease B (anti-DNase B) titre is more frequently elevated. Ninety percent of patients with acute glomerulonephritis following streptococcal pyoderma will have an elevated anti-DNase B titre, whereas only 50% will have an elevated ASO titre.

Impetigo contagiosa usually heals without scarring. Untreated disease may become widespread, but tends to resolve spontaneously over several weeks. It has not been proven that treatment with systemic antibiotics will prevent acute glomerulonephritis. Topical antibiotics alone are successfully used, especially in mild, localized infections. It appears that systemic therapy shortens healing time, results in fewer failures, and decreases the carrier state. Most cases of impetigo need not be routinely cultured.

Treatment

1. Systemic therapy with one of the following
   a. Benzathine penicillin, 300,000–600,000 units I.M. for children and 1.2 million units I.M. for adults
   b. Phenoxymethyl penicillin (Penicillin VK powder or tablets), 250 mg every 6 hours for 10 days
   c. Erythromycin, 30–50 mg/kg/day in four divided doses for children, and 250 mg four times a day for adults for 10 days
2. Local care
   a. Debridement with wet compresses of saline or Burow's solution, 1:40 (one Domeboro Powder Packet or Tablet in a pint of water) three times a day for 20 minutes
   b. Topical application of Betadine Ointment, Polysporin Ointment, or Neosporin Ointment between compresses
3. General measures
   a. An antibacterial skin cleanser should be used daily (Betadine Skin Cleanser, pHisoHex, Safeguard, or Dial soap)
   b. Separate towels and wash clothes should be used and changed after each use

ECTHYMA

Ecthyma is a bacterial infection of the skin characterized by deep crusted lesions which ulcerate. As in impetigo contagiosa, the primary organism appears to be group A β-hemolytic *S. pyogenes*, although *S. aureus* may also be cultured. The lesions begin as vesicles or pustules on an erythematous base, and enlarge and crust. The legs and buttocks are the areas most commonly involved. The infection extends deep into the dermis, producing a shallow ulcer with a "punched out" appearance. The ulcer may not be visible unless the grayish yellow crust is removed. The border is indurated and violaceous (Figs. 10.2 and 10.3).

This condition often occurs in children, and poor health and hygiene are predisposing factors. Ecthyma also occurs in debilitated alcoholics and has been reported in military personnel in Vietnam. Healing takes several weeks and may result in scarring. Postpyoderma nephritis is a potential complication.

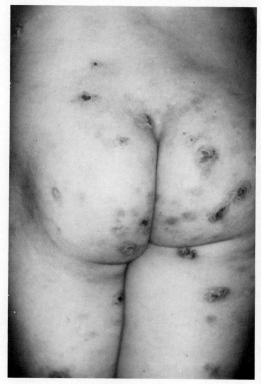

Fig. 10.2. Ecthyma

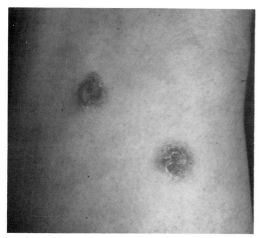

Fig. 10.3. Ecthyma

Systemic therapy with penicillin is recommended, and the treatment is the same as that outlined for impetigo contagiosa.

BULLOUS IMPETIGO

Bullous impetigo is a superficial infection of the skin producing large bullae. The causative organism is *S. aureus* phage group II, usually type 71, which elaborates an exfoliative toxin causing a blister to form below the stratum corneum. This organism is also responsible for the staphylococcal scalded skin syndrome.

Bullous impetigo occurs in infants and children. Early lesions are vesicular and rapidly progress to flaccid bullae. The Nikolsky sign is negative. Surrounding skin appears normal. The bullae rupture, and thin light brown crusts form. *S. aureus* can be cultured from the contents of intact bullae. The treatment of choice is a penicillinase-resistant penicillin.

Treatment

1. Systemic therapy
   a. Cloxacillin or dicloxacillin, 250–500 mg four times a day for 7 days
   b. Erythromycin, 250 mg four times a day for 7 days in penicillin allergic patients
2. Compresses with saline or Burow's solution, 1:40 three times a day for 20 minutes

ERYSIPELAS, CELLULITIS, AND LYMPHANGITIS

ERYSIPELAS

Erysipelas is a superficial cellulitis caused by group A β-hemolytic streptococci. It occurs in the very young, the aged, and the debilitated. About one-third of the patients have a history of a preceding upper respiratory tract infection, and this may furnish the bacterial source. Erysipelas is common on the face and scalp, but may occur anywhere. A small break in the skin provides access for infection.

Erysipelas begins as a small, bright red area, which becomes raised and spreads peripherally. The lesion is warm, tender, and indurated, with a peau d'orange appearance. The advancing margin is elevated and well demarcated as shown in Figure 10.4 (see color plate III). Small vesicles develop in more severe cases. The patient appears ill, and systemic manifestations of fever, chills, and malaise are usually present. The leukocyte count is elevated with a left shift, and streptococci can often be cultured from the pharynx and aspirates of the skin. The streptococci infiltrate lymphatics in the dermis, producing edema and vascular dilation. Bacteremia often occurs and can lead to endocarditis. Poststreptococcal nephritis is a potential complication. Some patients have a marked tendency to recurrence in the same area, possibly due to underlying chronic lymphatic obstruction. Antibiotic treatment with penicillin results in rapid improvement.

CELLULITIS

Cellulitis involves the dermis and subcutaneous tissue, and is distinguished by the lack of a sharp advancing margin and a less intense color. The area involved is red, warm, and edematous, and superficial vesicles may form. Often, there is a preceding wound, such as a stasis ulceration. Tender lymphadenopathy occurs, and systemic manifestations are usually present. Bacteremia may occur. Group A streptococci and *S. aureus* are causative organisms (Fig. 10.5).

LYMPHANGITIS

Lymphangitis is an infection that involves the subcutaneous lymphatic channels, caused primarily by group A β-hemolytic strepto-

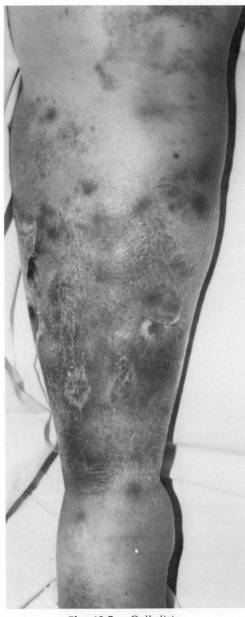

Fig. 10.5.   Cellulitis

cocci. A small break in the skin surface, such as a paronychia or tinea pedis, can serve as the entry point for infection. Tender, red, linear streaks extend from the local lesion to the regional lymph nodes. Regional lymphadenopathy is present and a leukocytosis occurs. Occasionally, an infection of the thumb or index finger drains directly to the axillary nodes and can lead to a subpectoral abscess.

The drug of choice for the above infections is penicillin. In patients with cellulitis, and chronic predisposing skin conditions such as stasis dermatitis, staphylococci may coexist, and a penicillinase-resistant penicillin should be used. Patients with extensive infections should be hospitalized and treated with parenteral antibiotic therapy. Appropriate cultures of skin aspirates and blood should be performed.

Treatment

1. Mild, early infections
   a. Phenoxymethyl penicillin (Penicillin VK Powder or Tablets), 250 mg every 6 hours for 10 days
   b. Erythromycin, 250–500 mg every 6 hours for 10 days
2. Extensive infections
   a. Aqueous penicillin G, 600,000 to 2 million units I.V. every 4–6 hours
   b. Cephalothin, erythromycin, or clindamycin may be substituted in the penicillin-allergic patient
3. Possible staphylococcal infections
   a. Dicloxacillin or erythromycin, 250–500 mg every 6 hours for early infections
   b. Oxacillin or nafcillin 1.0–1.5 g I.V. every 4–6 hours
   c. In the penicillin allergic patient, cephalothin, erythromycin, or clindamycin may be substituted. Staphylococci resistant to erythromycin may emerge during therapy and, in severe infections, vancomycin should be used in the patient with a strong penicillin allergy
4. Local care
   a. Immobilization and elevation of the involved area
   b. Application of moist heat

FOLLICULITIS, FURUNCLES AND CARBUNCLES

These conditions are caused by *S. aureus*, which is frequently carried in the nasal mucosa or perineum. Organisms may spread to normal skin and to other individuals.

FOLLICULITIS

Folliculitis is an infection of the hair follicle. Superficial folliculitis appears as dome-shaped pustules at the opening of hair follicles. Treatment with an antibacterial soap (pHisoHex, Betadine Surgical Scrub, Hibiclens Antimicrobial Skin Cleanser) and a topical antibiotic ointment (Neosporin Ointment, Polysporin Ointment) is effective. In moist areas, a drying sulfur lotion may be helpful (Sulfacet-R Lotion). A stye is an infection around a lid cilia resulting in an erythematous swelling, and is best treated with frequent warm, moist compresses and an ophthalmic antibiotic.

PSEUDOFOLLICULITIS BARBAE

Pseudofolliculitis barbae is a condition of the beard area, especially common in black patients, resulting from ingrown hairs following shaving. After close shaving, hairs may grow between the outer layers of the epidermis, or may penetrate the side of a follicle, causing a foreign body reaction or pustule (Fig. 10.6). Treatment of this condition is difficult. The beard should be allowed to grow for about 4 weeks to allow existing inflammation to subside. Treatment with a coarse sponge twice a day (Buf-Puf Cleansing Sponge) will help prevent hair tips from penetrating the skin. Patients should be instructed to shave in one direction and to avoid putting tension on the skin. Shaving with an electric barber clippers with a triple "O" head will allow a millimeter of hair to protrude from the skin and help prevent ingrown hairs. In some patients, an electric shaver or depilatory cream is effective. Application of benzoyl peroxide gel, 5%, following shaving and hydrocortisone cream, 1%, at night is helpful.

FURUNCLE

A furuncle, or boil, can arise from preceding superficial folliculitis. A furuncle is a deep,

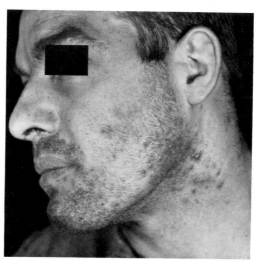

Fig. 10.6. Pseudofolliculitis barbae

painful, inflammatory nodule which forms around a hair follicle. Furuncles occur in hairy areas, especially in areas of friction and perspiration, such as the face, neck, axillae, and buttocks. Clinically, a furuncle is a firm, red, tender nodule which enlarges and becomes fluctuant. The lesion often ruptures, discharging purulent material. Treatment consists of local application of warm, moist compresses. Early antibiotic treatment with a penicillinase-resistant drug (dicloxacillin or erythromycin, 250 mg four times a day) can abort a lesion. A lesion that is fluctuant and pointing should be incised and drained. After drainage, only topical antibiotics are needed, although many physicians will also use oral antibiotics. A deep wound should be packed with iodoform gauze and removed in 24–48 hours. Moist dressings should not be applied after drainage because tissue maceration with spread of infection can occur.

CARBUNCLE

A carbuncle is a deep infection involving several hair follicles, and tends to occur in thick, inelastic skin such as the posterior neck and back. The lesion appears red and indurated, with pustules on the surface and multiple drainage points. Systemic manifestations of fever and malaise are often present, and the patient may appear ill. Bacteremia is a potential complication. Lesions over the upper lip, nose, and cheek area drain via the facial and emissary veins to the cavernous sinus. A penicillinase-resistant penicillin such as dicloxacillin, 250–500 mg every 4–6 hours is the treatment of choice. For severe infections, parenteral nafcillin or oxacillin should be administered. Cephalothin, clindamycin, or erythromycin may be substituted. Application of moist heat is helpful in localizing infection.

RECURRENT FURUNCULOSIS

Recurrent furuncles are a difficult problem. Most patients are otherwise healthy. Frequent close skin contact, especially sexual intercourse, can spread staphylococci. In many patients furunculosis is localized to the groin, perineum, or buttocks. Obesity, poor hygiene, hyperhidrosis, and exposure to oils are predisposing factors. Acne and seborrheic dermatitis frequently coexist. Infections may be more extensive in diabetics. Use of corticosteroids and cytotoxic agents can predispose to infections. Blood dyscrasias, defects in neutrophil function, and dysglobulinemia are rare underlying causes. Early treatment with dicloxacillin or cloxacillin, 250 mg four times a day for a week may abort a furuncle and decrease the incidence of recurrence.

Treatment

1. General care
   a. Cool, dry climate
   b. Bath and shampoo 1–2 times a day
   c. Antibacterial soap (pHisoHex, Betadine Skin Cleanser, Hibiclens Antimicrobial Skin Cleanser)
   d. Separate wash cloth and towel
   e. Clean linens daily
   f. For beard lesions, use a new blade daily, and soak razor or razor heads in alcohol between shaves
2. Antibiotic ointments. Daily application of bacitracin or Neosporin Ointment in the anterior nares may reduce carriage
3. Systemic antibiotics. Culture and sensitivity should be performed, and appropriate antibiotics given for 1–3 months, and as necessary
4. Bacterial interference. This procedure,

which has potential complications, has been limited to experimental study protocol, in which nonpathogenic staphylococci are inoculated on the skin after the patient's pathogenic strain has been eliminated by intensive antibiotic administration.

ERYTHRASMA

Erythrasma is a superficial bacterial infection caused by a Gram-positive rod, *Corynebacterium minutissimum*. Infection is localized to the intertriginous areas and may be chronic. These organisms are often part of the normal flora. This condition is common in the tropics, and heat and humidity seem to play a role in the development of infection. Clinically, lesions appear as slightly scaly, reddish brown plaques in the axillary, inguinal, or inframammary folds, and may be asymptomatic or pruritic. Lesions can easily be mistaken for a superficial fungal infection. The organisms produce a water-soluble porphyrin, and the lesions fluoresce a "coral red" under a Wood's lamp. Treatment with a 5–7 day course of erythromycin, 250 mg four times a day is effective.

SUPERFICIAL *PSEUDOMONAS* INFECTIONS

Pseudomonas aeruginosa is an ubiquitous Gram-negative bacillus which frequently causes cutaneous infection in moist areas, such as the external ear canal, toe webs, and nail folds. It is often cultured from cutaneous ulcers and thermal burns. *Pseudomonas* organisms produce a blue pigment, pyocyanin, and a yellow-green substance, fluorescein. Using a Wood's lamp, the presence of the organisms can be identified by the greenish color.

Pseudomonas paronychial infections occur in people who frequently immerse their hands in water, and infection produces a blue-green discoloration of the nail. Infection of the toe webs results in a macerated, scaling, greenish discolored area which may be mistaken for tinea pedis. The organism has been cultured

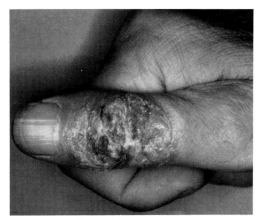

Fig. 10.7. Pyoderma

from whirlpools, and causes a self-limited papular eruption.

Minor infections usually heal rapidly with topical therapy and drying of the area. Application of 1% gentian violet or 5% acetic acid three times daily is antiseptic and drying. Involved nails should be trimmed short. Application of 4% thymol in chloroform is beneficial, but is not universally available. Polymyxin, 0.1% in acetic acid, or corticosteroids with polymyxin (Cortisporin Ointment) are useful in treating external otitis. Mafenide (Sulfamylon Cream) is bacteriostatic against many organisms, including *Pseudomonas*, and is used in the treatment of burn wounds.

SECONDARY INFECTIONS

Any area of damaged skin, such as contact dermatitis, atopic eczema, insect bites, traumatic abrasions, viral infections, and fungal infections, can become secondarily infected (Fig. 10.7). Proliferation of bacteria may prolong the underlying disease. *S. aureus* and group A streptococci, as well as a mixture of other organisms, often colonize the damaged skin. The appearance of the skin is not specific, and depends on the underlying condition. Treatment with a systemic antibiotic, such as erythromycin, in addition to the treatment of the underlying condition, is usually effective.

References

1. Aly, R: Effects of drugs on cutaneous microbial flora. In F. N. Marzulli and H. I. Maibach (Eds.) *Advances in Modern Toxicology*, Vol. 4, *Dermatotoxicology and Pharmacology*, p. 501. John Wiley and Sons, New York, 1977.
2. Dajani, A. S., Ferrieri, P., and Wannamaker, L. W.: Natural history of impetigo. II. Etiologic agents and bacterial interactions. *J. Clin. Invest., 51:* 2863, 1972.
3. Ferrieri, P., Dajani, A. S., Wannamaker, L. W., and Chapman, S. S.: Natural history of impetigo. I. Site of sequence of acquisition and familial patterns of spread of cutaneous streptococci. *J. Clin. Invest., 51:* 2851, 1972.
4. Fitzpatrick, T. B. et al, (Ed): *Dermatology in General Medicine*, Ed. 2. McGraw-Hill, New York, 1979.
5. Hoeprich, P. D., (Ed.): *Infectious Diseases*, Ed. 2. Harper and Row, Hagerstown, Md., 1977.
6. Kligman, A. M., Leyden, J. J., and McGinley K. J.: Bacteriology. *J. Invest. Dermatol, 67:* 160, 1976.
7. Musher, D. M., and McKenzie, S. O.: Infections due to *Staphylococcus aureus.* Medicine, *56:* 383, 1977.
8. Nissenson, A. R., (Moderator): Poststreptococcal acute glomerulonephritis: fact and controversy. Ann. Intern. Med., *91:* 76, 1979.
9. Peter, G., and Smith, A. L.: Group A streptococcal infections of the skin and pharynx. *N. Engl. J. Med., 297:* 311, and 365, 1977.

CHAPTER 11

DERMATOPHYTOSIS AND OTHER SUPERFICIAL MYCOTIC INFECTIONS

ALFRED D. HERNANDEZ

DERMATOPHYTOSIS

Dermatophytosis is a mycotic infection of the keratinous structures of the skin. This disease is caused by the genera *Trichophyton*, *Microsporum*, and *Epidermophyton* collectively known as dermatophytes. The clinical manifestations of dermatophytosis are dependent on the keratinous structure affected (stratum corneum, hair, or nail), the infecting organism, and the host-parasite relationship.

Since many dermatophytic fungi are capable of infecting more than one keratinous structure, dermatophytosis has been classified not by the infecting organism, but by the anatomical location involved. Regardless of the anatomical area involved, infection of a specific keratinous structure has essentially the same pathogenesis and clinical appearance. However, classification of the disease by anatomical location may not be adequate for determining the appropriate material for microscopic examination and culture, or for understanding the pathogenesis and, consequently, the therapy of the disease. Therefore, this chapter will first briefly examine the pathogenesis of infection of each keratinous structure and then, using this as a foundation, address each anatomical classification of dermatophytosis.

Pathogenesis

STRATUM CORNEUM INFECTION

The initiation of a dermatophytic infection is dependent on the virulence of the infecting organism and the physical state of the inoculation site. Of these factors, the later appears to play a critical role. Investigators have shown that contact with large numbers of viable organisms is not sufficient to initiate an infection (1). However, if the inoculation site is altered by hydration, maceration, abrasion, or minor trauma before or during the inoculation, the frequency of experimental infection is increased (2-4). How these alterations of the skin favor the initiation of dermatophytic infection is not clear.

Once the infection is established, two factors determine the size and duration of infection. The size of the affected area is related to the duration of infection. The duration of the infection is related to the rate at which the organism invades keratin, and the rate at which the stratum corneum is shed. If the fungal growth rate is less than the epidermal turnover rate, the disease will be terminated by sloughing the parasitized stratum corneum. As long as the fungal growth rate at least equals the epidermal turnover rate, the disease will persist. Our knowledge of the factors which affect fungal growth or epidermal turnover is limited. However, investigators have found that inflammatory infections are usually of short duration even if not treated. They also have found that the epidermal turnover rate is increased at the periphery of a dermatophytic lesion (5). Since there is probably a lag time between the presence of the organism, the host's inflammatory response, and the subsequent increased epidermal turnover, the organisms within the area of inflammation are shed, while those at the periphery are not significantly affected. As this process continues, the typical annular lesions of dermatophytosis are formed. This may explain why the best yields, when trying to culture or examine scale for organisms, are obtained from scales collected at the periphery of lesions.

Anti-inflammatory agents and cytotoxic agents may directly or indirectly decrease the epidermal turnover rate which, in turn, affects the duration, size, and spread of disease. Systemic and topical corticosteroids are reported to change the clinical appearance of the disease, increase the duration of infection, and cause widespread disease (6, 7). As might be expected, patients receiving these drugs have abundant organisms observed in scales obtained from infected areas.

HAIR INFECTIONS

Hair infections can be divided into two categories; ectothrix (spores surrounding the surface of the hair) and endothrix (spores within the hair). The pathogenesis of hair infection has been studied using primarily ectothrix models, and it is assumed that endothrix infections begin in a similar fashion.

Experimental ectothrix infection of scalp hair showed that the initial infection begins in the adjacent stratum corneum. As hyphae reach the follicular orifice, they descend along the hair's surface, form arthrospores, and penetrate the hair cortex. Intrapapillary hyphae then descend to the keratogenesis zone (the border between viable and nonviable tissue) forming Adamson's fringe. The intrapapillary hyphae proliferate most abundantly in this lower portion of the hair. As the hyphae reach the surface of the cortex, they segment into arthrospores which are then carried outward as the hair grows. Few intrapapillary hyphae are observed in the upper portion of hair. Because the hyphael proliferation in the lower portion of the hair dispute the hair's structural integrity, traction on the hair causes it to fracture just above the hyphael proliferation. Examination of the infected hair under the microscope shows ectothrix spores surrounding the hair. The infection of the stratum corneum is relatively short-lived compared to that of hair (3). Therefore, examination of scale from the scalp may not reveal hyphae, whereas examination of hair is positive for arthrospores. Failure to examine hair may lead to an erroneous diagnosis.

During a scalp infection, not all hair within a diseased area becomes infected. Although hyphae surround and descend follicles indiscriminantly, penetration of hair occurs almost exclusively in anagen rather than telogen phase of hair growth (3).

Since hair from areas other than scalp and beard have comparatively shorter anagen and longer telogen cycles, this may account for their short-lived and infrequent infection.

The pathogenesis of endothrix infection is not well understood. It is assumed that infection is initiated in a similar fashion as ectothrix infections. However, once the hair is penetrated, the hyphae form arthrospores within the hair. As the infection continues, the arthrospores replace the structural stability of the hair. In the lower portion of the follicle, the hair is supported by the internal root sheath and walls of the follicle but, as it reaches the area where the root sheath ends and the follicle dilates, the hair fractures just below the surface of the skin. This results in what has clinically been called "black-dot" tinea capitis. Since most infected hairs do not surface intact, potassium hydroxide (KOH) examination of plucked hair from this type of infection has a low yield. However, removal of the "black-dot" with a needle gives a very high yield in identifying endothrix spores.

Unlike ectothrix infection, endothrix infections do not appear to regress when the hair enters telogen. This, along with the poor inflammatory response seen in these infections, may explain why these infections tend to be very chronic unless treated.

NAIL INFECTIONS

Dermatophytic involvement of the nail may be classified as primary or secondary infection of the nail plate. The most common type of infection affects the nail plate secondarily. Initial infection begins in the stratum corneum of the hyponychium or lateral gutters. The associated hyperkeratosis beneath the nail plate causes the nail to lose its translucency and, if extensive enough, it causes the nail plate to rise. Infection from the stratum corneum extends to the nail plate and, as the structural stability of the nail plate is affected, it may become brittle and friable.

Primary infection of the nail plate is less common. The nail plate may be affected on the surface, causing what is clinically known as white superficial onychomycosis, or it may affect the inner aspect of the nail plate, so that the surface appears normal except for a whitish discoloration within the nail plate. This later disease is known as proximal subungual onychomycosis (8). The infecting organism in this type of disease is thought to descend along the proximal nail fold and to penetrate the nail plate close to the matrix in a manner analogous to hair infections. Whether the infrequent reports of this infection are due to the disease being rare, or to the lack of its recognition, is not clear.

Fungal infections of the nail plate are not limited to dermatophytes. In fact, only 23% of clinical onychomycosis of toenails could be shown to be caused by dermatophytes (8). This observation stresses the importance of culture in making the diagnosis of dermatophytic onychomycosis since examination of affected material may show hyphae but it may be due to nondermatophytic fungi.

INFECTING ORGANISM

Dermatophytes may be grouped according to their primary reservoir. This classification is useful in determining the epidemiology of the infection and correlates with the degree of inflammation elicited in the normal uncompromised host. Dermatophytes isolated primarily from soil are grouped under the category of geophilic. When a geophilic fungus infects an animal or human, the infection usually evokes marked inflammation. Zoophilic fungi are those primarily adapted to animals. These fungi usually elicit little inflammation in their primary host, but cause a greater degree of inflammation in other animals or humans. Anthropophilic fungi are predominantly isolated from humans. This group causes a greater degree of inflammation when infecting animals than when infecting humans. However, *Trichophyton schoenleinii* and *Trichophyton violaceum*, which are anthropophilic fungi, may also cause marked inflammation in some humans. In general, as the fungus becomes adapted to a particular host, it tends to cause little inflammation and the infection tends to become chronic. (Table 11.1).

HOST-PARASITE RELATIONSHIP

The factors which determine the host-parasite relationship appear to be related to the host's ability to mount an adequate inflammatory response. As previously noted, certain categories of fungi are capable of eliciting varying degrees of inflammation in a "normal" human host. Some apparently "normal" humans, when infected with organisms capable of eliciting marked inflammation, show a minimal amount of inflammation. These patients tend to have chronic infections. Investigation of these individuals has implicated their lack of a delayed hypersensitivity response to soluble fungal antigens or the presence of an immediate hypersensitivity response to such an antigen as possible factors causing chronic disease (9, 10). There is some evidence that the cell-mediated immune system may be directly or indirectly responsible for an increased resistance to infection and for limiting the duration and extent of infection (11). It is not clear whether these observations are due to direct products of the immune reaction or are secondary to the inflammatory response. In humans, there is no evidence that the level of circulating antibodies induced by dermatophytic infection correlates with disease activity or resistance (12).

Table 11.1
Classification of Dermatophytes by their Primary Reservoir

Anthropophilic	Zoophilic	Geophilic
Trichophyton concentricum	*Trichophyton equinum*	*Trichophyton ajelloi*
Trichophyton mentagrophytes, var. *interdigitale*	*Trichophyton mentagrophytes,* var. *mentagrophytes*	*Microsporum fulvum*
Trichophyton megninii	*Trichophyton simii*	*Microsporum gypseum*
Trichophyton rubrum	*Trichophyton verrucosum*	
Trichophyton schoenleinii	*Microsporum canis*	
Microsporum audouinii	*Microsporum distortum*	
Trichophyton soudanense	*Microsporum gallinae*	
Microsporum ferrugineum	*Microsporum namum*	
Epidermophyton floccosum	*Microsporum persicolor*	

Stratum Corneum Infections

TINEA CORPORIS

Tinea corporis is a dermatophytic infection of glabrous skin which manifests itself classically as a well demarcated, red, scaly-to-vesiculopustular, circinate lesion accompanied by pruritus (Fig. 11.1).

Etiology and Epidemiology. Tinea corporis may be caused by any species of dermatophyte. However, *Trichophyton rubrum*, *Trichophyton mentagrophytes*, and *Microsporum canis* are most frequently isolated in the United States.

The disease may be transmitted by direct contact with infected humans, animals, or fomites. It may affect individuals of either sex and of any age.

Clinical Features. The clinical presentation of tinea corporis is quite varied, so that almost any papulosquamous lesion may be suspect. The classical lesion may begin as an erythematous papule which enlarges to form a well demarcated annular lesion. The border of the lesion is red and may have scales, vesicles, or pustules. Lesions may increase in size to form large gyrate patterns. Within these lesions, the skin may appear relatively normal, dappled with erythematous scaling papules, or be entirely erythematous and covered with scales. Pruritus is almost always present. Other constitutional symptoms are usually absent.

Other presentations include a marked inflammatory response with fluctuant pustular lesions similar to those seen with kerions. This type of disease is known as Majocchi's granuloma, and occurs primarily on the legs of females. The lesions are caused by a foreign-body response to hair and fungus which has invaded the dermis secondary to the rupture of a hair follicle. Some lesions have a granulomatous clinical appearance without histologic evidence of granuloma. A rare presentation of tinea corporis is that of a mycetoma (13). Clinically, these patients have fluctuant nodules without sinus tracts or evidence of fungal "grains." The histopathology of these lesions is similar to that observed with mycetoma, i.e. granulomatous response, and microcultures of compact organisms (grains). This disease has been reported primarily in blacks with extensive cutaneous and/or hair infection.

The differential diagnosis of tinea corporis is extensive because of its varied presentation. The classical lesion may resemble psoriasis, lichen planus, the healed patch of pityriasis rosea, seborrheic dermatitis, or contact dermatitis. Kerion-like lesions are most frequently confused with bacterial infections, especially staphylococcal furuncles. Granulomatous lesions must be differentiated from other causes of granulomas such as sarcoidosis and foreign body reaction. They may also resemble various panniculitides.

Diagnosis. The diagnosis of tinea corporis is made by identifying fungal hyphae in the KOH examination of infected scale and by culture confirmation. Only 40–60% of KOH examinations are positive even though the patient does have dermatophytosis. Therefore, the diagnosis is confirmed by a positive culture on Sabouraud's agar. Addition of antibiotics to the agar will prevent bacterial contamination.

Treatment. For a single or a few accessible lesions of tinea corporis, topical antifun-

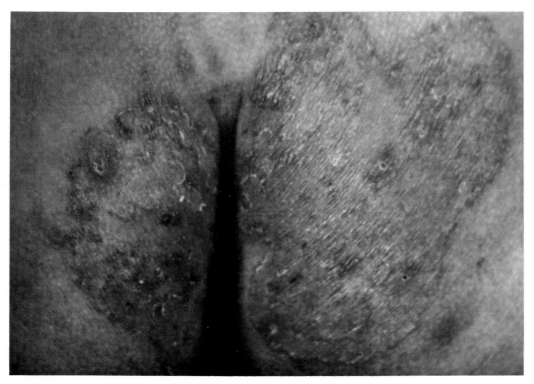

Fig. 11.1. Tinea corporis showing a well defined circinate scaly lesion. Areas within the lesion appear relatively clear of scale.

gals are recommended. Although there are a wide variety of prescription and nonprescription topical antifungals, the most effective appear to be imidazole derivatives, i.e. clotrimazole (Lotrimin Solution 1%) and miconazole (MicaTin Brand Miconazole Nitrate 2%). These agents are applied twice daily for 2–4 weeks. They are equally efficacious. Since these agents also are effective against *Candida* infection, they are particularly useful when awaiting the confirmatory culture of infections which are suspected of being caused by either a dermatophyte or a yeast. With the exception of occasional skin irritation when used in intertrigenous areas, these agents have no side effects.

For multiple lesions, the use of a systemic antifungal is usually recommennded. The only noninvestigational, systemic, antidermatophytic agent currently available is griseofulvin. The recommended dose for the micronized form is 500 mg twice a day for adults, 750 mg in two divided doses for children weighing 50–90 lbs, and 250 mg twice a day for children weighing 30–50 lbs. The dose schedule for the ultramicronized form (Gris-PEG Tablets) is one-half of the dose stated above. There is no significant therapeutic advantage of one form over the other. The treatment should be continued for 4 weeks even if the infection appears clinically clear before that time since the frequency of reinfection is higher in those treated under 4 weeks. The cure rate for this dose schedule is greater than 90%. The side effects of griseofulvin are usually mild and transient. Headache, skin rashes, and gastrointestinal distress are among the most common side effects. Because griseofulvin interferes with porphyrin metabolism, it may precipitate attacks of porphyria cutanea tarda (14, 15). Since it also increases microsomal activity in the liver, it should be used with care in patients receiving medications metabolized by this system such as warfarin sodium (Coumadin) and phenobarbital. It may be contraindicated in patients with liver disease (16, 17).

TINEA CRURIS

Tinea cruris is a dermatophytic infection of

the groin. Its pathogenesis and clinical manifestation are similar to tinea corporis.

Etiology and Epidemiology. Although any species of dermatophyte may cause tinea cruris, the most frequently isolated organisms are *Epidermophyton floccosum, Trichophyton rubrum,* or *Trichophyton metagrophytes.* This type of infection occurs predominantly in males. Factors which predispose to infection are moisture, occlusion, and trauma. Wet bathing suits, athletic supporters ("jock itch"), tight-fitting apparel, and obesity frequently contribute to the initiation or recurrence of infection.

Clinical Features. The clinical manifestations of tinea cruris are similar to those of tinea corporis. The area of involvement is most frequently the inner thighs. In males, the penis and scrotum are usually spared (in contradistinction to candidiasis where these sites are frequently involved).

The differential diagnosis includes candidiasis, erythrasma, psoriasis, and seborrheic dermatitis.

Diagnosis and Treatment. The diagnosis and treatment of tinea cruris is similar to tinea corporis. In order to decrease the rate of recurrence in treated patients, preventive measures directed at decreasing the predisposing factors should be instituted, such as decreasing moisture and chaffing by the use of powders, or by wearing loose fitting clothing.

TINEA PEDIS AND TINEA MANUUM

Tinea pedis and tinea manuum are dermatophytic infections of the plantar and palmar aspects of the feet and hands (Figs. 11.2–11.4). Interdigital infection as well as infection of the dorsal aspect of the hands or feet are also included under this classification (Fig. 11.5). The clinical presentation runs a spectrum from a fine scaling process to a vesiculopustular eruption. Pruritus is usually present.

Etiology and Epidemiology. As in other infections of the stratum corneum, any species of dermatophyte is capable of causing disease. The most frequently isolated organisms are *T. rubrum, T. mentagrophytes,* and *E. floccosum.*

Tinea pedis occurs primarily in people who wear shoes. Although this type of infection

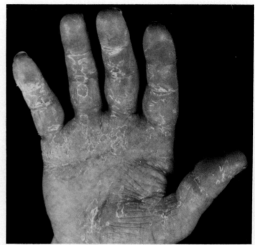

Fig. 11.2. Tinea manuum. This patient also had tinia pedis. The extent of disease had worsened when the patient was treated with topical steroids for a presumptive diagnosis of dyshydrosis.

may occur in any age group, there is an increased frequency of infection with age. There is no sexual predominance. Tinea manuum is most frequently associated with concurrent tinea pedis.

Clinical Features. Tinea pedis may be divided into three clinical presentations. The most common is infection of the intertrigenous area between the toes (Fig. 11.5). This type of disease presents with red scaly lesions which may go on to fissure and become macerated. Pruritus is the most common symptom.

In the hyperkeratotic presentation of tinea pedis (Fig. 11.3), there is a fine to coarse scale which may be localized or extended over the entire plantar aspect of the foot. Recurrent or chronic infection is common with this type of tinea pedis. There are usually minimal signs of inflammation. Symptoms, when present, are usually confined to mild pruritus.

The third type of clinical presentation is characterized by tense vesicles filled with a clear exudate. As the vesicles rupture, they leave a collarette of scale. An ulcerative vesticulopustular form of this type of tinea pedis occurs occasionally. It may be accompanied by secondary bacterial infection and, if severe, will progress to ulceration. Most frequently, ulceration occurs adjacent to the plantar as-

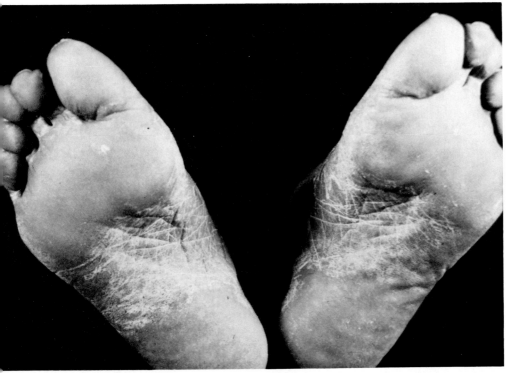

Fig. 11.3. Tinea pedis. Hyperkeratosis primarily of the arch of the foot.

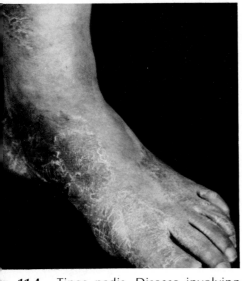

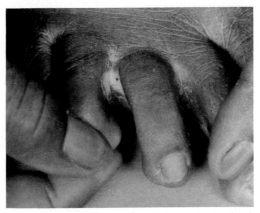

Fig. 11.5. Tinea pedis. Patient only had interdigital disease. This clinical presentation must be differentiated from candidiasis, erythrasma, and some Gram-negative bacterial infections.

g. 11.4. Tinea pedis. Disease involving ›th plantar and dorsal surfaces.

·cts of the toes. Symptoms may vary from ·uritus to pain severe enough to hamper ·alking.

The manifestations of tinea manuum are similar to those of tinea pedis. However, there is a greater frequency of unilateral infection in tinea manuum.

The differential diagnosis for intertrigenous

infection includes candidiasis, erythrasma, and infections caused by *Pseudomonas* (18) and other Gram-negative bacteria. The hyperkeratotic type of infection must be distinguished from psoriasis, chronic contact dermatitis, hyperkeratosis palmaris et plantaris, and pityriasis rubra pilaris. The vesiculopustular form may be confused with acute contact dermatitis, pustular psoriasis, dyshidrosis and occasionally keratosis blennorrhagica.

Most, though not all, fungus infections of the foot involve mostly the sole, toe webs or sides of the foot. Inflammatory reactions on the dorsum of the foot, especially over the big toe, are often an allergic contact dermatitis due to chemical used in shoes.

In some patients with tinea pedis or tinea corporis, an "-id reaction" may occur. This type of reaction may involve any cutaneous site, but most frequently occurs on the hands. It may be clinically indistinguishable from a dermatophytic infection. However, KOH examinations of scale and cultures do not reveal a dermatophyte.

Diagnosis. The diagnosis is made by KOH examination and culture. In the vesiculo-pustular type, the root of the vesicle must be examined or cultured. No organisms will be seen in the exudate. When severe desquamation and ulceration have occurred, KOH examination and culture may be negative.

Treatment. Tinea pedis and manuum should be treated like other stratum corneum dermatophytic infections, except that the duration of therapy should be lengthened to 6–8 weeks. When concurrent dermatophytic nail infection is present (Fig. 11.6), griseofulvin should be used until the nail infection is cured in order to prevent reinfection of the skin. However, the treatment of toenail infection in patients with tinea pedis, may not be practical because of the prolonged duration of therapy required to cure toenails and the high incidence of toenail reinfection.

As with dermatophytic infection of stratum corneum elsewhere, the factors which increase susceptibility to infection are humidity, trauma, and occlusion. Preventive measures which decrease these factors may be useful in limiting the frequency of reinfection.

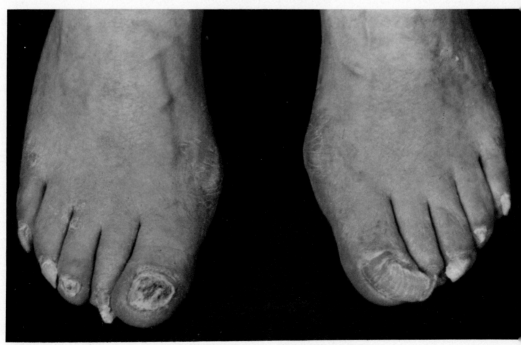

Fig. 11.6.   Patient with recurrent tinea pedis which probably recurred from a reservoir of organisms harbored in his onychomycotic toenails.

Hair Infections

TINEA CAPITIS

Tinea capitis is a dermatophytic infection of scalp hair characterized by alopecia and varying degrees of scale and inflammation.

Etiology and Epidemiology. Tinea capitis is caused by species of the genera *Trichophyton* and *Microsporum*. The major cause of infection is anthropophilic fungi. Primarily a disease of childhood, tinea capitis infection has its highest incidence in the 3- to 10-year age group. The incidence of *Microsporum* infections drops sharply after age 10. However, this drop in the incidence of infection is not as marked in *Trichophyton* infections. Tinea capitis does occur in adults. There is little evidence to directly support the hypothesis that tinea capitis heals spontaneously at puberty due to changes in the chemical composition of sebum (19).

The factors influencing transmission of tinea capitis are not well understood. There is an increased frequency of transmission when there is poor hygiene and overcrowding. Contaminated combs and barbers' instruments have been implicated in the transmission of this disease. There is experimental evidence that minor trauma increases the establishment of infection (3). Even during epidemics of tinea capitis, the number of infections is usually between 5–20% of the population at risk. Therefore, keeping patients with tinea capitis from attending school until they are disease free is unwarranted.

Clinical Features. Tinea capitis may be clinically divided into inflammatory and non-inflammatory types. Inflammatory tinea capitis is characterized by single or multiple areas of alopecia accompanied by varying degrees of erythema and scaling. They are caused primarily by ectothrix infections (Table 11.2). Folliculitis also may be present. If extensive inflammation occurs, areas of folliculitis may form fluctuant, suppurating nodules (kerion). These nodules are due to an allergic response to the infecting organism and are not usually due to bacterial secondary infection. A rule of thumb is that in children alopecia accompanied by pustules or fluctuant nodules is due to a dermatophyte until proven otherwise.

Severe inflammatory tinea capitis may be associated with fever, malaise, and regional lymphadenopathy. If inflammation is severe enough and/or chronic enough to destroy hair follicles, permanent alopecia will result. Kerions usually result in rapid loss of hair and the short stubby hairs usually seen in tinea capitis may not be present by the time the patient visits the physician.

Noninflammatory tinea capitis may be caused by ectothrix or endothrix infections. This type of disease usually presents with multiple well delineated areas of alopecia. In noninflammatory ectothrix infection, the areas of alopecia show broken, stubby hair with varying degrees of scaling. Endothrix infection usually produces little or no inflammation. This type of infection is characterized by "black dots" which are the result of infected hairs breaking just below the follicular orifice. There are usually no associated signs or symptoms in noninflammatory tinea capitis.

Diagnosis. The diagnosis of tinea capitis is confirmed by finding infected hair on KOH examination and by culture. The most fre-

Table 11.2
Classification of Dermatophytes Causing Tinea Capitis

Fluorescent Under Wood's Light	Not Fluorescent Under Wood's Light	
Ecthothrix Small Spores (2–3 μm)	Ectothrix Large Spores (5–10 μm)	Endothrix Spores (5–8 μm)
Microsporum canis	*Trichophyton verucosum*	*Trichophyton tonsurans*
Microsporum audouinii	*Trichophyton mentagrophytes*	*Trichophyton violaceum*
Microsporum distortum	*Trichophyton megninii*	*Trichophyton soudanense*
Microsporum ferrugineum	*Microsporum gypseum*	*Trichophyton yaoundei*
	Microsporum fulvum	
	Microsporum nanum	

quent mistake made is to examine only the scale. Since the stratum corneum infection is relatively short-lived in comparison to the hair infection, examination of scales instead of hair may lead to false negative interpretation. An adjunct to making the diagnosis is illuminating the scalp with a Wood's light. In certain dermatophytic infections (Table 11.2), Wood's light reveals yellow-green fluorescent infected hair.

The highest yield of positive KOH examinations from endothrix infection is obtained by removing the "black-dot" with a needle and not by plucking hairs at random. Direct observation of an infected hair not only makes the diagnosis but helps determine which species may be causing the infection (Table 11.2).

The differential diagnosis of tinea capitis includes most causes of alopecia. Mild noninflammatory tinea capitis, where there is minimal hair loss, may be difficult to differentiate clinically from seborrheic dermatitis or mild psoriasis. When there is considerable alopecia in tinea capitis, alopecia areata, trichotillomania, and secondary syphilis may be included in the differential diagnosis. Inflammatory tinea capitis may be confused with pustular psoriasis, and especially bacterial folliculitis of the scalp. Tinea capitis in adults may appear clinically similar to discoid lupus erythematosis.

Treatment. Tinea capitis is treated with griseofulvin. The optimum dose schedule is not known. A daily dose similar to that used in tinea corporis is commonly used. The duration of therapy ranges from 1 to 3 months in most cases, but should be determined by clinical and mycological assessment. Weekly (20) and single (21) dose schedules also have been found effective. A single dose of 3 g of griseofulvin has been shown effective in curing 80% of the cases. Of the 20% not responding to this dose schedule, most were endothrix infections caused by *Trichophyton tonsurans*. This regimen has been used for patients who cannot afford or cannot be relied upon to take daily medication.

Since inflammatory tinea capitis is capable of causing permanent hair loss, it should be treated with griseofulvin without the delay caused by a trial of antibiotics for a presumed bacterial infection.

Topical antifungals are not effective in ti-nea capitis nor do they appear to increase the cure rate of patients taking griseofulvin.

TINEA BARBAE

Tinea barbae is a dermatophytic infection of beard hair. Its pathogenesis and clinical presentation is similar to tinea capitis.

Etiology and Epidemiology. The most common cause of tinea barbae is *T. mentagrophytes* and *T. verrucosum*. Organisms less frequently isolated include *T. violaceum*, *T. rubrum*, and *M. canis*.

This is predominantly a disease of rural men who acquire it from infected animals.

Clinical Presentation. Tinea barbae, like tinea capitis, may be divided clinically into an inflammatory and noninflammatory type. Inflammatory lesions are characterized by pustules and hair loss (Fig. 11.7). There may be symptoms of fever, malaise, and regional lymphadenopathy with this type of disease.

Noninflammatory tinea barbae shows little if any folliculitis. The lesions are circinate and scaly and appear more like tinea corporis than a hair infection. There are no constitutional symptoms. Pruritus is sometimes present.

The differential diagnosis includes bacterial folliculitis, contact dermatitis, herpes zoster, and herpes simplex.

Diagnosis. The diagnosis is made by KOH examination and culture of hair and purulent material. Purulent material will frequently show arthrospores. Hair which can be removed with little resistance gives the highest yield of positive KOH examinations. A Wood's light is seldom helpful in making the diagnosis.

Treatment. The treatment of tinea barbae is similar to that of tinea capitis.

Nail Infections

TINEA UNGUIUM

Tinea unguium is a dermatophytic infection of the nail bed or nail plate. Clinically, it may be divided into three types of disease: distal subungual, proximal subungual, and white superficial onychomycosis.

Etiology and Epidemiology. *T. rubrum* and *T. metagrophytes* are the frequent causes of tinea unguium. Species of *Microsporum* or *Epidermophyton* rarely cause nail infection.

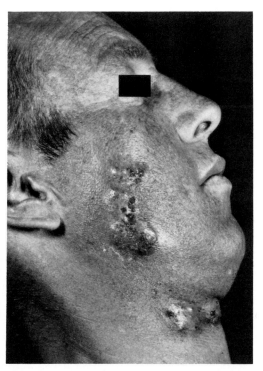

Fig. 11.7. Tinea barbae caused by *Trichophyton mentagrophytes.* This patient had many pustules and fluctuant nodules and was initially treated for a bacterial infection without any improvement. Examination of hair showed ectothrix spores. Patient was then started on griseofulvin. Within 2 weeks, there was a marked clinical improvement and after 6 weeks of therapy the patient was clinically and mycologically cured.

Recurrent tinea pedis is associated with toenail infections. The incidence of tinea unguium increases with age.

Clinical Features. Distal subungual infection of the nail is the most common form of tinea unguium. It begins as a white to yellow discoloration at the distal or lateral aspect of the nail plate. As the disease continues, there is increased hyperkeratosis which may cause the nail plate to rise and separate from the nail bed. The nail plate may become secondarily infected causing it to become friable. There are usually no symptoms unless the distorted nail plate impinges on the surrounding soft tissue.

Irregular white bands that may traverse the entire width of the nail plate are seen in proximal subungual infection. The white discolorations begin in the proximal portion of the nail plate. As the nail plate grows outward, the areas of leukonychia move with it. The surface of the nail plate is not affected. This type of disease is due to a primary infection occurring within the nail plate.

In white superficial onychomycosis, the surface of the nail plate is covered with a whitish yellow material which is a colony of the infecting organism. Localized or widespread involvement of the nail plate may occur.

The differential diagnosis of distal subungual and white superficial onychomycosis includes disease caused by other nondermatophytic fungi such as *Cephalosporium, Aspergillus,* and *Fusarium,* and some bacteria. Other nail diseases which may be confused with these types of tinea unguium include lichen planus, psoriasis, and mucocutaneous candidiasis. Proximal subungual infection must be differentiated from other causes of leukonychia, the most common of which is trauma.

Diagnosis. The diagnosis of tinea unguium is dependent on culture confirmation. A positive KOH examination is not sufficient since hyphae are seen in other nondermatophytic nail infections. The importance of mycologic confirmation is obvious since infection due to other nondermatophytic fungi will not respond to griseofulvin therapy.

The most appropriate material for culture and KOH examination is the hyperkeratotic debris in distal subungual disease, pieces of nail plate within the areas of leukonychia in proximal subungual disease, and scrapings from the white material in white superficial onychomycosis.

Treatment. Griseofulvin is required for the successful treatment of distal and proximal subungual tinea unguium. The dose schedule is the same as for tinea corporis but the duration of therapy ranges from 3–4 months for fingernail infections and 6 months or more in toenail infections. The duration of therapy may be shortened by avulsion of the affected nail plate. The cure rate in fingernails is greater than 80% with a recurrence rate of almost zero (22). The recurrence rate for toenail infection is significantly greater than fingernails (23).

Since the organism is limited to the surface

of the nail plate in white superficial onycho-mycosis, this type of infection may be cured by paring the infected portion or by topically applying dilute solutions of gluteraldehyde (24).

OTHER SUPERFICIAL MYCOTIC INFECTIONS

TINEA VERSICOLOR

Tinea versicolor is caused by the lipophilic yeast *Malassezia furfur.* Infection is confined to the stratum corneum and commonly presents as asymptomatic, hypopigmented to fawn-colored lesions covered with a fine scale.

Epidemiology.   Tinea versicolor is world-wide in distribution, although it is most commonly seen in tropical and subtropical climates.

Clinical Features.   Tinea versicolor classically begins as perfollicular hypopigmentation. As the infection progresses, the areas of hypopigmentation coalesce producing irregular patches covered with fine scale. The scale is not always clinically evident. However, it is easily demonstrated by scraping the lesions. The degree of hypopigmentation is related to sun exposure because the unaffected skin darkens in response to ultraviolet light while the infected areas do not. Less frequently, the disease may present as pink- to fawn-colored lesions (Fig. 11.8). Occasionally the lesions are papular.

The lesions of tinea versicolor are usually asymptomatic although they may be accompanied by mild pruritus. They may affect any cutaneous area, although they are most commonly seen on the upper trunk.

The differential diagnosis may include dermatophytosis, pityriasis rosea, and occasionally seborrheic dermatitis when the lesions are erythematous, or pityriasis alba and vitiligo if the lesions are hypopigmented.

Diagnosis.   The diagnosis of tinea versicolor is established by finding the hyphae and cluster of yeast cells when the scale is treated with 20% KOH and examined microscopically. The addition of blue ink to the KOH may increase the ease of identifying the organism (25). A yeast or hyphal form may

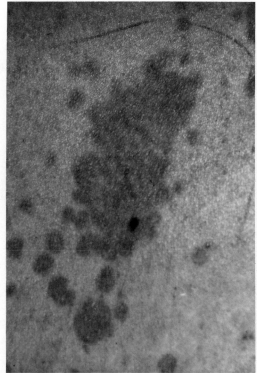

Fig. 11.8.   Tinea versicolor. This patient had tinea versicolor which caused erythematous scaly lesion as opposed to the more common hypopigmented lesions.

predominate in rare cases. Culture is not feasible without special media, and it is not required for diagnosis.

Treatment.   There are various treatments to tinea versicolor. A relatively inexpensive treatment is to use 2.5% Selenium sulfide (Selsun Lotion shampoo) (26). The patient is instructed to lather the entire body with the shampoo, leave it on for 10–20 minutes and then wash it off. This is done every other day for 1–2 weeks. The topical imidazoles (MicaTin Brand Miconazole Nitrate 2%, Lotrimin Cream 1%) have also been shown to be effective in the treatment of tinea versicolor. However, these agents are more expensive, especially if large areas are involved. An older form of therapy is a solution of 20% sodium thiosulfate. However, most patients object to the odor of this preparation. Tinver Lotion is a better smelling sodium thiosulfate preparation.

Repigmentation of the affected area is dependent on sun exposure and may require several weeks depending upon the geographic location and season. Although the cure rate for this disease is high, recurrence is frequent.

TINEA NIGRA

Tinea nigra is a superficial mycotic infection of the stratum corneum, caused by *Exophiala werneckii*, previously known as *Cladosporium werneckii*. It most frequently affects the palmar and plantar skin. Tinea nigra is characterized by a light brown to black, nonscaly macule which is asymptomatic.

Epidemiology.   The geographic distribution of this disease is primarily tropical and subtropical climates. However, it is not limited to these climates. The disease occurs most frequently in children and young adults, girls outnumbering boys 3 to 1 in most reports.

Clinical Features.   The initial lesion of tinea nigra is a well defined, light brown macule which spreads peripherally and darkens. The lesions are found primarily on palmar and plantar surfaces. As the lesion enlarges, its color may become darker or mottled. These macules produce no scale, nor are they symptomatic. The importance of tinea nigra is that it may be misdiagnosed as malignant melanoma (27). In some cases, this has resulted in extensive local excision and scar production. Other diagnosis which must be differentiated from tinea nigra include junctional nevus, postinflammatory hyperpigmentation and stains due to chemicals or dyes.

Diagnosis.   The diagnosis of tinea nigra is made by finding pigmented hyphae in scrapings treated with KOH and examined microscopically, as well as by culture confirmation of *E. werneckii*.

Treatment.   Manual removal of the infected stratum corneum is the treatment for tinea nigra. Since the organism is harbored in the upper portion of the stratum corneum, scraping the lesion with a blade, or repeated stripping with adhesive cellophane tape is curative (28). Keratolytics such as 4% salicylic acid (Keralyt Gel) or Whitfield's ointment may also be effective. This infection does not respond to griseofulvin.

References

1. Baer, R.L., Rosenthal, S.A., Rogachefsky, H., and Litt, J.Z.: Newer studies on the epidemiology of fungous infections of the feet. Am. J. Public Health, *45:* 784, 1955.
2. Huppert, M., and Keeney, E.L.: Immunization against superficial fungous infection. J. Invest. Dermatol., *32:* 15, 1959.
3. Kligman, A.M.: The pathogenesis of tinea capitis due to *Microsporum audouini* and *Microsporum canis*. I. Gross observation following the inoculation of humans. J. Invest. Dermatol., *18:* 231, 1952.
4. Reiss, F., and Leonard, L.: Experimental *Microsporum lanosum* infection in dogs, cats and rabbits. II. Studies on the course of reinfection. J. Invest. Dermatol., *24:* 589, 1955.
5. Berk, S.H., Penneys, N.S., and Weinstein, G.D.: Epidermal activity in annular dermatophytosis. Arch. Dermatol., *112:* 485, 1976.
6. Ive, F.A., and Marks, R.: Tinea incognito. Br. Med. J., *3:* 149, 1968.
7. Kligman, A.M., Baldbridge, G.D., Rebell, G., and Pillsbury, D.M.: The effect of cortisone on the pathologic response of guinea pigs infected cutaneously with fungi, viruses and bacteria. J. Lab. Clin. Med., *37:* 615, 1951.
8. Zaias, N.: Onychomycosis. Arch. Dermatol.., *105:* 263, 1972.
9. Jones, H.E., et al.: Immunologic susceptibility to chronic dermatophytosis. Arch. Dermatol., *110:* 213, 1974.
10. Jones, H.E., et al.: Model dermatophytosis in naturally infected subjects. Arch. Dermatol., *110:* 369, 1974.
11. Jones, H.E., et al.: Acquired immunity to dermatophytes. Arch. Dermatol., *109:* 840, 1974.
12. Grappel, S.F., Blank, F., and Bishop, C.T.: Circulating antibodies in human favus. Dermatologica, *143:* 271, 1971.
13. Kwon-chung, K.J., and West, B.C.: Mycetoma caused by dermatophytes: A review. *Primer Simposis Internacional de micetoma.* Barquismeto, Venezuela, 1978.
14. Berman, A., and Franklin, R.L.: Precipitation of acute intermittent porphyria by griseofulvin therapy. JAMA, *192:* 1005, 1965.
15. Simon, N., Berko, G., Polay, A., et al.: Der einfluss der griseofulvin-therapie auf die liberfunktion und den prophyin-stoffwechsel. Arch. Dermatol. Forsch., *241:* 148, 1971.
16. Griseofulvin and porphyrin metabolism. Lancet, *1:* 870, 1963.
17. Steagall, R.W., Jr.: Severe reaction to griseofulvin. Arch. Dermatol., *88:* 218, 1963.
18. Amonette, R.A., and Rosenberg, E.W.: Infection of toe-webs by Gram-negative bacteria. Arch. Dermatol., *107:* 71, 1973.
19. Burgoon, C.F., and Keiper, R.J.: Tinea capitis. Pediatr. Clin. N. Am., *8:* 759, 1961.
20. Friedman, L., Derbes, J.V., Newell, B.L., and Lee, E.: The control of tinea capitis among indigent populations. Am. J. Public Health, *54:* 1588, 1964.
21. Vanbreuseghem, R., Gatti, F., and Ceballos, J.A.:

Mass treatment of scalp ringworm by a single dose of griseofulvin. Int. J. Dermatol., *9:* 59, 1970.

22. Russell, B., and Frain-Bell, W., et al.: Chronic ringworm of the skin and nails treated with griseofulvin. Report of a therapeutic trial. Lancet, *1:* 1141, 1960.

23. Stevenson, C.J., and Djavahiszwili, N.: Chronic ringworm of the nails: Long-term treatment with griseofulvin. Lancet, *1:* 373, 1961.

24. Suringa, D.W.R.: Treatment of superficial onychomycosis with topically applied glutaraldehyde. Arch. Dermatol., *102:* 163, 1972.

25. Popkess, F.G.: A practical office method for the diagnosis of tinea versicolor. Ann. Allergy, *22:* 42, 1964.

26. Albright, S.D., and Kitch, J. M.: Rapid treatment of tinea versicolor with selenium sulfide. Arch. Dermatol., *93:* 460, 1966.

27. Vaffee, A.S.: Tinea nigra resembling malignant melanoma. N. Engl. J. Med., *283:* 1112, 1970.

28. Falabella, R., and Caplan, R.M.: Cure of tinea nigra by epidermal stripping. Arch. Dermatol., *91:* 637, 1965.

CHAPTER 12

PARASITES

JAMES E. RASMUSSEN

A discussion of insects and parasites is difficult to organize because of the diversity of the vectors and the broad spectrum of the lesions they produce. I have chosen to divide this chapter into two parts, based on the usual physical distances between host and parasites. From near to far, we will discuss the "creatures that live 1) on in or near the skin, and 2) at some distance from the skin."

CREATURES THAT LIVE ON OR IN THE SKIN

Scabies

Tuberculosis and syphilis were the masqueraders of the 1940s and 1950s. Today, that role has been assumed in part by scabies (1, 2). It is a disease with protean manifestations which include papules, nodules, vesicles, blisters, and scale. The hallmarks of nearly all of these disguises, however, is pruritus. Listen to your patients: "they itch, their children itch, other family and friends itch." Listen again: "soap and water doesn't help," and "I think I have scabies."

In this, as in most clinical situations, it is important to look first with your ears, and use the suspicions so generated to direct your examination. Pruritus is the watchword. Whenever it is mentioned, think scabies. This eternal vigilance is justified because of the resurgence of the mite *Sarcoptes scabei*. It has once again become a common pathogen and any clinician who is not making the diagnosis frequently, is missing the diagnosis frequently.

Scabies is spread predominantly when flesh meets flesh so it is routinely found among families and close friends. The mite pays no regard to the sex, age, or social stations of its host, but scabies *is definitely* less common in American blacks. A common clinical history is exposure to an infected patient (spouse, parent, friend, lover) followed in 2–4 weeks by a crescendo pattern of itch and dermatitis.

Many texts suggest that the nocturnal pruritus of scabies is an important clue to the diagnosis, but most diseases that itch do so at night. Also misleading is the patient's suggestions that they can "feel" something crawling on the skin. The *Sarcoptes* mite is almost too small to see without magnification and burrows within the skin, rather than on the surface.

If the patient's history of itch has aroused an appropriate suspicion, search the entire surface of the skin for confirmation. *Look first from a distance for the distribution of lesions*: web spaces of fingers, flexor surfaces of wrists, periumbilical area, and penis. The face and scalp are invariably spared except in infants and there are usually very few lesions below the knees. The most suggestive lesions occur in the webs, wrists, elbows, penis, and periumbilical region but infants and young children may have severe involvement of the palms and soles.

Then, a few steps closer to the patient, search for primary and secondary lesions: the most characteristic are serpiginous burrows which are found in the webs and on the penis. These are not found in all patients; some have only small vesicles and scaly papules on the webs (Fig. 12.1), wrists, penis, and waist. The palms and soles of children are frequently involved with crops of small vesicles. Total number of lesions may be small in recent cases on patients who are fastidious but, frequently, they are so numerous that they superficially resemble atopic eczema, psoriasis, or ichthyosis. The most severe involvement occurs in the mentally ill or retarded, institutionalized patient where scratching may not be as prominent as expected. Equally severe disease can be seen during therapy with topical or systemic corticosteroids.

In addition to the above scabetic stereotypes, nodular lesions are also quite common (1). They are seen almost routinely on the upper back and chest of young children (Fig. 12.2) as well as the male genitals and the axillary folds. Initially, the nodules may be crusted, suggesting impetigo, but following antiscabetic therapy they assume a smooth surface with a red or brown color. They are generally assumed to represent a granulomatous reaction to the mite and can persist for months.

An attempt *should always be made to confirm a diagnosis of scabies*, no matter how suggestive the history and physical examination. Clinicopathological correlations are important for accuracy, education of patient and physician, personal satisfaction, and safety. In at least 85–90% of cases, mites can be readily identified in scales collected from the web spaces

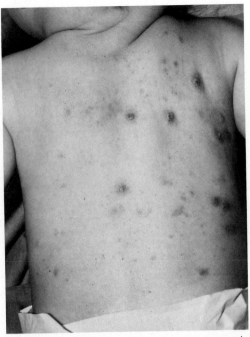

Fig. 12.2. Nodular lesions are commonly found in babies with scabies, especially on the upper back and chest, genitals, and axillary folds.

with potassium hydroxide (a "KOH prep"). The technique (3) is simple: 1) select the "best" patient from among those infected. Do not scrape small children, they rarely cooperate. Look for a hand with numerous papules, vesicles, and burrows in the web spaces. Moisten *every* web with water or immersion oil so that the scraped scale will adhere to the blade! Scrape *every* web space with a round-bellied No. 15 blade, taking care to completely remove the top of all the vesicles, papules, and burrows. Then, transfer the scale to a glass slide and complete the search by gently scraping the entire area of each web to pick up any itinerant mites. By this time, you should have considerable scale on the glass microscope slide. *The most common error is to collect too little scale from one web space.*

Add 1 drop of 20% KOH (or immersion oil if it was used in the webs), a coverslip, and *examine under reduced light and low power (× 100).* Look systematically, as if using a hemocytometer. Your careful search will be excitingly rewarded with adult mites, eggs, or egg cases. Figure 12.3 demonstrates the striking appear-

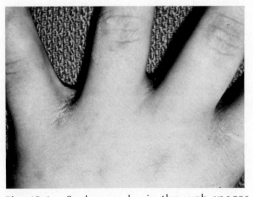

Fig. 12.1. Scaly papules in the web spaces are suggestive of scabies. Burrows, while characteristic, are not always seen.

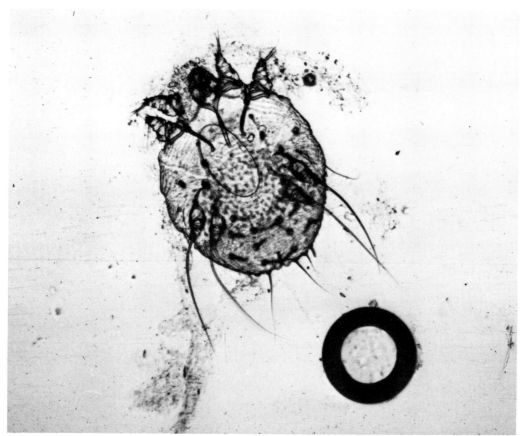

Fig. 12.3.   Adult female mite with an egg (×100). Note the graceful arching spines on each of the four hind legs.

ance of the adult *S. scabei*; note the characteristic arching spines on the back paired legs. Occasionally, the adult will be vivisected during the scraping, but an accurate diagnosis can still be made from the leg and spine.

Treatment.   The treatment of choice of scabies is γ-benzene hexachloride (GBH), (Kwell Lotion). Other drugs (Eurax Cream, sulfur, benzyl benzoate) are less effective and are distinctly second choices, useful primarily when Kwell is not indicated. The manufacturer currently recommends a single 24-hour application, repeated in 1 week only if necessary. Apparently, these are emperical suggestions because, frequently, a single overnight application (6–10 hours) is quite satisfactory. Although not often stressed, it is important to currently treat all "family" members who occupy the same living area, whether they itch or not, and treat all areas of the body from neck to toes (not just the areas with visible lesions or symptoms). *Kwell does not produce an immediate relief of symptoms or resolution of signs*; clinical healing may take 1–2 weeks, even longer with severe infection and nodular lesions. Some patients may even need topical (or systemic) corticosteroids to carry them through this gradual resolution.

There has been much recent discussion about the acute safety of topical GBH (4–6). Some have suggested that it should not be used in infants and small children. It is difficult, however, to find a solid basis for this reasoning—the number of reported reactions to Kwell is extremely small and usually have occurred after substantial misuse, such as frequently repeated applications. There is no doubt that GBH is absorbed through the skin (7, 8) but this is true of nearly all topical agents. The continued use of GBH in all patients with scabies seems justified (except pregnant women).

For those who are concerned about the potential hazards of GBH, consider: 1) 3–6% precipitated sulfur, 2) Eurax Cream, or 3) 10–20% benzyl benzoate. The reader should remember that the safety and efficacy of these products are far from proven and that experience with their use is limited. Benzyl benzoate and sulfur have been reported to cause toxicity when used as a scabiticide, although Eurax Cream appears quite safe.

Animal Scabies and Other Mites

Animal scabies is only rarely confused with human scabies, partly because the host specificity prevents person-to-person transmission. Mites from dogs (sarcoptic mange), cats, sheep, goats, and horses, and even more exotic forms, have been reported to cause a dermatitis in man. Inability to complete its life cycle limits the infection to sites of contact (thighs and lower abdomen in pets) eliminating the presence of burrows and eggs. Facial lesions are common in children. The invading mite usually produces erythematous papules and vesicles but chronic exposure generates eczematous scaly areas.

DO NOT APPLY GBH TO ANIMALS— they lick it off and become seriously ill. Consult a veterinarian for appropriate advice.

OTHER MITES

In general, other mites (grain mites, harvest mites (chiggers), avian mites, rodent mites, etc.) are not normally human parasites but accidentally contact skin while in search of a protein meal. Areas of contact will determine the pattern of disease but in general it is limited to the exposed parts of the body. Cutaneous reaction to the mite is usually a red macule but chronic exposure or hypersensitivity can produce eczematous patches or wheals, vesicles, and bullae. Occasionally, the mite can be seen on the skin surface with a magnifying glass.

Treatment. Therapy is frustrating if exposure continues; topical or systemic corticosteroids and oral antihistamines are helpful. Insect repellants (see next section) help prevent cutaneous contamination.

DEMODEX

Demodex folliculorum is an obligate human parasite whose entire life cycle is limited to follicules, primarily on the face and scalp. Its pathogenicity is doubtful but it has been considered to be one cause of rosacea and marginal blepharitis. In suspected cases, the mite can be identified in scrapings of inflammatory papules or around eyelashes.

Treatment. Two to four percent sulfur in cream or ointment base is usually successful; topical antibiotics (such as tetracycline, erythromycin and clindamycin) may also be helpful.

Lice

Pediculosis (1) are: crab louse (pubic louse), is *Phthirus pubis*; body louse (clothing louse) is *Pediculus humanus*, var. *corporis*; and head louse (scalp louse) is *Pediculus humanis*, var. *capitis*.

PEDICULOSIS CAPITIS

Head lice are common parasites of the scalp and beard area. Children are most frequently infected, complaining of itching of the neck, ears, sides of the face, and upper shoulders. The adult louse lives on longer strands of hair, leaving this bushy jungle to feed on the nearby, less hairy, skin of the face, neck, and upper trunk. Its bite produces small erythematous papules which are commonly infected. Longer hair, pruritus, and infection produce the characteristic picture of matting, cervical adenopathy, and a purulent dermatitis which appears to be characteristic of economically and mentally marginal patients. Lice, however, have no respect for salary or social system and the diagnosis should be suspected in anyone who complains of pruritus of the head, neck, and shoulders. Let your ears (the history) direct your examination to the hair above and posterior to the ears where the concentration of lice and nits will be the greatest.

The adult louse is an elongated insect 3 mm in length; much more numerous are the smaller (0.5–15 mm) nits, found projecting from the sides of hair 2–10 cm from the scalp. Easily confused are hair casts and scales of dandruff which are: 1) not fixed to hairs, sliding easily with finger traction, and 2) do not project from the side of the hair. When in doubt, place the suspected nit on a glass microsocpe slide and view under low power (Fig. 12.4).

Treatment. GBH shampoo is preferred treatment but patients respond poorly unless all of the family members and personal social contacts are also treated. In some cases, the hair must be clipped short and all eggs removed with a very fine-toothed comb.

PEDICULOSIS CORPORIS

The body louse usually produces disease in

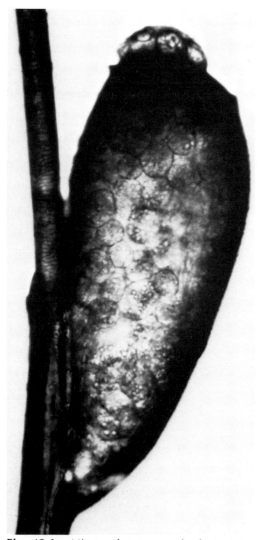

Fig. 12.4. Nit on human scalp hair. Nits will not slide on the hair shaft like the scales of dandruff or lint (×100).

vagrants, alcoholics, and poorly supervised institutional patients. Transmission is from person-to-person via clothing, bedding, furniture, or flesh-to-flesh contact. The adult lice usually live in the seams of shirts and undergarments where they deposit their eggs (Fig. 12.5). They feed primarily on the upper one-half of the trunk, their bite producing pruritic, erythematous papules. Excoriations are quickly infected and, if chronic, gradually yield a pattern of small round scars on the upper back which is quite suggestive of lice.

Patients with pruritus of the upper trunk should be suspected of harboring body lice— search the seams of clothing, but beware of the patient who just changed clothes for his visit to the doctor.

Treatment. GBH is the treatment of choice; all clothing and bedding must be washed thoroughly with very hot water or dry-cleaned. Secondary infection requires the systemic use of appropriate antibiotics.

PEDICULOSIS PUBIS

The pubic—"crab"—louse (Figs. 12.6–12.8) is one of the most common causes of venereal disease in the United States. "Crabs" are morphologically suited to life in the sparsely treed forest of the pubic areas. Their eggs are attached to pubic, or eyelash, hairs in a fashion similar to body lice. The adults are usually inconspicious; most patients noticing only pruritus and nits. Occasionally, sec-

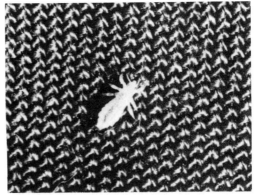

Fig. 12.5. Adult body louse on clothing. This may be a knit sweater. Notice the elongated body as compared to the compact crab louse.

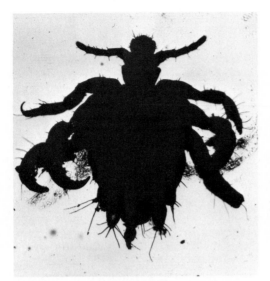

Fig. 12.6. An adult crab louse on clothing (×50).

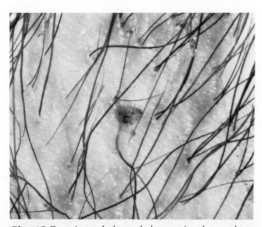

Fig. 12.7. An adult crab louse in the pubes.

ondary infection complicates the clinical presentation but not as often as with body lice. An even rarer variation is the production of blue-gray macules of the lower abdomen and infra-axillary areas (maculae cerulae).

Treatment. GBH is the treatment of choice; lashes (Fig. 12.9) should not be treated with Kwell because of ocular toxicity. Applications of petrolatum four times a day for 3 days is usually effective; if not, use phisostigmine (Eserine), or yellow oxide of mercury, for 24–48 hours. Both of these drugs are potent, and the patient should be well ac-

quainted with their use before prescribing them.

CREATURES THAT ENCOUNTER THE SKIN ONLY TO FEED OR STING OR BITE

Fleas (Pulicidae)

Three species of fleas commonly feed on man (9): *Pulex irritans* (the human flea) (Fig. 12.10), *Ctenocephalides felis* and *canis* (cat and dog fleas). Adult fleas do not ordinarily live on the human host, returning only to feed. They are prodigious leapers and use this ability to attack a host from some distance. Fleas shun the light and quickly crawl under clothing until their progress is restricted. Their bites are relatively painless, characteristically producing clusters of erythematous papules (breakfast, lunch, dinner, and a snack, (Fig. 12.11) on arms, legs, and waist areas. Children in a family seen to be more severely afflicted than adults, often developing hundreds of 4–8 mm edematous papules (papular urticaria). This sensitivity is presumed to be a transient allergic reaction but proper definition of the etiology has yet to be forthcoming.

The most severe parasitization commonly occurs among groups who have recently

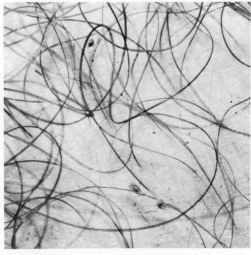

Fig. 12.8. Nits on the pubic hair.

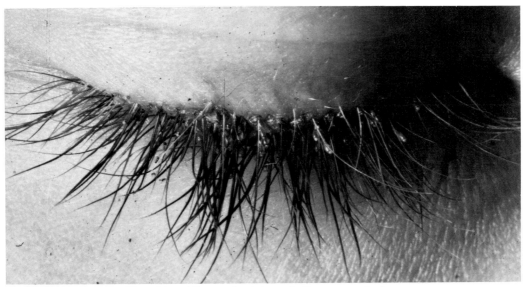

Fig. 12.9. Nits and adult crab lice on eyelashes.

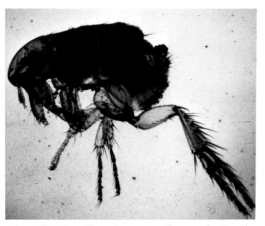

Fig. 12.10. The human flea, obviously equipped for jumping.

moved into a house whose owner previously had dogs and cats. In this situation, fleas can easily be found between the cracks in floors and at the perimeter of rooms near the baseboard. Less severe infestations are acquired from a domestic pet dog or cat).

Treatment. Inflammatory papular lesions resolve spontaneously within 5–10 days; topical steroids and/or local or systemic antipruritics provide some symptomatic relief. Insect repellants such as diethyltoluamide (OFF, and others) are partially effective but

eradication of fleas from the home is the most effective therapy. If they are found in the flooring, use insecticides safe for use in the home (pyrethrum flowers, etc.). Do not remove the pets from the house; the fleas will

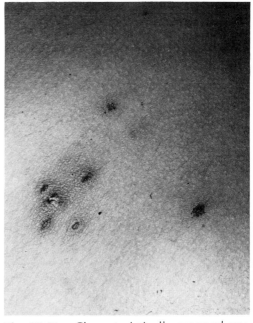

Fig. 12.11. Characteristically grouped erythematous papules of flea bites.

then be forced to parasitize humans. A more rational approach is to use a commercial "flea collar" on the pet, *not on the patient!* There are no effective systemic repellents.

Note: Certain species in certain locations may transmit plague or typhus.

Ticks (Acarines)

Ticks have eight legs, two body divisions, and no wings. (Insects have six legs, three body divisions, and wings). Ticks are large, blood-sucking acarines with either hard or soft bodies, Ixodidae or Argosidae, respectively. "Hard" tick larvae or adults attach themselves to the skin of animals (including man) and feed for several days before dropping off; "soft" ticks feed rapidly and may parasitize several hosts, making them more important vectors of disease such as erythema chromicum migrans, Lyme arthritis, relapsing fever, and tick paralysis as well as a variety of other rickettsial and viral disease.

Hard ticks present clinically as a gray-brown papule—the tick's body (Fig. 12.12 and 12.13). The head is firmly anchored to the skin, resisting most attempts at removal. Local fold literature contains many "pearls" for removing these pests (heat, ether, chloroform, clockwise rotation, mineral oil) but most have a more impressive appearance than outcome. Complete removal should be accomplished surgically if head or mouthparts remain in the skin.

Treatment.   Insect repellants are partially helpful if occupational exposure is a problem. More controversial is the prophylactic use of appropriate antibiotics in areas where tick-borne rickettsial diseases are common.

Mosquitos and Flies (Diptera)

These winged insects are vectors of malaria, yellow fever, dengue, trypanosamiasis, and other serious diseases in many areas of the earth. In the United States, however, they are more notable for their painful or pruritic bites. Lesions are usually distributed over exposed body areas (arms, legs, head) but the pattern will very according to the type of insect and amount of clothing. Individual lesions range from small urticarial papules to painful erosions. Occasionally, larger papules and blisters are seen when the victim is sensitized.

Treatment.   Insect repellants (diethyltoluamide) are quite helpful where exposure cannot be avoided. Antihistamines may benefit the more urticarial papules. Thiamine is not an effective systemic repellant.

Spiders (Araneida)

Spider bites produce two syndromes—arachnidism and loxoscelism.

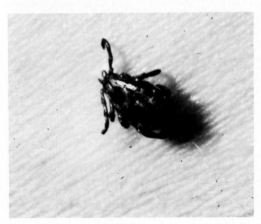

Fig. 12.12.   A tick before a meal with relatively thin body.

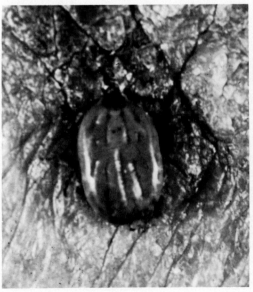

Fig. 12.13.   A tick after eating with a thicker body.

ARACHNIDISM

Latrodectus ma·tans (black widow spiders) are notably feared because of the systemic muscle cramping and abdominal pain that rapidly follows its bite. The cutaneous manifestations are trivial, usually only a small red punctum, which require little or not treatment.

LOXOSCELISM

Loxosceles reclusus (brown recluse). These spiders are occasionally found in the homes and outhouses of the southern and midwestern United States. Victims are frequently bitten while sleeping or sitting; the bite rapidly becomes painful and edematous. Within 3–10 days, a necrotic eschar can be found covering a much larger area than the original bite (Fig. 12.14). Systemic toxicity can also occur with hemolysis, hematuria, and high fever.

Treatment. Treatment of the local necrotic reaction is controversial; suggestions that systemic antihistamines and corticosteroids are effective have been challenged by others. Intralesional steroids may be effective.

Larva Migrans

Creeping eruption (sand itch, cutaneous larva migrans). Man is the unfortunate and ineffective host for a variety of hookworm larvae in the southeastern region of the United States and in many tropical countries. These "worms" parasitize the intestines of dogs and cats, depositing their eggs in animal stool. With proper temperatures and humidity, the larvae hatch and can survive for some time in warm, moist, sandy soil. When the opportunity presents itself, the larvae penetrate the patient's skin, hoping to complete their life cycle. They roam randomly through the dermis for a few weeks and then die. Their characteristic tracts are serpiginous, erythematous, and quite pruritic. The location of the lesions depends upon the areas exposed—arms, legs, buttocks, abdomen, and back are characteristic sites. While southerners are quite familiar with these patterns, northern physicians may see patients who have recently vacationed in the southern states and tropical countries.

Ancylostoma braziliense is the most common pathogen but at least eight other "worms" have been implicated in larva migrans. *Strongyloides stercoralis* whose life-style includes a definitive human phase, produces a characteristic clinical presentation somewhat different from creeping eruption. This human gut parasite's eggs hatch rapidly, often before they are evacuated with the stool. The larvae crawl from the rectum and penetrate the skin of the buttocks, thighs, and lower abdomen. Here, their tracts lengthen much more rapidly than larva migrans, giving rise to the appropriate nomenclature, larva currens (running eruption).

Treatment. Larva migrans and currens respond rapidly to topical thiabendazole (Mentizole 500 mgm/5 ml), applied topically three times a day for 1–2 days. Alternate therapy includes thiabendazole, after means (high incidence of gastrointestinal side effects) and cryotherapy directed to the advancing end of the tract including 2–4 cm of normal skin surrounding this terminus. *Strongyloides* must also be treated systemically (Vermox Chewable Tablets, 100 mgm twice a day for 3 days, Mentizole).

Avian Bloodflukes

Swimmer's itch is an acute pruritic, papular, dermatitis that occurs soon after exposure to sea water or freshwater contaminated with the cercaria of avian bloodflukes. Their nat-

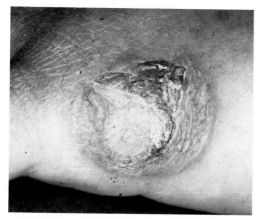

Fig. 12.14. A necrotic spider bite. This took 8 weeks to heal.

ural hosts are mollusks, but man is invaded in a futile attempt at fulfillment. Both exposed and covered areas can be infected with this intensely pruritic, papular dermatitis, which fortunately is self-limited and resolves in 5–10 days. There is no definitive therapy but topical steroids may provide symptomatic relief.

References

1. Orkin, M., Maibach, H., Parish, L., and Schwartzman, R. (Eds): *Scabies and Pediculosis*, J. B. Lippincott Co., Philadelphia, 1977.
2. Orkin, M.: Today's scabies. JAMA, *233:* 882, 1975.
3. Muller, G., Jacobs, P., and Moore, R.: Scraping for human scabies. Arch. Dermatol., *107:* 70, 1973.
4. Gamma benzene hexacloride alert. FDA Drug Bull., *6:* 28, 1976.
5. Lee, B., Grath, P., and Turner, W.: Suspected reactions to gamma benzene hexachloride. JAMA, *236:* 3846, 1976.
6. Solomon, L., Fahrner, L., and West, D.: Gamma Benzene Hexachloride Toxicity. Arch. Dermatol., *113:* 353, 1977.
7. Ginsburg, et al.: J. Pediatr., *91:* 998, 1977.
8. Solomon, L., et al.: J. Invest Dermatol., *68:* 310, 1977.
9. Rook, A.: Skin diseases caused by arthropods and other venomous or noxious animals, In A. Rook, D. S. Wilkinson, and F. J. G. Ebling, (Eds.) *Textbook of Dermatology*, Ed. 2, p. 847. Blackwell Scientific Publications, Oxford, 1972.

CHAPTER 13

WARTS

FRANK E. DUNLAP

"A collection of hard, rough material beneath the skin, rarely larger than a bean, rarely solitary, usually seen in children and may disappear suddenly. The wart splits at the top readily, bleeds easily and is hard to eradicate."

Celus, 50 AD

ETIOLOGY

The papovaviruses were defined in 1962 by Melnick and include the SV-40, polyoma and papilloma groups. They resist the effects of heating, desiccation, and ether. They contain no lipid and all are inactivated by formaldehyde. The papilloma group in which wart virus is included is responsible for infectious papillomas in horses, dogs, cattle, monkeys, and goats as well as man. They are spherical bodies consisting of DNA chains, and are intranuclear pathogens. The human strain has at least 4 subtypes identified to date and antigenic typing may separate out several more. There is some indication that the various clinical wart types may be related to a specific virus subtype.

The number of virus particles demonstrable in a lesion decreases with the age of that wart and varies with the type of wart: plantar warts having the largest number of particles with condylomata having the least.

A premalignant viral condition related to plane warts (epidermodysplasia verruciformis) is fortunately extremely rare.

Viral bodies have not been found in giant condyloma acuminatum of Buschke and Löwenstein and this may, indeed, be a low grade form of squamous cell carcinoma.

CLINICAL PRESENTATION

As the infected keratinocyte multiplies, carrying the human papilloma virus (HPV) with each division, the tumor that develops has the appearance of a fan in cross section. The folded surface provides the verrucous look so easily recognized by the clinician. Initially, the various clinical types of warts were presumed to be due solely to the underlying nature of the tissue infected. More recent research has differentiated several subtypes of human papilloma virus and has shown some to be associated with one clinical wart type.

The clinical presentation of infection with HPV must be a combination of both factors. A patient with warts on the palm and dorsae of the fingers can be presumed to have the same virus subtype but the warts have a different appearance. If this same patient bites the wart, or is a child who sucks its fingers, moist warts may appear on the mucous membrane. One does not see this type of patient develop plane or flat warts however, and the two types are seldom seen in the same patient at the same time.

Plantar warts and palmar warts are more keratinized, tend to grow deeper, and can be explained by the tissue type and the pressure applied to the area. In a patient with plantar warts, any wart appearing on the nonweight-bearing areas is indistinguishable from a common wart on glabrous skin elsewhere.

Condylomata are probably more influenced by the area of the infection than by the underlying tissue. Those arising from the mucous membrane areas cannot be distinguished clinically from those arising from adjacent glabrous skin. As the infection moves toward a drier area, more keratinization is evident. Thus, warts on the penile shaft are more resistant to podophyllin treatment than those on the glands. As with herpes simplex type I and type II infections, the localization of warts in the past may have been due more to social or sexual practices than to the ability of the virus to infect a certain epidermal area.

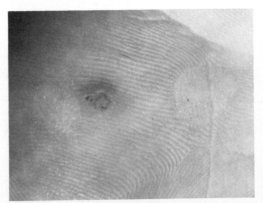

Fig. 13.3.   Palm wart. Note two *scars*. Warts previously removed 2, and 4, years before.

EPIDEMIOLOGY

Culture of the wart virus has been difficult and this has retarded the progress of research. Although warts have been transmitted by inoculating humans with wart tissue extract, only one report of warts resulting from inoculating cell culture material appears in the literature (11). The viral particles have not been identified in any but wart tissue and thus, to date, we must presume direct transmission of the virus from a wart to each new site of infection as shown in Figure 13.1 (see color Plate III). That the infecting virus can be carried on an inanimate object is confirmed by multiple reports of accidental injury with contaminated tools, by the spread of plantar warts among swimmers, and by the unusual incidence of warts in meat cutters (Fig. 13.2).

The rather long incubation period for the wart to appear after inoculation may be explained by the work of Murray, Hobbs, and Payne (14). Knowing that individuals who are heterozygous for the X-linked enzyme glucose 6-phosphate dehydrogenase have two populations of cells which contain either the A or B electrophoretic form of the enzyme, they studied wart tissue from such subjects. They found that any one wart contained only one electrophoretic form of the enzyme. This leads to the conclusion that warts do not grow by spread of the virus from cell to cell but are the result of proliferation from a single infected cell (Fig. 13.3).

Few patients live their lives without experiencing warts. The incidence in the general population at any one time is probably in the area of 7–10% with some surveys in patients showing twice that figure.

Massing and Epstein (10) followed the natural history of warts for 2 years in an institution for mentally defective children. The overall incidence of warts increased from 18 to 25% during the 2-year period. Sixty-seven percent of the lesions noted on initial exami-

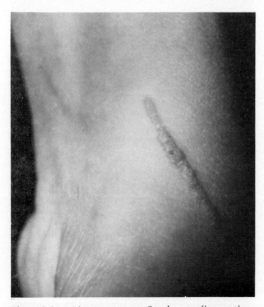

Fig. 13.2.   Linear warts. Such configuration helps confirm innoculation by inanimate objects.

nation involuted but only 46% of the patients were free of all warts at the end of the study due to new warts appearing. Regression occurred almost twice as often in boys (56%) as in girls (32%). One-third of the patients developed new warts while old ones were disappearing. The authors concluded that each wart has a life cycle of its own, independent of the host or neighboring warts.

A large series of studies do, however, point to some immunological activity. Pyrhonen and Johansson (20) found 80% of patients had wart virus antibodies measured by immunodiffusion and 20% also were positive by complement fixation techniques. The later were associated with rapid healing.

Perhaps most important in the spontaneous regression of warts, or their regression under treatment, is the development of a cell-mediated immune response (CMI). Most patients show a positive cell-mediated response at the time of resolution of their warts but the detectable immunity is short-lived. The exact relationship, and its importance between this CMI and antibodies of the circulating type, has not been clarified. Every clinician is familiar with the sudden death, drying up, and falling off of multiple warts. One can not help but think this represents some immunological phenomenon.

TREATMENT

Nothing humbles the physician like a humble wart. A pest to mankind since antiquity, it continues to be one of the most common reasons for office visits.

Perhaps the oldest therapy is the "wart charmer." They seem to rely on the high rate of spontaneous disappearance, but even here there is controversy. Can suggestion influence warts? The success described with hypnosis seems primarily dependent on the depth of the hypnosis. Sinclair-Gieben and Chalmers (22), using good hypnotic subjects, were able to remove warts only on one side of the body in 9 out of 10 patients. The 10th subject lost warts on both sides of the body. Their apparent success at using the patients as their own controls is fascinating in view of the subsequent findings on circulating and cell-mediated immunity. A combination study is warranted.

The newest of wart therapies is the use of a potent antigen notably dinitrochlorobenzene (DNCB) to sensitize the patient and then apply eliciting doses of the sensitizer to the warts. This method seems to carry about the same cure rate as more destructive modes of therapy.

The destructive approach to wart therapy has withstood the test of time and practicality. Since warts are an epidermal lesion, it is theoretically possible to remove them without leaving a scar. This is usually not the case. Most recurrences are at the edge of the scar and carrying any destructive treatment in a more lateral direction, rather than deeper, provides a better cure rate and a softer, less noticeable scar. The older hot tip cautery seems more proficient at accomplishing this than a spark gap machine (Fig. 13.4).

Freezing with liquid nitrogen has gained considerable popularity for treating warts (Fig. 13.5). No needles are involved and the amount of scar tissue is less than with cautery. There is discomfort both on freezing and

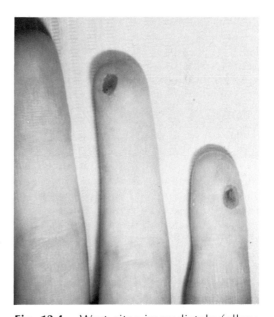

Fig. 13.4. Wart sites immediately following removal by cautery and currette. Note shallow depth of wounds.

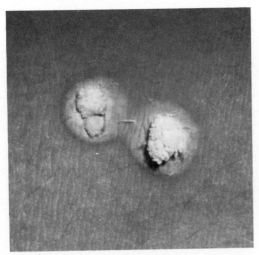

Fig. 13.5. Wart sites immediately after liquid nitrogen application. Resulting blisters will match the frozen area.

thawing, to the point where it is not often used on periungual or subungual lesions.

Cantharidin as a blistering agent has been used alone and mixed with other chemicals in various wart remedies. Painless at application, large bullae produced later, especially if bloody, can frighten the patient. With cantharidin, and also with liquid nitrogen, one occasionally encounters a ring-shaped recurrence of the treated wart where the virus has floated to the edge of the blister (Fig. 13.6).

Before radiation for benign conditions fell out of favor, the use of radiation with careful shielding was often a painless and successful wart therapy especially for plantar warts.

The use of formaldehyde in treating warts predated the discovery that papilloma viruses are so sensitive to it. The problem is to deliver the chemical to the intranuclear location of the virus and, perhaps, will ultimately be solved by the use of more penetrating solvents. Formaldehyde is a sensitizer, and indiscriminate exposure of surrounding tissue should be avoided. Exposure of the wart to aqueous formalin solution daily results in some hardening and fixation of the tissue. This can then be trimmed or abraded once or twice weekly to facilitate deeper penetration of the solution on subsequent application. This regimen is especially useful on large mosaic plantar warts.

Podophyllin is the mainstay of therapy for condylomata, or moist warts. A plant extract, it is a mitotic poison. Moist warts being less keratinized and more filiform allow good penetration. Various concentrations in different solvents have been recommended over the years. The most popular is 25% in tincture of benzoin which enhances adhesion. The painted areas are washed 4–8 hours later to remove the podophyllin.

Maximum reaction occurs in approximately 48 hours. The area is treated in a soothing manner and no further applications are made until complete healing has taken place—usually 5–7 days. Because of the delayed reaction and the poisonous nature of podophyllin, it must not be applied to large areas, applied too frequently, or used intravaginally. Applications are best made by the physician. In extensive cases of condylomata, literally 1 or 2 drops to a 1- or 2-cm area is an adequate beginning.

Podophyllin is not normally effective in verrucae vulgaris unless penetration can be obtained. A quick touch with the hot tip cautery will usually help accomplish this, and subsequent application of podophyllin solution results in the same delayed inflammatory reaction seen with moist warts (Fig. 13.7). The patient must be warned of this. Little, if any, residual scar results. In cases of multiple warts

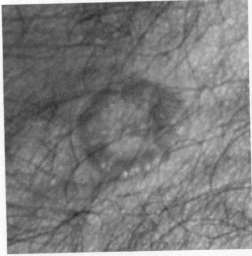

Fig. 13.6. Ring, or doughnut, wart. Not uncommon. Complication of blistering treatments (liquid nitrogen and cantharidin).

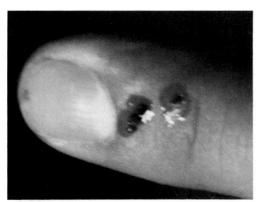

Fig. 13.7. Podophyllin applied after lightly touching the warts with a hot cautery. Subsequent inflammatory reaction often obliterates the warts with little or no scar.

in a cooperative patient, this technique can be used every 1–3 weeks. An added advantage is the possibility of stimulating the immune system of the patient, the likelihood of which seems higher with any treatment that creates inflammation.

Acids have been a mainstay of wart therapy. The most common is salicylic acid, used alone or in combination with lactic acid and/or zinc chloride in a flexible collodion base. The principle being controlled destruction, these wart paints require considerable sophistication on the part of the patient to be successful without discomfort.

Salicylic acid alone in a mastic base (40% salicylic acid pad) is the most effective and least traumatic treatment for keratinized warts. It is especially useful for plantar warts and periungual warts (Fig. 13.8). The pad is cut to size and shape and taped in place. Maximum migration of the salicylic acid occurs in 48–72 hours, at which time the pad may be replaced. No activities need be curtailed. Getting the area wet simply increases the acid activity. Often, on the second or third changing of the pad, a large segment of tissue separates painlessly. If the separation is to the level of pink tissue, the pad is not reapplied.

Salicylic acid acts by dissolving the intercellular fibrils and penetrates the tissue by simple diffusion. Salicylic acid is not caustic or poisonous and, where penetration occurs to vascular tissue, it is simply carried to the kidneys and excreted. Occasionally, on the

sole of the foot, one will see a sterile reaction where the area of the wart swells, becomes somewhat painful and, when the overlying keratotic tissue is pared away, a thick grayish liquid material escapes. This signals the death of the wart and no further treatment is necessary.

More aggressive acids are sometimes used in wart treatment. Mono-, di-, and trichloro-acetic acids are the most popular. They can be applied directly to filiform and condylomatous warts. On keratinized warts, the surface must be pared first, to the point of beginning capillary bleeding, and then the acid applied. The acid should be kept off the surrounding normal skin and, if this is difficult, petrolatum can first be placed around the wart. In cases such as meat cutters, where common verrucae may be numerous and the patient works with his hands, this paring technique is often useful. The acid seals the surface and no bandage is required. Applications should be made approximately once weekly.

Flat warts which frequently involve the dorsae of the hands and the face are troublesome to treat (Fig. 13.9). The physician must attempt to remove the warts without leaving scars. Most techniques used are attempts to create an inflammatory reaction and perhaps

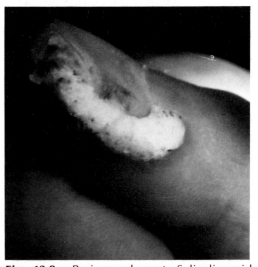

Fig. 13.8. Periungual wart. Salicylic acid and plaster has macerated and softened the wart. This tissue can be gently removed or will separate later. No pain is involved and no scar is created.

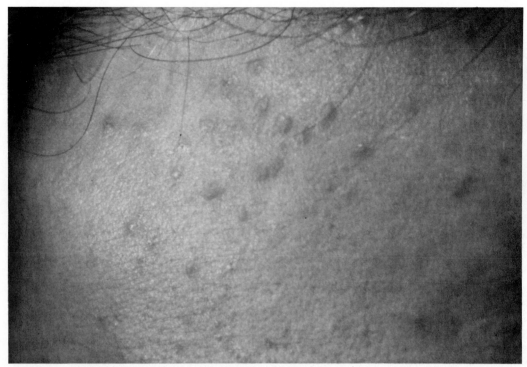

Fig. 13.9.   Plane warts on forehead. Cautery or acid in the area often leaves scars. Freezing or peeling with keratolytics often is the best approach.

stimulate the immune mechanism of the patient. Carbon dioxide and acetone slush, light liquid nitrogen spray, local retenoic acid cream, and even drying acne preparations may meet with some success. The concomitant peeling and redness created by this approach is often disturbing to the patient.

In view of the possible oncogenic role of viruses in man, wart vaccines may entail more risk than possible benefit.

The use of so many different treatments for warts serves to confirm that no one cure exists. Add to those mentioned here another score or so, and the list is still not complete. Remembering that there is considerable likelihood of spontaneous disappearance and tailoring, the therapy to meet the individual case seems by far the best approach.

References

1. Berman, A., and Winkelmann, R.K.: Flat warts undergoing involution. Arch. Dermatol., *113:* 1219, 1977.
2. DePewter, M. et al.: An epidemiological survey of virus warts of the hands among butchers. Br. J. Dermatol., *96:* 427, 1977.
3. DiGiovanna, J.J.: Condylomata acuminata. Dermatology, *1:* 6, 1978.
4. Eng, A., Morgan, N.E., and Blekys, I.: Giant condyloma acuminatum. Cutis, *24:* 203, 1979.
5. Gibbs, R.C., and Scheiner, A.M.: Long term follow-up evaluation of patients with electrosurgically treated warts. Cutis, *21:* 383, 1978.
6. Greenberg, J.H.: Warts: pest or pestilence. Dermatol., *1:* 29, 1978.
7. Haines, H.H., and Blank, H.: Viral infections. In A. Rook (Ed.) *Recent Advances in Dermatology,* Ed 3. Churchill Livingstone, London, 1973.
8. Jablonska, S., et al.: Epidermodysplasia verruciformis versus disseminated verrucae plana: is epidermodysplasia verruciformis a generalized infection with wart virus? J. Invest. Dermatol., *72:* 114, 1979.
9. Lubritz, R.R.: Cryosurgery of benign lesions. Cutis, *16:* 426, 1975.
10. Massing, A.M., and Epstein, W.L.: Natural history of warts: two year study. Arch. Dermatol., *87:* 306, 1963.
11. Mendelson, C.G., and Kligman, A.M.: Isolation of wart virus in tissue culture: successful reinoculation into humans. Arch. Dermatol., *83:* 559, 1961.
12. Morison, W.L.: In vitro assay of immunity of human wart antigen. Br. J. Dermatol., *93:* 545, 1975.
13. Morison, W.L.: In vitro lymphocyte stimulation by wart antigen in man. Br. J. Dermatol., *94:* 523, 1976.
14. Murray, R.F., Hobbs, J., and Payne, B.: Possible clonal origin of common warts (verrucae vulgaris). Nature, *232:* 51, 1971.

15. Niimura, M. et al.: Primary tissue culture of human wart-derived epidermal cells (keratinocytes). J. National Cancer Institute, *54:* 3, 1975.

16. O'Connor, J.J.: Perianal and anal condylomata acuminata. J. Dermatol. Surg. Oncol., *5:* 276, 1979.

17. Orth, G., et al.: Characterization of a new type of human papilloma virus that causes skin warts. J. Virol., *24:* 108, 1977.

18. Orth, G. et al.: Evidence for antigenic determinants shared by the structural polypeptides of (Shope) rabbit: papilloma virus and human papillomavirus Type I. Virology, *91:* 243, 1978.

19. Pringle, W.M., and Helms, D.C.: Treatment of plantar warts by blunt dissection. Arch. Dermatol., *108:* 79, 1973.

20. Pyrhonen, S., and Johansson, E.: Regression of warts. Lancet, *1:* 592, 1975.

21. Pyrhonen, S., and Penhinem, K.: Wart virus antibodies and the prognosis of wart disease. Lancet, *2:* 1330, 1975.

22. Sinclair-Gieben, A.H.C., and Chalmers, D.: Evaluation of treatment of warts by hypnosis. Lancet, *2:* 480, 1959.

23. Viac, J. et al.: An immunoelectron microscopic localization of wart-associated antigens present in human papilloma virus (HPV) infected cells. J. Invest. Dermatol., *70:* 263, 1978.

24. Whitlock, F.A.: *Hypnosis and the Skin in Psychophysiological Aspects of Skin Disease.* W.B. Saunders, London, 1976.

CHAPTER 14

NAIL DISEASES

RICHARD K. SCHER

It has been estimated that about 6% of new patients seeking medical advice from nondermatologists for cutaneous diseases appear for nail disorders. This means that a physician providing general medical care, whether a family practitioner, internist, or pediatrician, will be presented with a nail problem in about 1 out of 20 first-visit patients. This represents a high statistic and probably varies from doctor to doctor, according to his practice, but certainly suggests that a reasonable working knowledge of this anatomical site is important.

In this chapter, an attempt will be made to provide this information in a simple form, thereby permitting the physician to logically, systematically, and *correctly* approach the abnormal nail unit.

Onychomycosis makes up one-half of all nail maladies so that a large portion of the discussion will be devoted to this entity. The other half is comprised of psoriasis, lichen planus, and benign and malignant tumors as well as a variety of infrequently seen onychodystrophies. The latter will be omitted here, being beyond the scope of this discussion but, for those interested in additional material, suitable references are provided. Finally, there will be a short presentation of those nail changes that are a manifestation of systemic disease and often may be the first indication of such disorders, thereby enabling the internist to treat earlier than might otherwise have been possible.

ANATOMY

In order to understand the diseases that follow, a thorough knowledge of the anatomy (1) of the nail unit is essential. It consists of the following structures (Fig. 14.1):

Proximal nail fold
Lateral nail fold (one on each side)
Nail matrix
Nail bed
Hyponychium
Nail plate

The proximal nail fold represents a modified extension of the digit which is an actual fold of skin (epidermis and dermis without subcutaneous tissue) that overlies the matrix. It is continuous with the lateral nail folds that form the side boundary of the nail plate bilaterally. The cuticle is its horny end product, which is deposited on the surface of the newly formed nail plate where it soon desquamates.

The nail matrix, below the proximal nail fold, is the growth center that produces the nail plate. Any insults to the matrix will subsequently be reflected in the evolving nail plate. The distal portion of the matrix is called the lunula and often may be seen beneath the proximal nail plate, particularly in the thumb. The proximal portion of the matrix lies against the bony terminal phalanx, which many believe should be regarded as an additional component of the nail organ.

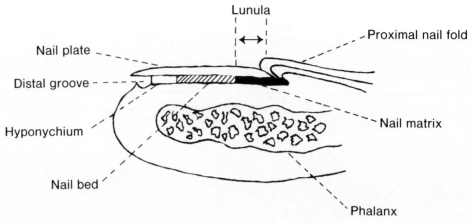

Fig. 14.1.   Anatomy of the nail unit.

The nail bed is that structure which begins where the matrix (lunula) ends distally and extends in an acral direction to the site of separation of the nail plate at which point the hyponychium commences. The epidermis of the nail bed is arranged in longitudinal ridge-and-groove fashion overlying its dermis. This construction explains the well known splinter hemorrhage, where a small amount of blood accumulates in the groove below the plate, resembling a wooden splinter. Glomus bodies are located here and, therefore, the benign but painful glomus tumor will likewise be found in this location.

The hyponychium is unattached to the overlying nail plate, and is histologically different from the nail bed. It extends a few millimeters further acrally to where the volar digit begins. Its significance lies in the fact that it is the source of entry of fungal organisms in the most common type of onychomycosis-distal subungual.

ONYCHOMYCOSIS

Onychomycosis, by definition, means infection of one or more components of the nail unit by fungal organisms (2). There are recognized, at this time, four main varieties:

Distal subungual onychomycosis
Proximal subungual onychomycosis
White superficial onychomycosis
Candida onychomycosis

Distal Subungual Onychomycosis

CLINICAL FEATURES

This is the most common type and develops secondary to invasion of mycotic organisms at the region of the hyponychium (Fig. 14.2). From here, they advance proximally so that the picture presented to the physician is one of a damaged distal portion of the nail appendage with a healthy proximal portion—except at a very advanced stage of the disease—when the latter may also become involved. The signs noted include separation of the nail plate from the nail bed (onycholysis), thickening of the epidermal horny layer of the nail bed (subungual hyperkerotosis), and actual destruction of the distal nail plate.

ETIOLOGY

Etiology is usually *Trichophyton rubrum*, although other species may also be responsible.

DIAGNOSTIC TESTS

KOH Wet Mounts.   Scrapings of the debris from the involved hyponychium and nail bed are placed on a glass slide. One or more drops of a 10% solution of potassium hydroxide (KOH) is applied and the slide warmed slightly. Microscopic examination is then carried out in an effort to locate the hyphae diagnostic of fungal disease.

Cultures.   A portion of the scrapings for microscopic study is placed on a suitable cul-

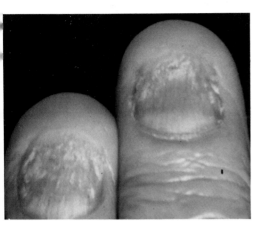

Fig. 14.2. Distal subungual onychomycosis.

ture medium (e.g. Sabouraud's) and examined in 1–2 weeks for fungus growth.

Biopsy. If, after several negative KOH mounts and fungal cultures, onychomycosis is still suspect, a nail biopsy may be necessary. It likely will confirm this diagnosis or possibly provide an alternative one. A periodic acid—Schiff stain—should be done on all nail biopsies to highlight any fungal organisms that may be present.

Many physicians may prefer to have a competent dermatologist perform these tests or a qualified laboratory do the KOH and culture evaluations.

TREATMENT

The same as for proximal subungual onychomycosis, below.

Proximal Subungual Onychomycosis

CLINICAL FEATURES

In this type, the fungal organisms attack below the proximal nail fold and move in a distal direction (Fig. 14.3). The acral portion of the digit—except very much later—is normal. There is destruction of the proximal nail plate and thickened whitish areas (leuconychia) in the deeper portions of the nail plate.

ETIOLOGY

Trichophyton rubrum predominates.

DIAGNOSTIC TESTS

KOH and culture.

TREATMENT

The therapy of both the distal and proximal subungual onychomycosis is the same. Oral griseofulvin should be administered. Usually 6 months of therapy is required for the fingernails and 1 year for the toenails. This systemic therapy should be given only after confirmation of dermatophyte infection! Because of the prolonged therapy required, periodic monitoring of the blood for hematologic and/or hepatic changes is necessary.

Griseofulvin, microsized. (Grisactin, Fulvicin U/F, Grifulvin V), 500 mg twice a day. An elixir of grifulvin is available for children at appropriately reduced dosage schedules.

Griseofulvin, ultromicrosized. (Gris-PEG Tablets, Fulvicin P/G Tablets), 125 mg three times a day.

Surgical nail avulsion or **chemical nail**

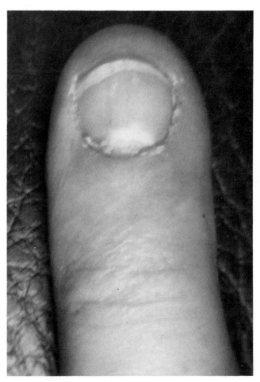

Fig. 14.3. Proximal subungual onychomycosis, early.

avulsion with 40% urea under an occlusive dressing may sometimes be needed as adjunctive therapy. These procedures, however, are best performed by the dermatologist.

Topical therapy is usually not effective in these types, but may be employed if oral therapy is contraindicated. Details will be given in the next section.

White Superficial Onychomycosis

CLINICAL FEATURES

Usually confined to toenails (Fig. 14.4); fingernails rarely. Organisms attack the surface of the nail plate and produce foci of leuconychia superficially only. When the foci coalesce, the nail plate may become rough, soft, and crumbly with yellowish discoloration.

ETIOLOGY

Trichophyton mentographytes.

DIAGNOSTIC TESTS

KOH and culture.

TREATMENT

Scraping or **vigorously abrading** the nail plate surface is usually all the therapy required. Topical therapy may also be added.

Topical Therapy. Miconazole (MicaTin Brand Micanozole Nitrate Cream and Lotion), Clotrimazole (Lotrimin Cream 1%, Mycelex 1% Cream), or Haloprogin (Halotex Cream/Solution).

Any one of these may be applied twice daily using gentle massage with a toothbrush.

Candida Onychomycosis

CLINICAL FEATURES

Chronic paronychia predominantly of the fingers is the hallmark of candidosis of the nail unit (Fig. 14.5). There is noted swelling, edema, and tenderness of the digit nail folds. The disorder occurs most frequently in persons whose hands are wet a significant proportion of the time (housewives, bartenders, waitresses). Nail plate involvement is secondary and shows longitudinal white strands with increased opacity. Onycholysis and Beau's lines (transverse ridging of the nail plate) also occur.

ETIOLOGY

Candida albicans is the great pathogen here with *Candida parapsilosis* being responsible a small percentage of the time.

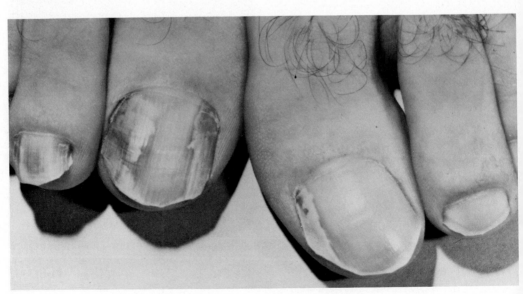

Fig. 14.4. White superficial onychomycosis.

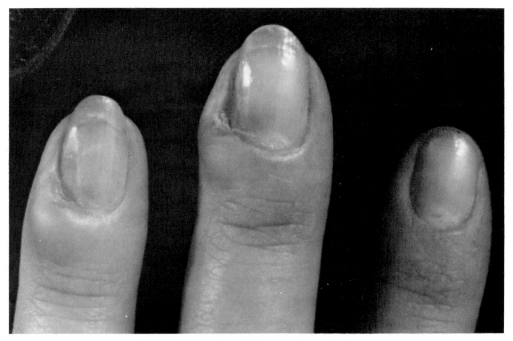

Fig. 14.5. *Candida* onychomycosis.

DIAGNOSTIC TESTS

KOH and culture; a blood sugar is also recommended because of the increased incidence of candidosis in diabetes mellitus. Women should have a gynecologic examination to rule out this site as a possible source of yeast organisms.

TREATMENT

Keep hands as **dry** as possible.

Nystatin. (Mycostatin Oral Tablets), 500,000 units four times a day for 2 weeks. Although not absorbed, this drug will eliminate the organism from the gastrointestinal tract.

Topical therapy is the same as with white superficial onychomycosis. In addition, Mycolog Ointment twice daily has also been used with some success.

Onychomycosis may occasionally be caused by saprophytic fungi or a variety of molds. These infections do not respond to oral therapy but are treated locally, similar to white superficial onychomycosis. Because of their occurrence, the need for culture identification of organisms is further stressed. Successful therapy is dependent upon accurate diagnosis! Nail avulsion may also be required.

PSORIASIS

CLINICAL FEATURES

Diagnosis of psoriasis of the nails is a relatively simple matter in the patient with extensive cutaneous involvement. If, however, no skin lesions are present (2–6% of the time) the situation is more difficult. The earliest change noted occurs when only the nail bed is involved (3). Here, one sees distal onycholysis (Fig. 14.6) and, somewhat later, a brownish discoloration of the nail bed itself, proximal to the site of separation. This discoloration is due to abnormally high accumulations of glycoprotein and has been termed the "oil drop" change because of its resemblance to a drop of oil beneath the nail plate. It is virtually pathognomonic of nail psoriasis. Small, random indentations of the nail plate (pitting) is a very characteristic change due to focal psoriasis of the nail matrix itself. More advanced changes include subungual hyperkeratosis, nail plate crumbling, destruction, and yellowish discoloration. Psoriasis may also present with splinter hemorrhages—an example of this phenomenon in the absence of systemic disease. Leuconychia and transverse grooving are also a feature.

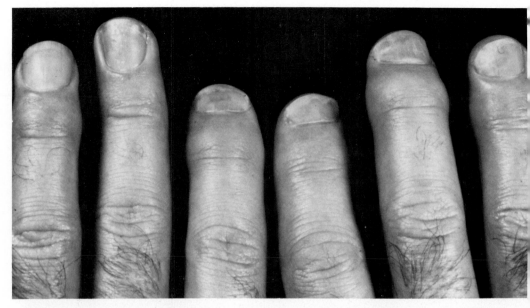

Fig. 14.6. Psoriasis: pitting, distal onycholysis, "oil drop" change, psoriatic arthritis.

ETIOLOGY

The cause of psoriasis is unknown.

DIAGNOSTIC TESTS

Multiple KOH studies and cultures should be performed—once weekly for 3 weeks. Should these be consistently negative, a nail biopsy (4) would be advisable to ascertain the diagnosis.

TREATMENT

Topical corticosteroids under occlusion with saran wrap at bedtime is often effective. Diflorasone diacetate, 0.05%, (Florone Cream) or 0.5% triamcinolone acetonide ointments (Aristocort High Potency Cream) work most consistently. When there is matrix involvement, intralesional steroids may be employed. For example, triamcinolone acetonide suspension (Kenolog-40 Injection) injected into the nail folds once monthly, in a concentration of 2–5 mg/cc is often used. This treatment and other specialized modalities such as x-ray, PUVA, (oral psoralens, plus black long wave ultraviolet light) and 5-flurouracil are best administered by a dermatologist qualified in their use.

LICHEN PLANUS

CLINICAL FEATURES

Diagnosis of lichen planus of the nails, as with psoriasis, is not difficult if typical cutaneous or mucous membrane lesions are also present. When, however, there is only nail involvement (1–4% of the time) the diagnosis becomes a problem to establish. The changes seen depend on the pathologic site. Lichen planus of the matrix results in accentuated longitudinal grooving and splitting (Fig. 14.7) of the nail plate (onchorrhexis (5)) with subsequent thinning (hapalonychia). If more destruction of the matrix ensues with permanent scarring, the characteristic pterygium (Fig. 14.8)—almost pathognomonic of lichen planus—results.

The latter is due to direct attachment of the proximal nail fold to the nail bed without the intervening nail plate. The latter cannot be produced because of matrix destruction. The nail fold then grows distally with the nail bed giving rise to the triangular pterygial defect. Changes noted as a consequence of nail bed lichen planus include atrophy, onycholysis, subungual hyperkeratosis, and subungual hyperpigmentation (6).

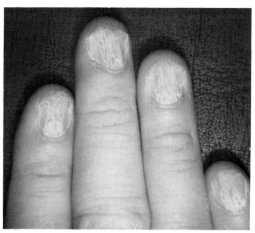

Fig. 14.7. Lichen planus: onychorrhexis.

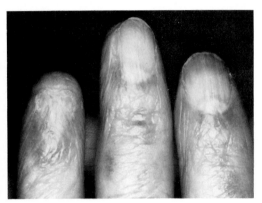

Fig. 14.8. Lichen planus: pterygium of index finger.

ETIOLOGY

The cause of lichen planus is unknown. Some drugs, however, such as thiazides, phenothiazines, and benzodiazepines have been reported to produce a clinical eruption indistinguishable both clinically and histologically from lichen planus.

DIAGNOSTIC TESTS

Nail biopsy confirms the diagnosis of lichen planus after fungal studies have been negative.

TREATMENT

At this point in time, the only effective treatment for the destructive lichen planus described above is intralesional corticosteroids. In the event no response occurs, oral corticosteroids may be required in doses of 20–40 mg daily of prednisone. This treatment should not be used if medically contraindicated, and close observation of the patient for steroid side effects is mandatory. Suffice it to say that these modalities should only be considered in biopsy proven lichen planus!

TUMORS OF NAIL APPENDAGE

VERRUCA VULGARIS

The most frequent neoplastic lesion of the nail unit is verruca vulgaris (Fig. 14.9), or the common wart (7). When this growth involves the nail folds, the tenacious periungual wart is produced. Clinically, it appears as a mass of varying size with a corrugated surface. There is often associated tenderness and bleeding points. The lesion also may undergo fissuring.

Its etiology is viral and generally a clinical diagnosis may be made. If there is doubt,

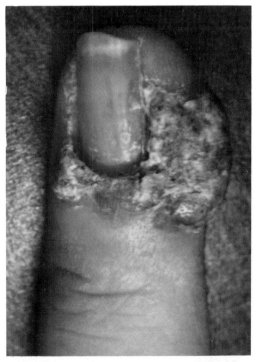

Fig. 14.9. Periungual verruca vulgaris.

however, or if the wart fails to respond or behave as anticipated, a biopsy may have to be performed. Bowen's disease and squamous cell carcinoma have been reported with verrucous wart-like surfaces.

Simple treatment methods, such as salicylic acid and lactic acid (Duofilm) may be tried at first but, generally, more vigorous attacks are required.

Electrofulguration and curettage under local anesthesia and cryotherapy with liquid nitrogen have been successfully employed.

MYXOID CYST

This is not a true tumor but rather a collagenous degeneration of the extensor tendon presenting as a small mass. Often, the only evidence of its presence is a unilateral longitudinal notch of the nail plate (Fig. 14.10) due to pressure of the lesion on the underlying matrix.

Intralesional steroids have been used but the best treatment is probably surgical removal.

GLOMUS TUMOR

This neoplasm is characterized by pain in the nail bed accompanied by a small erythematous focus made more prominent after lateral pressure. Surgical excision with biopsy is the only treatment.

PIGMENTATION

Pigmentation of the nail plate is due to a focal pigment producing lesion of the nail matrix (Fig. 14.11). When this is a solitary finding, unaccompanied by mucous membrane lesions, particularly in a caucasian patient, biopsy is mandatory. This may be the first indication of acral lentiginous melanoma (8) which requires vigorous early therapy. Pigmented streaks of the nail plate are a frequent occurrence in black patients and, here, biopsy may not be required. In addition to melanoma of the nail, Bowen's disease, squamous cell carcinoma, and keratoacanthoma have been seen.

A wide range of other neoplasms, benign and malignant, may involve the nail appendage less frequently. The reader is referred to the References for additional material, as a discussion of all of them is beyond the scope of this chapter (9).

NAIL IN SYSTEMIC DISEASE

Any systemic disease that affects the skin may produce nail changes. The purpose of this section is to alert the physician to a few of those nail changes that may be the first indication of generalized illness. For a comprehensive treatise of all nail signs of systemic disease refer to any standard dermatologic text.

Periungual erythema may precede the onset of connective tissue disease. It is particularly common as a manifestation of lupus erythematosis. Telangiectasia of the proximal nail fold is highly suggestive of scleroderma and such patients should be evaluated accordingly.

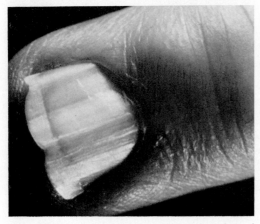

Fig. 14.10. Myxoid cyst of proximal nail fold with longitudinally notched nail plate.

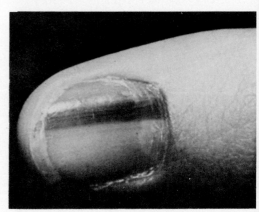

Fig. 14.11. Linear pigmentation of nail plate: acral lentiginous melanoma, early.

Yellow nails may signal the syndrome of lymphatic anomalies with edema as well as chronic bronchitis with bronchiectasis. Severe sub- and periungual hyperkeratosis with nail plate destruction resembling psoriasis is known as paraneoplastic acrokeratosis. It heralds the subsequent development of respiratory or gastrointestinal malignancy.

Clubbing of the digits as a precursor to bronchogenic carcinoma is well known and, when this phenomenon occurs unexplained, the latter should be looked for. Heart disease, thyroid disease, and ulcerative colitis also have been reported to occur concomitantly with clubbed digits.

Koilonychia, or spoon nails, has been reported in iron deficiency anemia. Here, the normal contour of the plate is lost so that it becomes concave in appearance as well as softer and thinner than normal. Other etiologies beside iron deficiency may also be responsible such as Raynaud's syndrome with or without impaired peripheral circulation.

White nails (leuconychia (10)) may be associated with liver disease and hypoalbuminemia, whereas the half-and-half nail is associated with renal disease. In the latter, the proximal half of the nail bed is white and the distal half is red.

References

1. Scher, R.K.: Nail surgery. In E. Epstein and E. Epstein, Jr. (Eds) *Techniques in Skin Surgery*, p. 164. Lea and Febiger, Philadelphia, 1979.
2. Zaias, N.: Onychomycosis. Arch. Dermatol., *105:* 263, 1972.
3. Zaias, N.: Psoriasis of the nail: a clinical-pathological study. Arch. Dermatol., *99:* 567, 1969.
4. Scher, R.K.: Punch biopsies of nails: a simple valuable procedure. J. Dermatol. Surg. Oncol., *4:* 528, 1978.
5. Scher, R.K., Fischbein, R.M., and Ackerman, A.B.: Twenty nail dystrophy: a variant of lichen planus. Arch. Dermatol., *114:* 612, 1978.
6. Zaias, N. The nail in lichen planus. Arch. Dermatol., *101:* 264, 1970.
7. Samman, P.D.: *The Nails in Disease.* William Heinemann Medical Books, London, 1979.
8. Reed, R.J.: *New Concepts in Surgical Pathology of the Skin,* p. 89. Wiley, New York, 1976.
9. Norton, L.A.: Disorders of nails. In S.L. Moschella, D.M. Pillsbury, and H.J. Hurley, Jr. (Eds.) *Dermatology,* p. 1222. W. B. Saunders, Philadelphia, 1975.
10. Baran, R. Pigmentations of the nails (chromonychia). J. Dermatol. Surg. Oncol., *4:* 250, 1978.

CHAPTER **15**

LUPUS ERYTHEMATOSUS

NANCY L. FUREY

Lupus erythematosus (LE) is a complex illness with an insidious onset and a variable clinical presentation and prognosis. Symptoms of the disease may be expressed as a rash and a mild, nondeforming arthritis or they may be severe, with inflammation of vital organs such as the kidney and brain, eventuating in death. Most commonly, patients with LE have a chronic, smoldering, persistent inflammation of several target organs for many years. Although LE occurs at all ages, 85% of patients are females in their reproductive years. In childhood and in old age, when the disease is less common, the male-female ratio is about equal.

The disease was first discussed at medical meetings about 1828 and named "érythémé centrifuge" by Biett. Later, in 1851, Cazenave wrote "this disease which Biett first described and named érythémé centrifuge is a type of lupus." The term "lupus" derived from the Latin word for wolf, was used figuratively to describe a variety of destructive processes that attacked the face and lower legs. During the Middle Ages, legends detailed the attack of the wolf, which would slash open the skin and eat the flesh of its living victims. The comparable ravages of such disease processes as skin cancer, tuberculosis of the skin, and syphilis were all included under the designation of lupus. Gradually, as the chronic destructive skin diseases were differentiated, specific qualifying words were added to distinguish each disease. Cazenave, after studying several cases, including those discussed by Biett, noted that the erythematous eruption often

resulted in severe scarring. He felt the disease should be classified as a variety of lupus and coined the name "lupus érythémateux" to emphasize both the specific erythema and the erosive-scarring characteristics of the disorder.

Moriz Kaposi first recognized and recorded the acute form of LE. In 1875, he wrote that, " ... lupus erythematosus appears in two forms: In the form of characteristic discs—Lupus erythematosus discoides in the form of peculiar, isolated and aggregated spots—Lupus erythematosus discretus et aggregatus. It, for the most part ... has a very chronic course, and, ... does not exercise any injurious influence whatever on the constitution. Lupus erythematosus may, however, make its appearance and continue its course accompanied by acute or subacute eruption attended by fever, and ... may ... affect the whole organism and endanger the patient's existence, or even prove fatal." Kaposi went on to stress that lupus erythematosus discoides " ... has a regular and chronic course, and is unattended by any severe complications but may, nevertheless, now and then, be complicated with erysipelas, or with the aggregated form and its acute symptoms ... " One hundred years later, Kaposi's concept of an acute, subacute, and chronic form of LE is still widely accepted.

Sir William Osler unequivocally established LE as a multisystem disease, when he discussed the "visceral complications of erythema exudativum multiforme" in 1895 in the *American Journal of Medical Science*. "By exudative erythema is understood a disease of

149

unknown etiology with polymorphic skin lesions—hyperaemia, oedema, and hemorrhage—arthritis occasionally, and a variable number of visceral manifestations, of which the most important are gastrointestinal crises, endocarditis, acute nephritis and hemorrhage from the mucous surfaces. Recurrence is a special feature of the disease and attacks may come on month after month or even throughout a long period of years. Variability in the skin lesions is the rule, and a case may present in one attack the features of an angioneurotic oedema, in a second of a multiform or nodose erythema, and in a third those of peliosis rheumatica. The attacks may not be characterized by skin manifestations; the visceral symptoms alone may be present, and to the outward view the patient may have no indications whatever of erythema exudativum." Analysis of numerous cases during subsequent decades resulted in expansion of the clinical spectrum of the disease. In 1941, Klemperer and his colleagues introduced the term "collagen disease" to emphasize the characteristic pathologic abnormality in the connective tissues.

Hargraves' discovery of the "LE cell" in bone marrow preparations of LE patients, and the subsequent modification of the test using serum from these patients, provided the first laboratory marker of the disease. Recently, a multitude of antinuclear antibodies have been identified in sera from patients with LE and the less specific but more sensitive fluorescent antinuclear antibody (ANA) test is routinely used in clinical laboratories. Patients with early and milder forms of the disease can be identified and the concept of the clinical spectrum and prognosis of LE has been broadened. The majority of cases are not life threatening and most patients with careful management can lead nearly normal lives. Patients with more severe disease now lead better quality lives due to better control of infections, extensive experience with corticosteroid and immunosuppressive therapy, and renal dialysis.

DIAGNOSIS

In 1971, the American Rheumatism Association (ARA) published preliminary criteria for the classification of systemic lupus erythematosus (SLE). The criteria were based on data collected from patients with unequivocal LE, probable LE, and classic rheumatoid arthritis as well as from nonrheumatic patients. The data were analyzed, and 14 major manifestations of LE were delineated (Table 15.1).

These criteria have been widely accepted and are considered helpful guidelines for diagnosis. However, there are LE patients who do not fulfil four of the criteria on initial presentation but do so only with evolution of the disease. The criteria rely on data collected in the early 1960s by rheumatologists and are derived from patients with more severe disease. The criteria were developed before the widespread use of tests for antinuclear antibodies, anti-DNA antibodies, and serum complement levels. Recent studies suggest that the criteria should be revised and should include high titer ANA and anti-DNA antibodies and depressed C3 levels.

From a purely dermatologic viewpoint, the criteria pertaining to the cutaneous manifestations are inadequate. Only acute facial erythema and the chronic discoid lesion have been included. Only a very few erythematous, scaly eruptions in the central portion of the face are due to LE. The acute erythema and edema on the nasal bridge and malar eminences (butterfly rash) are uncommon and usually occur only in the toxic, febrile, or acutely ill LE patient. Subacute, red, scaly lesions without follicular plugging, which can heal with minimal, if any, scarring, are not recognized. In addition, the common, telangiectatic, papular, infarctive lesions of the fingertips are not included. The morphology of the mucous membrane lesions is not specifically diagnostic for LE, and other conditions can cause mouth ulcerations. Rapid loss of scalp hair by the patient's history is not a reliable criteria in a young female who subjects her hair to a variety of hair care products or who might have experienced androgenetic or estrogen-related alopecia. The most characteristic alopecia in SLE is the diffuse loss of hair that occurs in conjunction with the clinical exacerbation of the disease. Photosensitivity is also a notoriously unreliable symptom since it is a common complaint in any dermatologic practice. The criteria of photosensitivity should be based upon the observation

Table 15.1
Preliminary Criteria for Classification of Systemic Lupus Erythematosus[a]

A person shall be said to have systemic lupus erythematosus (SLE) if any four or more of the following 14 manifestations are present, serially or simultaneously, during any interval of observation:

1. *Facial erythema (butterfly rash)*. Diffuse erythema, flat or raised, over the malar eminence(s) and/or bridge of the nose; may be unilateral.
2. *Discoid lupus*. Erythematous raised patches with adherent keratotic scaling and follicular plugging; atrophic scarring may occur in older lesions; may be present anywhere on the body.
3. *Raynaud's phenomenon*. Intermittent severe pallor of the fingers, toes, ears, or nose. Requires a two-phase color reaction, by patient's history or physician's observation.
4. *Alopecia*. Rapid loss of large amount of the scalp hair, by patient's history or physician's observation.
5. *Photosensitivity*. Unusual skin reaction from exposure to sunlight, by patient's history or physician's observation.
6. *Oral or nasopharyngeal ulceration.*
7. *Arthritis without deformity. One or more peripheral joints involved with any of the following in the absence of deformity: (a) pain on motion, (b) tenderness, (c) effusion or periarticular soft tissue swelling.* (Peripheral joints are defined for this purpose as feet, ankles, knees, hips shoulders, elbows, wrists, metacarpophalangeal, proximal interphalangeal, terminal interphalangeal, and temporomandibular joints.)
8. *LE[b] cells*. Two or more classic LE cells seen on one occasion or one cell seen on two or more occasions, using an accepted published method.
9. *Chronic false positive reaction to serological test for syphilis (STS)*. Known to be present for at least six months and confirmed by TPI or Reiter's tests.
10. *Profuse proteinuria*. Greater than 3.5 gm per day.
11. *Cellular casts*. May be red cell, hemoglobin, granular, tubular, or mixed.
12. *One or both of the following: (a) pleuritis,* (history of pleuritic pain, rub heard by physician, or x-ray evidence of both pleural thickening and fluid), (*b*) *pericarditis*, documented by EKG or rub.
13. *One or both of the following: (a) psychosis, (b) convulsions*, by patient's history or physician's observation in the absence of uremia and offending drugs.
14. *One or more of the following: (a) hemolytic anemia, (b) leukopenia* (WBC less than 4000 per cu mm on two or more occasions), *(c) thrombocytopenia* (platelet count less than 100,000 per cu mm).

[a] Reproduced with permission from: A. L. Cohen, W. E. Reynolds, and C. E. Franklin, et al.: Bulletin of Rheumatic Diseases, *23:* 643, 1971.
[b] The abbreviations used are: LE, lupus erythematosus; TPI, *Treponema pallidum* immobilization; and WBC, white blood cell count.

of new LE lesions or toxic systemic manifestations of LE after sun exposure. All other causes for a photodermatitis should have been excluded.

In spite of these and other shortcomings of the SLE criteria, they have been invaluable to the clinician, to define groups of similar patients and to classify patients, and to compare data from different sources regarding the epidermiology, prognosis, and response to therapy of the disease. SLE criteria were created for the purpose of "classification of systemic lupus erythematosus" and not for the diagnosis of the disease, and absolute diagnostic criteria are unlikely while the etiology

and pathogenesis of the disorder are unknown.

Attempts are currently being made to define a combination of laboratory tests that would select the great majority of SLE patients and exclude patients with other connective tissue diseases. A recent study evaluated three new but widely used tests 1) antibodies to native DNA, 2) antibodies to Sm, and 3) immune deposits at the dermal-epidermal junction of normal skin. No single one of these tests is positive in a high enough percentage of patients with SLE to serve alone as a criterion. When applied to a SLE population with over one-half the population with clinical evidence of renal disease, it was found that 80% of the SLE patients had abnormal values for at least two of these three tests and none of the patients with other connective tissue diseases had more than one abnormal value. These laboratory criteria cannot be substituted for the "preliminary clinical criteria" introduced by the ARA in 1971 but they are helpful in making the diagnosis of SLE in patients who do not meet the clinical criteria because they are evaluated early in the course of the disease or because they have a limited form of LE. Thus, some patients with nephritis, optic neuritis, "idiopathic" thrombocytopenic purpura, and autoimmune hemolytic anemia will meet these laboratory criteria for SLE but not the ARA criteria. Ideally, such patients can be identified and appropriate therapy can be initiated.

CUTANEOUS MANIFESTATIONS

Skin changes occur in over 70% of patients with systemic lupus erythematosus and are the initial manifestation in 20% of patients, second only to arthritis as the earliest sign of the disorder. Skin lesions found in association with LE may be specific or nonspecific. The specific cutaneous LE lesions can be classified as chronic discoid, subacute, and acute. The morphological appearance of the lesions reflects the host response and the severity and duration of the cutaneous eruption.

Chronic discoid LE lesions begin as simple patches of erythema, evolve into well circumscribed, red-to-violaceous, scaly, indurated plaques, and eventually heal with atrophy, telangiectasia, and postinflammatory areas of hyperpigmentation and hypopigmentation. The scales are most often yellowish gray and thick. On the face and scalp, where the pilosebaceous apparatus is well developed, the scales may plug the dilated follicular openings, giving rise to the descriptive term "carpet-tack scale." With chronicity, some lesions may become hypertrophic and elevated, but usually they become atrophic and scarred. A typical discoid LE plaque is a mosaic of changes, owing to the progression of the inflammatory process in some areas and its regression in others. A single lesion may display healed atrophic areas coexistent with an acute process, erythema, scaling, and active inflammation (Fig. 15.1)

Chronic discoid LE lesions occur most commonly on the face and scalp and have a peculiar propensity for the outer ear. Scarring lesions on the inner surfaces of the conchae are virtually diagnostic of discoid lupus. Similarly, when such lesions affect the palms and fingers, they appear as small, patchy, atrophic depressions filled with thick, tenacious scales and surrounded by a halo of bright erythema. Lesions in the mucous membranes of the nasal or oral cavity, where the stratum corneum is absent, are complicated by ulceration, particularly if they occur in areas of trauma. Less than 15% of patients with chronic discoid cutaneous LE will have extracutaneous manifestations of SLE or serological abnormalities of SLE, such as circulating antinuclear anti-

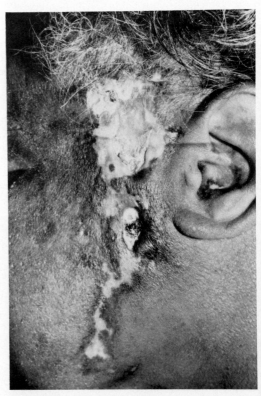

Fig. 15.1. Chronic discoid lupus erythematosus. Severe scarring and ulceration of a lesion present for 10 years. The patient also has a hypopigmented scarring lesion in the inner surface of the conchae.

bodies, anti-DNA antibodies, or depressed serum complement levels.

At the opposite end of the spectrum, in acute systemic LE, the cutaneous manifestations are quite varied. The most widely acclaimed eruption, the acute erythema of the central face or the so-called butterfly rash, is relatively uncommon and occurs in less than 10% of SLE patients. These patients have pronounced redness and edema of the nasal bridge and malar eminences. The entire face may be erythematous, the periorbital area edematous, and the skin over the nose and malar eminences raised and scaly.

Similar changes may occur in the skin of the anterior neck and chest especially with a red-violaceous hue and subtle telangiectasia after sun exposure (Fig. 15.2). These patients almost always have arthritis and fever and have a high incidence of vital organ involvement. When the eruption is typical, it can be differentiated easily from the eczematous eruption of seborrheic dermatitis, the pustular and papular telangiectatic lesions of acne rosacea, and the erythematous, telangiectatic skin changes of iatrogenic Cushing's disease. However, atypical LE rashes do occur, and a careful evaluation is required to differentiate these more benign conditions.

Subacute cutaneous LE lesions are commonly encountered in SLE and include a variety of inflammatory lesions of moderate intensity (Fig. 15.3). Some patients develop persistent, well demarcated, erythematous-to-violaceous scaly plaques, which resolve after treatment with no scarring or with only minimal telangiectasia and atrophy. Others have persistent erythematous or violaceous smooth plaques that resemble unremitting urticaria. These also may disappear without residual damage. The lesions most often erupt symmetrically, in sun-exposed areas, i.e. the forehead, cheeks, nose, V of the neck, upper arms, forearms, and dorsa of the hands. When these

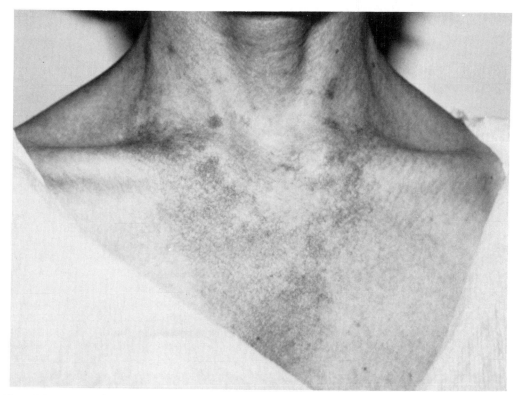

Fig. 15.2. Acute lupus erythematosus rash. Erythema and edema limited to area exposed to sunlight. The patient also had similar changes in the skin of her cheeks and nose.

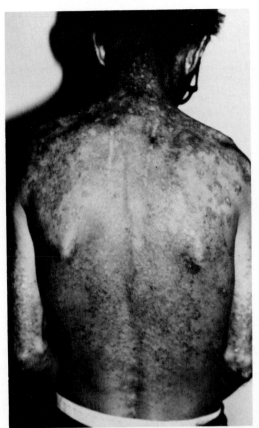

Fig. 15.3 Subacute cutaneous lupus erythematosus (LE). Generalized symmetrical, erythematous, telangiectatic, scaling eruption in a patient who also had LE nephritis and pleuritis. After therapy, this eruption resolved with only minimal hypopigmentation and telangiectasia.

lesions begin to appear, they are difficult to distinguish from the lesions of early chronic discoid LE. Only with complete resolution in a few months does their subacute character become obvious. The clinical course of the disease in these patients is variable and can be mild or relatively severe. The majority of patients with subacute cutaneous LE lesions have four or more ARA criteria for systemic LE and have serum antinuclear antibodies. Renal disease and central nervous system (CNS) abnormalities have been described in such patients but usually the prognosis in patients with this type of eruption is quite good.

Lupus panniculitis (lupus profundus), an unusual manifestation of LE, has a predilection for the subcutaneous tissue of the upper arms and cheeks but may occur on the buttocks, thighs, and trunk as well. Typical lesions are firm, slightly tender, erythematous nodules, which may be smooth or scaly and at times ulcerate and heal with severe atrophic scarring (Fig. 15.4). The nodules are often associated with overlying skin changes of discoid LE. Most of these patients have chronic cutaneous lesions with few systemic manifestations; however, a few patients with widespread systemic disease have been reported.

Widespread inflammation of the vascular system in SLE is expressed in a variety of cutaneous lesions. Urticaria-like lesions, with and without purpura can be seen in association with LE. Chronic intractable urticaria with arthralgia is occasionally the presenting feature of SLE. Urticarial lesions in LE are similar to "idiopathic" urticaria except that the SLE lesions tend to persist for days instead of hours. Light microscopic examination of biopsy specimens usually show a necrotizing vasculitis and the cellular infiltrates consist mainly of polymorphonuclear leukocytes with some mononuclear cells. Some patients with these lesions also have an associated intermittant angioedema of the face and lips. The extracutaneous manifestations are variable, but most often these patients are hypocomplementemic and have nephritis or severe SLE.

Prominent erythema and telangiectasia of the proximal nail fold is seen in patients with multisystem disease, especially during acute flare-ups. Patients occasionally also have subungual splinter hemorrhages. Scaly red telangiectatic plaques on the palmar aspect of the hands and fingertips may sometimes become ulcerated (Fig. 15.5). Occasionally, if the angiitis is very severe, infarctive fingertip ulcerations occur.

Some patients develop livedo reticularis and/or widespread papular telangiectatic lesions which result in extensive small ulcerative lesions of the extremities, especially the legs. These lesions heal with depressed white porcelain centers simulating atrophic blanche or malignant atrophic papulosis.

Chronic ulceration of the legs is not uncommon. The ulcers are sharply demarcated and usually occur just above the malleoli or on the

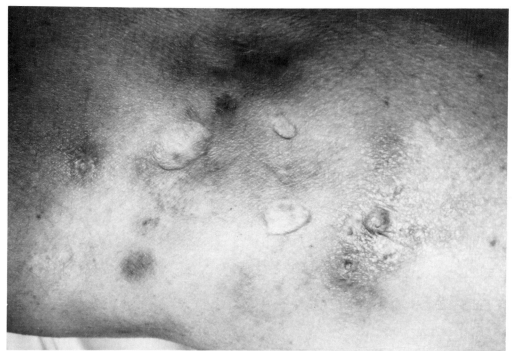

Fig. 15.4. Lupus profundus. Multiple tender erythematous nodules and severe atrophic scarring of the skin and subcutaneous tissue of the upper arm in a patient with lupus erythematosus.

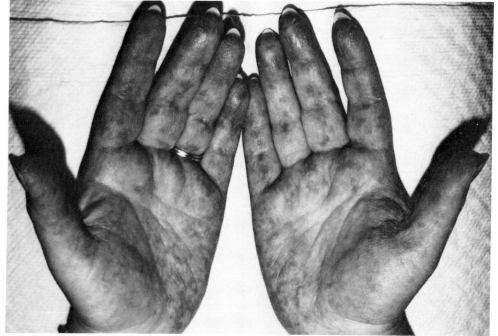

Fig. 15.5. Scaly, erythematous, telangiectatic skin of the palms of a patient with systemic lupus erythematosus.

lateral aspect of the dorsum of the foot (Fig. 15.6). They are indolent and recurrent. Hemorrhagic bullous lesions may precede ulceration.

Another peripheral vascular syndrome seen in LE is recurrent thrombophlebitis with and without subsequent venous stasis and ulceration. In some instances, this complication has preceded the onset of other manifestations of LE by many years. Abnormalities in coagulation and fibrinolytic activity have been documented. Endothelial cell damage may result in decreased synthesis of both factor VIII and plasminogen activator.

Raynaud's phenomenon occurs in about 40% of SLE patients. When SLE patients without Raynaud's phenomenon are compared to SLE patients with Raynaud's phenomenon, it has been determined that patients with Raynaud's have a greater incidence of arthritis, malar rash, and photosensitivity and a lesser incidence of severe renal disease. In general, patients with Raynaud's phenomena are less likely to have severe, life threatening disease.

Several types of hair loss can occur in LE. Scarring permanent alopecia is the end result of untreated chronic discoid LE lesions of the scalp. The cosmetic disfigurement may be mild, with only a few small areas of baldness easily covered by surrounding hair, or may be

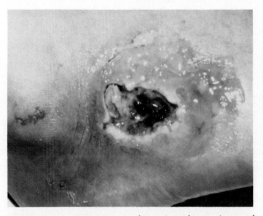

Fig. 15.6. Persistent chronic ulceration of the skin of the foot of a young woman with lupus erythematosus. She also had urticarial lesions, positive antinuclear antibody, arthritis, leukopenia, hemolytic anemia, hypocomplementemia, and recurrent episodes of thrombophlebitis.

so severe as to involve almost the entire scalp, necessitating the wearing of a hair piece.

There are two forms of nonscarring alopecia. In acute active LE, especially if the patient is febrile, a telogen effluvium may occur, resulting in diffuse thinning of the hair. The scalp is usually erythematous, although it may appear normal. This loss is generally reversible, and hair regrows with remission of the disease. This type of hair loss is the alopecia described as a criterion for the ARA classification of LE.

Another type of hair loss that may be encountered in the LE patient is characterized by the presence of numerous, fine, short hairs of irregular length, especially along the frontal hairline. Studies of these hairs indicate that the short hair, termed "lupus hair," may be caused by growth retardation rather than by breakage. Lupus hair is frequently noted coincidentally with clinical and laboratory evidence of increased disease activity. Recovery of hair growth is usually slow after the activity subsides.

PATHOLOGY AND IMMUNOPATHOLOGY OF CUTANEOUS LESIONS

In acute, subacute, and chronic cutaneous LE, the primary site of injury occurs near the vessel walls and at the dermal-epidermal junction, as demonstrated by light, immunofluorescence, and immunoelectronmicroscopic studies. The early erythematous, edematous, malar rash occurring in patients with acute SLE may not be diagnostic histologically. In the very early stages, the changes may consist only of dilated blood and lymphatic vessels in the upper dermis. In biopsy specimens from the fully developed eruption, the epidermis is atrophic, and there is extensive intracellular edema in the basal cell layer. Occasionally, lymphedema becomes so severe that intraepidermal or subepidermal vesicles are formed. In the upper dermis, the vessel walls are swollen, with extravasation of leukocytes and erythrocytes and only a sparse infiltrate of lymphocytes. The elastic fibers initially are normal but eventually become fragmented. Collagen bundles appear spongy and become thickened and eosinophilic.

In subacute cutaneous LE lesions, these pathologic changes are more pronounced and, in addition to destruction of elastic tissue and collagen, atrophy of sebaceous glands and hair follicles occurs. These histological features correlate with the clinical features of subacute LE lesions in which resolution is variable, with little or no scarring in some cases but with definite residual atrophy in others.

Early lesions of chronic DLE may appear similar to subacute LE. As the lesion progresses, the pathologic changes become diagnostic, owing to the dense infiltration of lymphocytes along the dermal-epidermal junction and around dermal blood vessels and appendageal structures. There is prominent hyperkeratosis with keratotic plugging of dilated follicular orifices. The malpighian layer is usually atrophic, but there may be areas of acanthosis. A variable degree of degeneration by liquefaction of the basal cell layer is present. At the dermal-epidermal junction, there is a band of *p*-aminosalicylic acid (PAS) positive material, unless inflammation has been so intense that only edema and amorphous material remain. In patients with dark skin, incontinence of pigment is characteristic and the melanin is engulfed by dermal macrophages. The elastic fibers degenerate, and hair follicles, sebaceous glands, and sweat glands atrophy and disappear. The histological changes of old, inactive, healed, scarred lesions of chronic discoid LE (CDLE) predictably are not diagnostic. Such lesions cannot be differentiated from other diseases of the skin that terminate in scarring.

Deposition of immunoglobulin along the dermal-epidermal junction can be demonstrated in active acute, subacute, and chronic cutaneous LE lesions and also in the clinically uninvolved skin of patients with systemic LE (Fig. 15.7). Patients with discoid LE lesions typically do not have immunoglobulin deposits in uninvolved skin. In lesional and clinically normal skin, both IgM and IgG are frequently found, alone or together. IgA is found less often and only in conjunction with IgG or IgM. Both classic and alternate pathway complement components are present in specific LE skin lesions. Early LE lesions may not have deposits of immunoglobulin. Serial biopsies of ultraviolet (UV)-induced lesions in

LE patients have demonstrated a time lag of several weeks between induction of the inflammatory response and detection of subepidermal immunoglobulin.

Examination of lesional skin by immunohistochemical methods is useful in patients who have cutaneous lesions that are compatible with, but not specific for, LE. Such disorders as polymorphic light eruption and drug eruption can simulate LE clinically and histologically but are negative when examined by the direct immunofluorescence technique.

Immunofluorescence studies of normal skin (lupus band test) is helpful in patients in which the suspected diagnosis of LE cannot be confirmed by specific serologic tests or by satisfying ARA criteria and who do not have LE specific skin lesions. Sun-exposed forearm skin is more likely to be positive than light-protected buttock skin.

Patients with chronic discoid skin lesions have a negative lupus band test. Exceptions are seen, however, in the occasional patient with chronic discoid lesions who also has clinical and serological manifestations of systemic disease. Patients with subacute cutaneous lesions do have immunoglobulin deposition, especially in sun-exposed skin. Approximately 50% of patients who satisfy at least four of the ARA criteria for the diagnosis of systemic LE and 85% of patients with LE nephritis have a positive band test.

Studies of serial biopsies of normal skin in SLE patients have shown that clinically active patients have more than four proteins (IgG, IgA, IgM, C3, C4, Clq) at the dermal-epidermal junction. This finding correlates with serially determined low levels of C3 and C4 and high levels of antibody to DNA. Cutaneous deposition of Clq, alone or in combination with other proteins, also correlated with clinical evidence of disease activity. The lupus band test, however, cannot be employed as a routine test to follow patients with SLE if more convenient, less expensive, serologic tests are available. Simultaneous immunofluorescence studies of biopsy specimens from the skin and kidney in SLE have shown conflicting results regarding the correlation of the deposition of immune reactants in the skin and the severity of nephritis. The majority of the studies conclude that the type of renal injury cannot be predicted on the basis of the

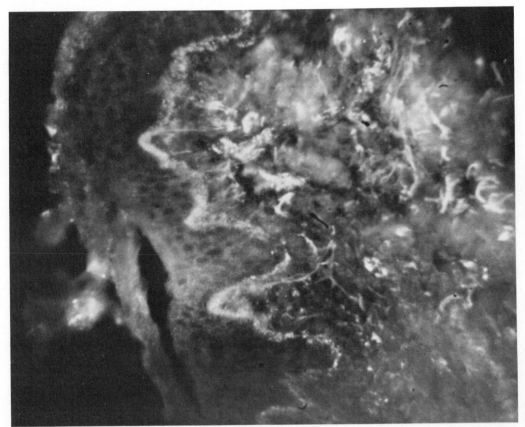

Fig. 15.7. Deposition of IgM is demonstrated in a granular pattern along the dermal-epidermal junction and in dermal vessel walls in a section of a skin lesion of a patient with lupus erythematosus.

lupus band test and this test cannot be used for evaluation of nephritis.

Immunofluorescence studies of biopsy specimens from normal skin are very helpful, however, as a diagnostic test, for example in the diagnosis of lupus nephritis when there are no extra renal manifestations of SLE or in any other single organ system involvement in SLE when serologic tests may be equivocal. Occasionally, a facial eruption that is not distinctive can best be evaluated by immunofluorescence studies.

SEROLOGICAL MANIFESTATIONS

Antibodies to Tissue Components

Patients with active systemic LE develop antibodies to nuclear material. This phenom-

enon is detectable by the antinuclear antibody (ANA) test, which essentially has replaced the LE cell test because it is more sensitive. During the 1960s, many investigators described multiple morphological patterns of nuclear staining, depending on the tissue substrate used, the type of lupus serum tested, and the attention paid to detail. Most laboratories recognize three patterns in lupus sera: peripheral, homogeneous, and particulate ("speckled" or "thready"). Using sera from patients with scleroderma and a human tissue substrate, two more specific patterns are seen: nucleolar and finely speckled. Additional patterns may be recognized if special substrates are used and the technician is experienced. Complicating the laboratory interpretation of staining patterns is the fact that some lupus sera contain a variety of nuclear antibodies and exhibit more than one pattern. The pattern can change with varying dilutions, and sometimes adjacent cells may exhibit different patterns. The individual morphological patterns reflect specific antibodies directed toward different antigens within the nucleus.

The fluorescent ANA test is the single most useful test for confirming a clinical diagnosis of LE, if it is properly interpreted. Unfortunately, at the present time, the test has not been standardized. Clinical laboratories employ many techniques including a variety of commercial kits that render the test relatively nonspecific. The physician must evaluate the quality and sensitivity of the test as performed in the laboratory before interpreting the results for the patient. Many patients have endured needless anxiety and expense because of an incorrectly interpreted ANA test. It should be remembered that a positive test alone is not conclusive evidence for a diagnosis of SLE. Positive tests occur in other rheumatic disorders, such as rheumatoid arthritis and scleroderma, as well as in malignancy and drug reactions. Relatives of SLE patients also may show positive test results.

Ideally, the ANA report should state the substrate used, the titer, and the pattern. In active SLE with murine liver or human spleen, or human cell cultures, the titer usually exceeds 1:40. The peripheral pattern is characteristic of a SLE patient with antibody to DNA and the titer of this pattern may reflect disease activity. A particulate, coarse, speckled pattern suggests that the patient may have antibodies to extractable nuclear antigens (ENA). Homogeneous patterns are nonspecific and are usually significant only in titers greater than 1:80. Nucleolar staining and fine speckles are seen most commonly in scleroderma. Except for the titer of the peripheral pattern, the titer of ANA in a lupus patient does not correlate with severity of disease and is not a useful guide for therapy. Aged, chronically ill patients, or patients with malignancy, rheumatoid arthritis, or other hypergammaglobulinemic states may have a positive ANA, but the titer is usually low.

The multiple autoantibodies detected in the serum are probably responsible for the direct cellular cytotoxicity and immune complex-mediated injury seen in SLE (Table 15.2). Antibodies to nuclear antigens can be divided into four main groups: 1) to DNA, 2) to deoxyribonucleoprotein, 3) to basic pro-

Table 15.2
Autoantibodies in Systemic Lupus Erythematosus (SLE)

To nuclear antigens
  DNA
  Nucleoprotein
  Histones
  Acidic proteins

To cytoplasmic antigens
  RNA
  Ribosomes and RNA·protein complexes

To T lymphocyte cell surface antigens
To B lymphocyte cell surface antigens
To red cell antigens
To platelet antigens

teins (histones), and 4) to acidic proteins. These main groups can be further subdivided and new antibody systems are constantly being identified and defined (Table 15.3).

Antibodies to DNA may react only with double-stranded or native DNA (dsDNA) or with single-stranded DNA (ssDNA), or they may react in immunologic identity with double-stranded and single-stranded DNA (dsDNA-ssDNA). Antibodies to ssDNA are found in SLE but are also found in other rheumatic diseases and in malignancy and chronic infection. Antibodies to dsDNA are highly specific for SLE. Antibodies to dsDNA-ssDNA are found in high titers in patients with active disease especially those with nephritis. Low titers can be found in other rheumatic disorders. This is the antibody system commonly referred to as "antibody to DNA." More than 50% of the time, active disease is associated with high DNA antibody and low total hemolytic complement. Complement-fixing DNA antibodies are associated mainly with episodes of renal disease. CNS disease often occurs without high DNA binding or depressed CH50 levels. The finding of antibody to DNA, although an important laboratory marker, should not be considered an indication for instituting more vigorous therapy, unless it is associated with a decrease in complement or with clinical evidence of activity. There is no evidence that early treatment to suppress antibody to DNA prevents later problems. About one-third of the patients with DNA antibody continue to be clinically stable in spite of multiple positive tests.

Table 15.3
Antibodies to Nuclear Antigens in Systemic Lupus Erythematosus (SLE)[a]
State of the Art

Antibody	Associated Disease
To DNA	
To dsDNA (nDNA)	SLE
To ssDNA	Rheumatic disorders, malignancy
To dsDNA-ssDNA	SLE (high titer), rheumatic disorders (low titer)
To deoxyribonucleo-protein (complex of DNA and histones)	SLE and drug induced LE (LE cell antibody)
To histones	SLE and drug induced LE
To acidic proteins	
To Sm	SLE: highly diagnostic
To RNP	SLE: (low titer), MCTD (high titer)
To Ma	SLE: severe
To SS-A (Ro)	SLE, Sjögren's syndrome
To SS-B (Sjt, La, Ha)	SLE, Sjögren's syndrome

[a] The abbreviations used are: SLE, systemic lupus erythematosus; ds, double-stranded; n, native; ss, single-stranded; LE, lupus erythematosus, and MCTD, mixed connective tissue disease.

Antibodies to deoxyribonucleoprotein produce the LE cell phenomenon. Antibodies to histones are found in both drug-induced and idiopathic SLE. In contrast to SLE in which antibodies to histones are found along with other nuclear antibodies, in drug-induced SLE, antibodies to histones are often the only nuclear antibodies present.

The list of antibodies to acidic nuclear proteins is expanding. Antibody to Sm antigen was first described in 1966 and was named for the patient in whom this antibody was first detected. Antibody to Sm is highly diagnostic of SLE and patients with Sm antibody tend to have very active disease.

Antibody to RNP is present in SLE, discoid LE (DLE), and in patients who have been classified as having mixed connective tissue disease (MCTD). The nature of MCTD and its relationship to the presence of high titers of antibody to RNP is still controversial. These patients sometimes present with a combination of clinical features similar to SLE, scleroderma, and polymyositis. They respond favorably to steroids and have a relatively benign course. Unfortunately the clinical features of these rheumatic disorders overlap, for example Raynaud's is common to both SLE and scleroderma and myositis and can be a feature of all three disorders. The typical clinical presentation of MCTD is thought to be characterized by Raynaud's phenomenon, arthralgia or arthritis, inflammatory myositis, esophageal hypomotility (usually asymptomatic), impaired pulmonary diffusing capacity, and swelling of the hands with sausage-like appearance of the fingers. Antibodies to DNA, deoxyribonucleoprotein (LE cells), hypocomplementemia, renal disease, and CNS disease are reported to be uncommon in MCTD.

Other investigators argue that MCTD is best seen as part of the spectrum of SLE. Most (85%) of these patients satisfy at least four of the preliminary criteria of the ARA for SLE. These patients do have a high incidence of Raynaud's phenomenon but only a few (15%) have symptoms of polymyositis or skin changes of scleroderma. This high incidence of Raynaud's phenomemon is associated with the presence of RNP and not to the presence of other clinical features. Patients with anti-RNP alone and Raynaud's have a low incidence of renal disease and a favorable prognosis. Many clinicians find that the number of patients with RNP who lack overlap features actually is greater than the number of patients with overlap features. Patients with antibody to RNP with clinical features of MCTD are only a small fraction of the total number of patients with anti-RNP antibody. It is interesting that a large proportion (70%) of patients with anti-Sm also have antibodies to RNP although the titer of RNP is usually low. It is difficult to classify these patients with both Sm and RNP if patients with Sm have SLE and patients with RNP have MCTD. The issue of whether MCTD is a separate disease entity or part of the spectrum of SLE cannot be resolved with the current data available. Careful longitudinal, clinical, and serologic studies over a prolonged period of time of patients who are producing these antibodies should help resolve this issue.

Two additional antibody systems directed to acidic nuclear proteins designated SS-A (Ro) and SS-B (SjT, La, Ha) have been identified in 90% of patients with Sjögren's syndrome and approximately 20% of patients with SLE. The incidence of antibody to SS-A in patients fulfilling ARA criteria for SLE is about 20%. Of these patients, 50–75% of them will have keratoconjunctivitis sicca. Serial studies have demonstrated the presence of SS-A before the onset of dry eyes or an abnormal Shirmer's test. Patients with antibodies to SS-A have been reported to have a high incidence of polyarthritis, rheumatoid factor, and photosensitive skin rashes. These patients can develop serious renal disease. The kidneys were studied from two patients who died from complications of SLE and the acid elutes from the renal homogenates contained SS-A anti-SS-A immune complexes.

Antibody to SS-B antigen is found almost exclusively in patients with sicca syndrome and in those with sicca and SLE. About 20% of patients with SLE and 70% of patients with Sjögrens syndrome have SS-B antibody. The antibody is only rarely found in patients with SLE without sicca and in patients with rheumatoid arthritis and sicca. This antibody is not found in patients with rheumatoid arthritis. The clinical significance of anti-SS-B antibody aside from the association with sicca syndrome has yet to be defined.

Recently, another distinct antibody to an acidic nuclear protein designated as MA antigen has been described in SLE patients with very severe disease. It has not been detected in patients with other rheumatic disorders or control groups. Patients with MA antibody have recalcitrant skin rashes (several had bullous eruptions), a high incidence of hypocomplementemia, serious renal disease, hypertension, hepatosplenomegaly, lymphadenopathy, and neurologic disease. The pathogenic role of the MA system has not yet been demonstrated.

There is currently much interest in the identification of these and other antibody systems in SLE and rheumatic disease patients. It is hoped that not only will these antibodies

and antigens provide insight into the pathogenesis of SLE but, also, that they may be useful as a guide to predicting flares of disease and subsets of SLE patients who have life threatening disease, so that these patients may be selected early to receive more aggressive therapy.

Complement Levels

Depressed levels of serum complement have been recognized for many years as a reliable marker for severe SLE, especially LE nephritis. Low total hemolytic complement and high titers of antibody to DNA indicate active disease, especially disease involving the kidney. Although therapy is often based on the results of these laboratory findings, it should be recognized that some patients will have hypocomplementemia with no clinical signs of disease activity. Randomly discovered abnormalities in anti-DNA antibody and complement levels are of no predictive value, and hypocomplementemia has frequently resolved spontaneously with no recognizable exacerbation of the disease. Serial evaluations of clinical features should be correlated with laboratory abnormalities to assess disease activity before therapy is altered.

Individual complement components can be measured quantitatively. In active LE, levels of early reacting components (C1, C4, C2) and late-reacting components (C3 to C9) may be reduced. There also may be a reduction of alternate pathway components. Investigations of LE patients with low C3 levels have demonstrated variability in C3 synthesis. Synthesis is sometimes decreased, but hypercatabolism accounts for the low serum level in untreated patients with active disease.

In many hospital laboratories, it is only possible to obtain serum C3 levels by radioimmunodiffusion methods. This test provides a simple, reliable, and accurate assessment of clinical activity. The determination of total hemolytic complement is difficult and often unnecessary since C3 levels usually correlate with CH50 values. However, to detect patients who have a hereditary deficiency of a complement component, which can predispose to the development of LE, a total hemolytic complement determination is essential on the initial evaluation. Such patients may have normal levels of C3 but show no lysis on functional assays for total complement and have total absence, for example, of C2. Many individuals with hereditary deficiency of C2 and LE have been reported. Many of these patients have had a photosensitive, chronic, cutaneous erythematous, facial rash (Fig. 15.8).

EXTRACUTANEOUS MANIFESTATIONS

The major extracutaneous manifestations of LE will be discussed only briefly, since the focus of this chapter is the dermatological aspects of the disease. The reader is referred to several monographs and reviews in the References at the end of the chapter for an in-depth discussion.

Arthritis is the most common initial symptom expressed in LE. Typically, patients have a nondeforming polyarthritis with inflammation of synovial tissues and minimal destruction of cartilage and bone. However, deforming arthritis of the hands with ulnar deviation has become more frequently recognized in a subgroup of patients with long-standing SLE polyarthropathy.

Serositis, with inflammation of the pleural, pericardial, and peritoneal membranes, is also a common manifestation of SLE and is a clinical guidepost of active disease. Pleural effusion, interstitial pneumonitis, focal alveolar hemorrhage, and diffuse pulmonary fibrosis are characteristic complications in the lung. Pericarditis, myocarditis, and endocarditis may occur, rarely, with cardiac tamponade and constrictive pericarditis. Scarring of the heart valves with thickening of leaflet tissue can lead to valvular regurgitation and insufficiency. Inflammation of parietal and visceral peritoneum may produce acute abdominal pain. Pancreatitis and ileitis severe enough to require surgical intervention have been reported.

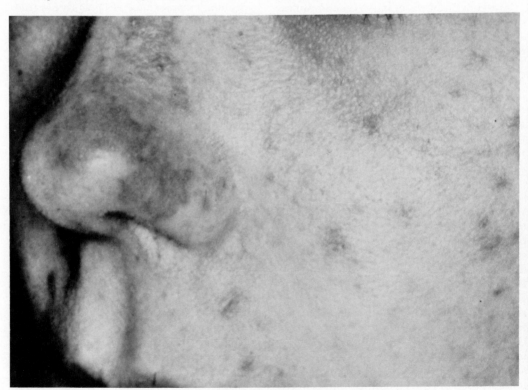

Fig. 15.8. A young patient with photosensitive chronic erythematous, edematous, facial lesions and a selective deficiency of the second component of complement.

Central nervous system involvement is probably related to immune complex-mediated vasculitis, and IgG, IgM, and C3 deposits have been identified in the choroid plexus of patients with CNS SLE and microinfarcts can be found in brains of patients who have died with the disease. However, a true necrotizing vasculitis is not invariably found and other nonspecific pathologic lesions of the brain and spinal cord are seen. Cranial nerve disorders, organic psychosis, seizures, status epilepticus, hemiparesis, and intracranial hemorrhage are among the highly variable clinical manifestations. Peripheral neuropathy with sensory deficits is not uncommon, and myelopathy with paraplegia may occur. Psychiatric disorders may be the result of vasculitis but, because mental disturbances may be complicated by the common problem of steroid-induced psychosis or mixed organic and steroid-induced psychosis, their etiology has yet to be defined. Serum complement levels and antibodies to DNA are not a measure of CNS activity. Unfortunately, there is no single consistent abnormality of the serum or cerebrospinal fluid that is diagnostic of central nervous system lupus. Electroencephalogram findings may be abnormal but cannot be depended upon to establish organic disease. Arteriography is not helpful in visualizing the small vessels of the brain. Radionuclide brain scan abnormalities can be detected in some patients with LE cerebritis and these abnormalities seem to improve with clinical remission. The computed tomography scan is not helpful. A noninvasive new technique using oxygen-15 brain scanning which permits the study of cerebral oxygen use and blood flow by inhalation of radioactive gas has been reported useful in detection of vascular abnormalities in the brain but, because of difficulty in production of the radioactive oxygen, this test will not be widely available. Also, this technique detects only vascular lesions. Therefore, no single procedure is consistently abnormal but measurement of cerebrospinal fluid (CSF) protein, CSF IgG, CSF anti-DNA, electroencephalogram changes, and flow brain scan abnormalities are all useful tests in assessing CNS involvement in SLE. Most important, in evaluating every LE patient with CNS symptoms, is obtaining adequate cultures of cerebrospinal fluid. Unrecognized and potentially treatable meningitis may be the underlying problem.

If lupus nephritis develops, it usually occurs during the first year of active multisystem disease and is less common after 5 years have elapsed. Controversy exists on the classification of lupus nephritis. Patients with lupus nephritis in the past have been classified according to Pollak's criteria as modified by Baldwin into three major categories: 1) mild or focal proliferative, 2) severe or diffuse proliferative, and 3) membranous glomerulonephritis. It was formerly considered rare for transitions to occur from one group into another, however, recent data indicate that changes in renal histology do occur. It is difficult to describe the degree of activity of the histologic lesions. Immunofluorescence studies have shown diffuse deposits of complexes in biopsies classified as focal by light microscopy. There is wide variation among pathologists and a broad range of criteria used to define focal disease, and it is doubtful if classification based on distribution of a lesion is important. There is no completely satisfactory classification but, currently, renal biopsies can be assigned to one of five groups—recognizing that at different times throughout the course of the disease one patient may show different features.

The five groups include: 1) mesangial lupus nephritis, 2) focal proliferative lupus nephritis, 3) diffuse proliferative lupus nephritis, 4) membranous proliferative lupus nephritis, and 5) membranous lupus nephritis.

Mesangial lupus nephritis shows proliferation of mesangial cells, increased mesangial matrix, and immune complex deposition only in mesangium by immunofluorescence and electron microscopy. These patients rarely develop renal failure. Focal disease shows less than 50% of the glomeruli with mesangial and segmental endothelial cell proliferation and irregular thickening of capillary loops. Immunofluorescence and electron microscopy show immune deposits in the mesangium and along the peripheral capillary loops, often subendothelial but, also, variable amounts can be found subepithelial and intramembranous. These patients frequently have microscopic hematuria and proteinuria but seldom develop azotemia and renal insufficiency. In diffuse glomerulonephritis, more than 50% of the glomeruli show extensive necrosis with marked proliferation of endothelial and mesangial cells obliterating the capillaries. Electron microscopy demonstrates extensive deposits of immune reactants that have been shown to contain DNA·anti-DNA complexes. These patients usually have gross hematuria and proteinuria and can develop azotemia, hypertension, edema, and renal failure. In membranous proliferative lupus nephritis there are uniform changes in the glomeruli. Capillary loops are regularly thickened, mesangial proliferation is prominent, and there is marked increase of mesangial matrix with extension around the peripheral capillary loops giving a double-contoured look to the glomerular basement membrane. Patients with diffuse proliferative and membranous proliferative nephritis have the worst prognosis. In membranous nephritis there is marked thickening of the glomerular capillary walls, with very little necrosis or leukocytic infiltration. The deposits of immunoglobulin and complement are subepithelial. These patients may have gross hematuria and proteinuria. They have a smaller risk of renal failure.

There has been controversy about the necessity for renal biopsy, and it is agreed that biopsy is not essential for diagnosis and management of lupus nephritis but is useful as a guide for staging the severity of the disease. Attempts are being made to classify renal biopsies not only according to the conventional system but according to pathologic findings that indicate activity of disease such as cellular proliferation, fibrinoid necrosis, nuclear karyorrhexis, hyalin thrombi, wire loops, and leukocyte infiltration. Chronic changes are indicated by sclerotic glomeruli, fibrous crescents, tubular atrophy, interstitial fibrosis. The combination of a high total of active lesions and advanced chronic changes indicates a poor prognosis for patients with proliferative glomerulonephritis. Most active pathologic lesions are potentially reversible after treatment of lupus nephritis but chronic sclerosing lesions are usually irreversible. This should be considered when selecting a therapeutic regimen. Renal function can change rapidly and can be judged most accurately by close clinical observation, serial profiles of complement and DNA antibody, urinary excretion of protein, and determinations of creatinine clearance.

Anemia occurs in more than 50% of patients and is the most common hematological abnormality in active lupus erythematosus. There are multiple causes, immune and nonimmune. The most common, the "anemia of chronic disease" is not life threatening and usually improves as the activity of the disease lessens. This anemia is normocytic and normochromic, with adequate bone marrow iron stores in spite of low serum iron values. There may be associated ferrokinetic abnormalities reflected by altered iron-binding capacity, plasma iron, iron utilization, and poor response to iron therapy. Occasionally, true iron deficiency does exist, owing to occult gastrointestinal blood loss and renal disease. There is some evidence that patients who develop anemia are more likely to deteriorate clinically and experience exacerbation of their renal disease. A positive direct Coombs' test, indicating the presence of immunoglobulin and complement on erythrocyte membranes, is common in lupus patients. However, less than 10% of these patients will have clinically significant hemolysis. Drug-induced (methyldopa, penicillin) Coombs' test-positive hemolysis also can be a complicating factor.

Thrombocytopenia is usually caused by peripheral destruction of platelets by antiplatelet antibodies but qualitative defects in thrombocyte aggregation have been described. Circulating anticoagulants rarely lead to spontaneous hemorrhagic crises but may be significant if invasive diagnostic procedures, such as renal biopsy, are performed. The anticoagulant antibody, usually IgG, is most commonly directed against factors XI, IX, and VIII, and against prothrombin and the prothrombin-converting complex.

The action of antibodies on erythrocytes, thrombocytes, and coagulation factors can usually be reversed by administration of corticosteroids. Splenectomy and immunosuppressive agents are selectively utilized in corticosteroid-resistant patients.

Leukopenia of both granulocytic and lymphocytic lines occurs commonly and is probably caused by a variety of mechanisms. Granulocytopenia can result from peripheral destruction by antigranulocyte antibody and from bone marrow suppression. Qualitative abnormalities of granulocyte function also have been noted. Lymphopenia, with marked reduction of the absolute number and alteration of the proportion of thymus-derived (T cell), bone marrow-derived (B cell), and null cells, is characteristic of active systemic lupus erythematosus. Patients with active SLE experience a generalized loss of regulatory mechanisms of the immune response, while those with less severe disease have only a moderate impairment. In limited forms of the disorder, such as DLE, immune regulation is generally intact.

PATHOGENESIS

Current research efforts are being directed in three main areas, immunologic, viral, and gentic. The viral hypothesis suggesting that a chronic C-type viral infection of thymic tissue could cause impairment of the immune response and emergence of LE is still an attractive theory but the evidence for a type C RNA virus infection is inconclusive. There is firm evidence that genetic characteristics are very important in permitting the expression of LE. SLE occurs in 5% of relatives of LE patients and there is an association between LE and HLA-A and HLA-B haplotypes within each family but different haplotypes are found in different families. Preliminary studies of the HLA-D region antigens on B lymphocytes of LE patients and their families have shown an increased risk for the disease if HLA-DRW2 or DRW3 antigens are present. In some families, it is apparent that the coexistence of two or more genes in the HLA-D region may be required for susceptibility. In the LE syndrome associated with hereditary deficiency of the second complement component there is a strong linkage disequilibrium between the C2-deficient gene and DRW2.

In virtually all patients with active systemic LE, there are defects in both B cell and T cell populations. Even in LE patients without active disease, there is an underlying B cell propensity for hyperactivity. When the disease is active, B cell abnormalities become florid and excessive quantities of antibody is produced. Most patients with LE cannot generate cells that can suppress the proliferation of B cells in response to pokeweed mitogen or the proliferation of T cells in response to allogeneic cells in the mixed leukocyte reaction. The defect in suppressor cells is selective and there appears to be distinct suppressor

cells for different immune functions. Anti-T cell antibodies are produced which preferentially eliminate suppressor cell precursors. Since LE patients have a functional defect in T suppressor cells and an increased B cell reproductive capacity, when insults to the body occur, polyconal B cell stimulation and production of anti-T cell antibodies with a loss of T cell regulation occurs, sufficient to turn inactive disease into active disease. A generalized B cell hyperactivity with production of a variety of antibodies including antinuclear antibodies leads to immune complex disease and tissue inflammation. The continued production of antibodies reactive with immature T cells can eliminate regulatory T cells and the B cell population can function autonomously. The result is a vicious cycle of autoantibody production (hypergammaglobulinemia) and inflammatory disease and further impaired T cell function until the cycle is suppressed with immunosuppressive therapy. Since the susceptibility to the cycle is ever present, when therapy is reduced or if another B cell stimulus occurs, e.g. an infection occurs in the patient, recurrence of the same cycle of events is to be expected.

Antibodies to DNA are found in the serum of almost all LE patients with significant disease. There are several major sources of continuous production of endogenous DNA in the body. In the bone marrow, nucleated red blood cells lose nuclear material. In the skin, the epidermal cells lose their nuclear material continuously during the process of keratinization. DNA has been found in vitro to be efficiently bound to isolated glomerular basement membranes and to connective tissue in the upper dermis. In a patient with antibody to DNA, it would be expected that DNA containing immune complexes would accumulate in these areas. There is also evidence that DNAase inhibitor levels are high in the serum of SLE patients and this may result in decreased degradation of normally released DNA.

Exposure to sunlight often causes skin lesions in SLE and, in fact, lesions have been produced in LE patients by using an artificial ultraviolet light source. Subepidermal deposition of immunoglobulins can subsequently be detected at the injured site. Ultraviolet light transforms DNA into antigenic thymine dimers. If this altered DNA is injected into mice, antibodies are produced. If the mice are then exposed to sunlight, antibody to altered DNA can be demonstrated at the dermal-epidermal junction similar to human cutaneous LE. The effect of ultraviolet light on cellular structures is not limited to the production of thymine dimers; many additional chemical complexes have been described. Accordingly, damage to skin by sunlight or other trauma could result in the production of a variety of altered nuclear macromolecules which, when released in the circulation, could induce antibodies of multiple specificities.

For a chronic immune complex disease to develop, there should be a constant source of antigen as well as an antibody response and defective clearing of complexes. There must be enough antibody to form immune complexes but not too rapid an elimination of antigen. Thus, an ongoing release of DNA nucleoprotein from tissue damage, could produce immune complex disease of SLE. Additionally, those patients who develop severe immune complex disease, such as nephritis, may be unable to remove complexes efficiently. The varying loss of T cell function is reflected in the clinical expression of the disease. If the host has severe T cell depletion and dysfunction, a state of T cell paralysis, loss of suppressor T cell activity, B cell escape, and hyperreactive antibody responses to a variety of antigens occurs. A state of perpetual T cell deficiency ensues until enough immune complex tissue damage occurs to destroy the involved organ. In the indeterminate and subacute forms of LE, reflected by recurrent and persistent skin lesions, arthritis, serositis, and mesangial lesions, with no detectable circulating immune complexes or antibody to DNA, a moderate impairment of T cell function is found. In patients with DLE, usually there is an intact T cell suppressor system, no B cell escape, and no hyperresponsives to DNA and other nuclear antigens.

MANAGEMENT

During the last 20 years, it has become apparent that SLE is more prevalent than was previously recognized and is most often a relatively benign disorder. A recent study disclosed an incidence of new cases of 7.6/ 100,000 using the ARA criteria for the diagnosis. The projected 10-year survival rate for these patients exceeded 90%. The prevalence of clinically important renal disease was only 11%.

Appreciation of the chronic nature of the disease is probably due in large measure to the detection of early and milder disease by wide application of the antinuclear antibody test. Heightened awareness by practitioners in all medical specialties of the extremely variable presentation of SLE has enlarged the clinical spectrum. Before 1960, SLE gained a reputation as a rare and vicious disease because mostly patients with severe forms were recognized. However, patients lacking CNS and renal involvement (80% of all SLE cases) have a chronic, smoldering course with periods of long remission. Some patients have only one or two episodes of active disease followed by complete remission. Ironically, one of the major problems encountered by patients today is overzealous therapy with corticosteroids and immunosuppressants, reflecting the mode of the early 1960s, when the disease was regarded as invariably fatal. Sometimes, problems such as sepsis, aseptic necrosis of the hip, and hypertension are encountered, making it difficult to determine whether the disease or the therapy is responsible for the complications.

The management of lupus rests solely on recognition of subtypes of the disease. Treatment must be tailored to the particular patient because of tremendous individual variation, and cannot be extrapolated from the therapy of poorly defined groups of patients described in the literature. Until multicenter long-term prospective studies are available, in which homogeneous populations of patients with lupus have been analyzed from a clinical immunological, and therapeutic standpoint all estimates of prognosis will be fraught with error. No patient should be given a pessimistic outlook.

General supportive measures and specific therapeutic measures must be considered in the care of each patient. Continued education of the patient is probably the single most important aspect of the overall program of management. Every LE patient needs to be informed not only that he or she has lupus but that there are many forms of the disease some requiring more careful monitoring and more medication than others. In fact, some patients with mild disease may be advised they need no specific treatment at that time. If the patient is an adolescent, the physician should outline the total management program for the patient and his parents, explaining the necessity for regular checkups or even the reason for less frequent checkups. If the family is oversolicitous, or the patient is unduly anxious about the disorder, sometimes it is helpful to refer him to one of the many organizations that have been formed to promote education and research and to give emotional support to patients with lupus. The physician who invests time in frank and open discussion with the patient is usually rewarded with active cooperation. Team effort in long-term management permits satisfying interaction between the patient and physician in dealing with a difficult disease.

Lupus patients should be encouraged to modify their life style to achieve an ideal balance between work, play, and rest. Since each patient differs, a fixed number of hours of sleep cannot be recommended. A patient should rest when tired and be as physically active as possible. Regular exercise, especially walking and bicycling, should be encouraged because neither requires special strength or skill, and both permit enjoyment of the outdoors. Strenuous competitive sports should be temporarily restricted for those patients with multisystem activity and those on high dose steroid or immunosuppressive therapy. Patients should not take unnecessary medications or contraceptive pills.

Direct exposure to the sun should be avoided. All clinicians have seen patients whose initial manifestations of the disease were related to sun exposure, and whose eruptions are limited primarily to sun-exposed skin. Sun exposure can also precipitate other clinical manifestations, such as fever and arthralgia. Until the pathogenetic mechanisms of UV-induced LE dermatitis and serositis are clarified, it is prudent for all lupus patients, even those who deny photosensitivity, to avoid direct sun exposure. Sunbathing is a current fad based on the highly questionable cosmetic desirability of being tan, a status symbol of leisure and affluence. Ultraviolet rays are destructive to the skin of light-complexioned

individuals and accelerate aging and the development of skin cancer. Patients should be advised not to take outdoor jobs but to swim and play outdoors after work when the sun's rays are less intense. If they are outdoors during the day, frequent applications of sunscreens containing p-aminobenzoic acid (PABA) are mandatory. These measures should not be psychologically crippling because they apply to anyone interested in preserving the integrity of the skin.

Most lupus patients can look forward to many functional years and should be encouraged to obtain education and skills that will permit them to lead a productive life. As with any chronic illness, job counseling is particularly important. The physician should note the interests and talents of the patient so that he can offer encouragement and practical advice. Obviously, physically stressful or outdoor labor cannot be encouraged. Patients with Raynaud's phenomenon should be warned against work that requires hard use of fingers (e.g. typing). There is no patient who is more time-consuming and difficult to manage than the patient who has been permitted by parents or physicians to indulge in boredom and self-pity.

Many patients with LE are women in the childbearing age and need advice about birth control and pregnancy. Oral contraceptives should not be used for birth control since there is an increased incidence of thrombosis and hypertension in women using these drugs. Intrauterine devices may precipitate dysmenorrhea and recurrent infections. The safest method is to encourage the use of both the condom and the diaphragm.

If pregnancy is desired, both husband and wife should be advised of the risks involved. There is a higher than normal rate of fetal death and of premature births. Disease activity may be exacerbated especially during the first 8 weeks postpartum. Although fetal complications are rare, neonates may have congenital atrioventricular block and may develop a transient cutaneous LE eruption and hematologic abnormalities.

Generally, if the patient does not have active disease at the time of conception, the mother and child do very well. SLE patients must be carefully monitored throughout gestation, with regular complete blood counts, urinalysis, serum complement, and anti-DNA levels. If there is evidence of exacerbation, prednisone can be used to suppress the activity. The dose should be the very lowest possible. At the time of labor, the mother should receive a "steroid prep" with high dose parenteral corticosteroids just as for a surgical procedure. After birth, the neonate should be monitored for signs of adrenal suppression. The 6-week postpartum period is sometimes difficult for the mother and she needs continued close supervision at that time. Induced abortions are of no therapeutic value for the mother since exacerbation of the LE is most common when the uterus is evacuated. Increased steroid therapy is indicated for disease suppression rather than induced abortion.

The most common pitfall in the general management of LE is overtreatment of a patient because of abnormalities revealed by laboratory tests. High sedimentation rates, low complement levels, mild anemia, mild leukopenia, and mild proteinuria are not indications for aggressive therapy if they are not accompanied by clinical symptoms. Far too often, high dosages of steroids have been maintained in anticipation of disease activity, when many times such exacerbations fail to appear or are mild. Indications of impending exacerbation are best appreciated by a careful history and physical examination at each visit. The physical findings of fever, rash, alopecia, pleuritic pain, and weakness are good indicators of disease instability. The extent of instability can be measured and confirmed by a host of laboratory determinations, but the most significant are the hemoglobin, white blood count, urinalysis, third component of complement level, and DNA antibody titer. Periodic laboratory studies are easily obtained and are essential to effective management. In these days of escalating health care costs, it is seldom justified to routinely order all available laboratory tests that reflect LE activity. The clinician should order tests appropriate to the type of LE and expand the cost of care only in instances of particular organ involvement, such as LE nephritis, when additional data such as creatinine clearance, 24-hour urinary protein excretion, and levels of several serum complement components are desirable. If CNS LE is suspected, a baseline brain scan, electroencephalogram, and spinal fluid examination for IgG, anti-DNA binding, culture, and cerebrospinal fluid may be indicated, as discussed previously.

Assessing fever in the lupus patient is a special problem. Although a flare in lupus activity commonly causes the fever, it is hazardous to increase steroid therapy before examining the patient for streptococcal pharyngitis, urinary tract infection, bacterial pneumonia, tuberculosis, and subacute bacterial endocarditis. Throat, blood, urine, and sputum cultures should be obtained when indicated. Unusual infections with opportunistic fungi and bacteria also must be considered in the critically ill patient. Sepsis is more emergent than SLE so it is sometimes justified, even in the absence of identifiable organisms, to treat the patient empirically with a broad-spectrum antibiotic and to institute increased immunosuppressive therapy a few days later if there has been no clinical response.

Patients with chronic scarring discoid skin lesions have a benign clinical course and seldom have multisystem involvement. In a recent analysis of 95 DLE patients, 80 were asymptomatic except for skin lesions and only 3 in this group had a positive ANA test. Of the 15 who had other manifestations of LE, 14 had a positive ANA, and 3 had a positive lupus band test. Two of these patients had membranous glomerulonephritis. The rare coexistence of chronic scarring skin lesions and lupus nephritis has not been studied enough to clarify the immunological status of the affected patients.

Although it is difficult to explain to an adolescent why the chronic scarring type of LE is preferable to other forms of the disease, the physician should try to convey its more favorable long-term prognosis. The skin lesions are never life-threatening, although they can be exceedingly destructive, psychologically crippling, and restrictive of many activities. Efforts should be made to arrest the local spread of lesions without disturbing the general immunological response of the patient, who may be localizing the disease in the skin. Daily administration of systemic steroids for nondisseminated chronic DLE is contraindicated since high doses for long periods are necessary for control. If there is rapid progression of the lesions, a short-term or alternate day course of oral corticosteroids is occasionally indicated. Intense local therapy with high potency topical corticosteroids, such as 0.5% triamcinolone acetonide cream or 0.05% fluocinonide cream or ointment, is administered seven or eight times daily. At night, some areas can be occluded with Saran Wrap held in place by nonirritating paper tape to enhance the local absorption of the steroid. The use of triamcinolone acetonide 0.5% in USP flexible collodion is helpful in sites where occlusive dressings are not practical. Intralesional injection of triamcinolone acetonide can be useful in selected patients. Injections generally are given at 3- to 4-week intervals to permit assessment of benefits before repeating the treatment. Occasionally, dermal atrophy results but it is usually reversible with time. However, noninjected lesions can heal with scarring, and some attempt should be made to decrease the inflammation in the lesion.

The use of antimalarials to control the cutaneous and articular manifestations of LE has been limited ever since the numerous reports of ocular toxicity that appeared in the 1960s. Chloroquine derivatives accumulate slowly in the tissues of the body and in the retina, causing secondary degeneration of rods and cones. If the macular area is damaged, visual acuity is markedly reduced.

The effectiveness of antimalarials has been well documented. There is a high incidence of relapse with discontinuation of therapy; thus, the majority of patients have required repeated courses or long-term maintenance. In selected patients, however, especially those with sudden flares of activity in old lesions accompanied by the development of new ones, it is tempting to offer the benefits of these drugs. Ocular toxicity using hydroxychloroquine is rarely encountered in a cooperative patient, if new low-dosage regimens are strictly adhered to and frequent ophthalmological evaluations are performed. Every patient is required to have a baseline opthalmological evaluation before initiation of therapy and at 4-month intervals thereafter. Protective sunglasses should be worn in direct sunlight. Quinacrine (Atabrine) has a low incidence of ocular toxicity, but many patients find the yellow discoloration of the skin cosmetically unacceptable. All these drugs also have to be monitored carefully to prevent other side effects, such as aplastic anemia and exfoliative erythroderma, which were more common years ago when higher dosages were employed.

Subacute, erythematous, scaly LE skin lesions respond more readily to topically applied high potency steroids than do chronic discoid lesions. Again, fluocinonide cream, ointment, or gel may be applied in a thin film at frequent intervals and covered with Saran Wrap at night when practical.

The erythematous, edematous eruption of the cheeks and bridge of the nose in acute SLE usually responds promptly to the daily high dosages of systemic steroids needed to suppress the extracutaneous activity. The topical application of high potency steroids often is not required. In fact, the use of these preparations is not advised because many patients continue to treat the residual slight erythema and telangiectasis present in the previously acutely involved area. After several months, these patients may develop a persistent steroid-induced, acneiform eruption that can be very resistant to therapy, requiring administration of low-dosage tetracycline and topical acne preparations for resolution. In addition, long-term topical, high potency, steroid preparations can induce further atrophic changes. Only low or medium strength steroid creams, such as 1% or 2.5% hydrocortisone should be used to suppress the erythema. Unscented, bland, lubricating skin lotions and creams should be prescribed if the patient complains of pruritus.

The use of appropriate cosmetic foundations and creams can effectively conceal residual damage to the face. An explanation and demonstration of the wide variety of lotions, creams, and gels available to achieve a natural look will usually be accepted even by the teenager who initially resists the idea of cosmetics. For those patients with marked alteration in pigmentation, a water-resistant cosmetic preparation (Cover Mark) can be compounded to blend with their normal skin color. Sometimes, it is very rewarding to realize that the few minutes invested in teaching the mechanics of camouflage can spare the patient some of the agonizing depression associated with the cosmetic problems induced by LE.

It is beyond the scope of this chapter to discuss the management of noncutaneous aspects of LE except to reemphasize the increasingly good prognosis of all forms of SLE. The arthritic manifestations often can be controlled by the administration of analgesics. Aspirin has been incriminated recently as a cause of toxic hepatitis in LE but this complication is reversible. In more severe arthritis, or with LE pleuritis and pericarditis, the more judicious use of steroids and the introduction of alternate-day steroid therapy have greatly reduced drug-associated mobidity. In lupus nephritis and vasculitis with CNS manifestations, many regimens are now under investigation. The addition of cytotoxic drugs, cyclophosphamide and azathioprine, with concomitant reduction of steroid dosage, has become a widely accepted therapy, although there are still treatment failures and considerable debate about the effectiveness of such combined programs. But just as it has taken many years to perfect the methods for optimally administering steroids, it may be that more successful regimens will be developed for immunosuppressive agents. A combination of chemotherapy and steroid "pulse" therapy, such as is used in the control of malignancy, may eventually be applicable to LE patients. In selected patients, plasmapheresis, dialysis, and renal transplantation have been used successfully, even with severe and rapid renal deterioration.

Since lupus erythematosus may reflect nonspecific tissue injury with release of endogenous antigens, such as DNA, which cannot be normally processed by the immunologically crippled host, current research efforts to improve therapy are now being directed toward a restoration of competent host response and a reduction of chronic antigen stimulation. Pharmacological manipulation of B and T cell populations (killer, memory, suppressor, regulator, and helper cells) may play a major role in combatting autoimmune, viral, and malignant disorders in the future. SLE may not have a single cause or a simple antidote. Future progress in overall management certainly will be facilitated by identification of subtypes of LE patients by specific clinical manifestations and serological markers. If these subtypes are homogeneous, it will permit a more appropriate selection of pharmacological agents, so that the end result of therapy will be more predictable.

References

1. Canoso, J.J., Cohen, A.S.: A review of the use, evaluations, and criticisms of the preliminary criteria for the classification of systemic lupus erythematosus. Arthritis Rheum., 22: 917, 1979.
2. Decker, J.L.: Systemic lupus erythematosus: evolving concepts. Ann. Intern. Med., 91: 587, 1979.
3. Dimant, J., Ginzler, E., Schlesinger, M., Sterba, G., Diamond, H., Kaplan, D., and Weiner, M.: The clinical significance of Raynaud's phenomenon in systemic lupus erythematosus. Arthritis Rheum. 22: 815, 1979.
4. Fries, J. F., and Holman, H.R.: *Systemic Lupus Erythematosus; A Clinical Analysis.* W.B. Saunders, Philadelphia, 1975.
5. Morris, R.J., Guggenheim, S.J., McIntosh, R.M., Rubin, R.L., and Kohler, P.: Simultaneous immunologic studies of skin and kidney in systemic lupus erythematosus. Arthritis Rheum. 22: 864, 1979.
6. Moses, S., and Barland, P.: Laboratory criteria for a diagnosis of systemic lupus erythematosus. JAMA, 242: 1039, 1979.
7. Reichlin, M.: Newly defined serologic systems in systemic lupus erythematosus and dermatomyositis. Int. J. Dermatol., 18: 602, 1979.
8. Small, P., Mass, M.F., Kohler, P.F., and Harbeck, R.J.: Central nervous system involvement in SLE. Arthritis Rheum., 20: 869, 1979.

CHAPTER 16

BLISTERING DISORDERS

NANCY L. FUREY

A variety of pathologic events can lead to the formation of blisters in the skin. Different pathophysiologic mechanisms result in a limited morphologic expression; therefore, classification based on clinical or histologic criteria alone give us little insight into the cause of these disorders. Such a classification, however, is useful in differential diagnosis. A diverse group of unrelated disorders that are associated with blister formation are listed in Table 16.1.

In some of these disorders, such as lichen planus and lupus erythematosus, blister formation is rare and these patients have other more characteristic skin lesions or physical findings. Other blistering eruptions are caused by infectious agents; most common are bullous impetigo and staphylococcal scalded skin syndrome. The onset of these lesions is abrupt and accompanied by fever and malaise suggesting an infection. Routine bacterial cultures quickly confirm the diagnosis. Viral agents, herpes zoster and herpes simplex, commonly induce vesicles in the epidermis. Disorders such as epidermolysis bullosa dystrophica are present at birth and are more properly discussed as a genodermatosis.

There remains, however, a specific group of vesiculobullous disorders of unknown etiology that has been recognized by clinicians for centuries as having similar clinical features and causing confusion in differential diagnosis (Table 16.2). Historically, pemphigus was the term used for all of these blistering eruptions and a variety of adjectives were added to the term to describe various clinical forms. Re-

cently, specific criteria have been recognized that have helped to define the disorders (Table 16.3). The nomenclature is changing even today as new laboratory methods are used to identify specific abnormalities characteristic of each disorder. For simplification, only the most current terminology of these disorders is given. This classification is arbitrary and many other classifications for this group are currently being used.

PEMPHIGUS VULGARIS

Very early, it was recognized that one type of blistering eruption differed from all others in that it had a fulminant course with a high mortality rate. In 1943, Civatte clearly distinguished this life-threatening eruption by one specific pathologic finding. He noted that the blister formed above the basal cell layer and single epidermal cells became detached and were seen lying free in the blister cavity (acantholysis). This finding was confirmed by others, and pemphigus vulgaris was the first of the chronic blistering disorders to be clearly defined by laboratory as well as clinical criteria. All the other disorders classified with the pemphigus group show similar pathologic and immunopathologic features.

Clinical Manifestations. Pemphigus vulgaris is rare and although it occurs worldwide in patients of many ethnic origins, it is more common in Jews. Almost all Jewish patients with pemphigus who have been studied are HLA-DRW4 positive. There is no sex predi-

Table 16.1
Histologic Classification of Blistering Disorders

Blisters	Classification
Intraepidermal	
Subcorneal	Pemphigus foliaceous, pemphigus erythematosus
	Bullous impetigo, staphylococcal scalded skin syndrome
	Subcorneal pustular dermatosis
	Miliaria crystallina
Prickle cell layer	Dyshidrotic eczema
	Viral blisters (herpes simplex, herpes zoster, varicella)
	Hailey and Hailey
	Miliaria rubra
Suprabasal	Pemphigus vulgaris, pemphigus vegetans
	Darier's disease
	Transient acantholytic dermatosis
Basal cell layer	Erythema multiforme (epidermal)
	Toxic epidermal necrolysis
	Lupus erythematosus
	Lichen planus
	Epidermolysis bullosa simplex
Dermalepidermal junction zone blisters	
	Bullous pemphigoid
	Cicatricial pemphigoid
	Herpes gestationis
	Epidermolysis bullosa acquisita
	IgA bullous dermatosis adult
	IgA bullous dermatosis child
	Dermatitis herpetiformis
	Erythema multiforme (dermal)
	Epidermolysis bullosa letalis (Herlitz type)
	Epidermolysis bullosa dystrophica
	Porphyria cutanea tarda
	Lichen sclerosis et atrophicus
	Steroid purpura
	Senile purpura

lection. Adults 40–60 years of age are most susceptible, but pemphigus has been reported in children. The initial lesions of pemphigus may be confined to small areas of skin or mucous membranes for months before generalized blistering occurs. About 60% of patients initially present with oral lesions and oral lesions are found in 90% of the patients at some time during the course of the illness. Other mucous membranes that may be involved include the pharynx, esophagus, larynx, conjunctiva, urethra, vulva, cervix, and rectal mucosa. No other organs except the skin and mucous membranes are affected. Characteristically, the blisters rupture easily, are very slow to heal, and result in denuded areas of skin (Fig. 16.1). If the clinically normal skin of a patient is rubbed with a finger, the epidermis may slide off (Nikolsky's sign). This phenomenon also may occur in extensive bullous pemphigoid, erythema multiforme, and toxic epidermal necrolysis and, thus, is not specific for pemphigus. Healing occurs with only slight atrophy and mottled hypopigmentation and hyperpigmentation.

Oral cavity blisters appear as painful persistent erosions or collapsed bullae, or both. There is usually considerable necrotic sloughed tissue still attached. The gingiva, palate, and buccal mucosa are the most se-

Table 16.2
Vesiculobullous Disorders of Unknown Etiology

Pemphigus
    Pemphigus vulgaris, pemphigus vegetans
    Pemphigus foliaceous, pemphigus erythematosus
Bullous pemphigoid
Herpes gestationis
Cicatricial pemphigoid and localized cicatricial pemphigoid
Epidermolysis bullosa acquisita
IgA bullous dermatosis
    Adult
    Child (chronic bullous dermatosis childhood)
Dermatitis herpetiformis
Erythema multiforme
    Erythema multiforme simplex
    Erythema multiforme major (Stevens-Johnson syndrome)
Toxic epidermal necrolysis

verely involved. Oral lesions are difficult to heal and sometimes persist even though the cutaneous disease has been completely controlled.

Pathology and Immunology. A biopsy of a skin blister shows a characteristic cleft above the basal cell layer. Acantholysis or breaking apart of the prickle cells caused by loss of cell adhesion is a prominent feature (Fig. 16.2). A Tzank preparation has been used as a screening cytologic test in the past. Scrapings are taken from the floor of the blister and stained to show the acantholytic cells. However, this procedure cannot be relied upon for diagnosis since acantholysis is not specific for pemphigus.

The diagnosis of pemphigus is confirmed by direct immunofluorescence (IF) studies. In this procedure, a skin biopsy is obtained from skin adjacent to a blister, where the epidermis is still intact. A blister should not be biopsied because the epidermis is usually lost in processing. The specimen is snap frozen in liquid nitrogen or put into a special transport medium and sent to an immunopathology laboratory. Sections of pemphigus skin stained with fluorescein-tagged antihuman IgG and the third component of complement show deposition of IgG and C3 on epidermal cell membranes producing a honeycomb-like staining referred to as intercellular staining (Fig. 16.3). Indirect immunofluorescence testing of the patient's serum or blister fluid detects a pemphigus antibody which reacts with epithelial cell membranes of most species; monkey esophagus is most commonly used.

Direct immunofluorescence testing is extremely valuable in patients without intact blisters and in patients with only erosive lesions of the mucous membranes. This latter group of patients with only mouth lesions may not have detectable serum antibody but will show typical staining if direct immunofluorescence antibody studies are done on mucous membrane tissue. Without the use of immunopathologic techniques, these patients with oral lesions may go unrecognized until more extensive skin involvement occurs. Early detection is desirable since the disease is easier to control in the initial stages.

Repeated measurement of the titer of serum antibody as a guide to therapy is advocated by many clinicians but challenged by others. A generalization may be made that patients without serum antibodies usually have milder disease and need less aggressive therapy. Those with very high titers have very extensive involvement and need close supervision. However, many exceptions have been demonstrated. The use of antibody titers to monitor therapy is very useful for most patients but may not be justified for all patients. Usually, with clinical control of the disease, the serum antibody titer falls. Repeated determinations of antibody titer help prevent continuation of high dose maintenance steroid and immunosuppressive therapy.

The cause of pemphigus remains elusive but specific immunologic mechanisms active in the production of the blisters have been identified. The antigens involved in pemphigus are epidermal cell surface-bound antigens and have specific physicochemical properties. The antigens are glycoprotein (MW 68,000) polypeptides with sulfur-hydryl residues. The pemphigus antibody sites are moveable in the cell membranes of the lower malpighian layers but are immobile in the upper layers.

Culture of skin explants enriched with serum from pemphigus patients results in the production of pemphigus-like lesions. The serum factor capable of inducing acantholysis or loss of epidermal cell adhesion is an IgG antibody. This process is not complement mediated. One theory is that the antibody causes epidermal cell death, leakage of hydrolytic enzymes and disintegration of cell-to-cell bridging. However, studies using mouse epidermal cell cultures show that, in the presence of IgG pemphigus antibody, the cultured cells do not stratify and normal cell-to-cell adhesion is lost. This in vitro destruction of cell-to-cell adhesion may be due to the activation of a normal epidermal neutral serine protease enzyme. The effect of pemphigus antibody on epidermal monolayers can be blocked by adding inhibitors of this enzyme. Thus a noncomplement-mediated, antibody-dependent pathogenic mechanism is capable of producing epidermal cell acantholysis.

Therapy. In the past few years, it has been demonstrated that most pemphigus patients are successfully managed and have a

Table 16.3
Bullous Disorders of the Skin: Diagnostic Features[a]

Disorder	Special Clinical Features	Histology of Blister	Direct IMF Staining of Periblister Skin	Serum Antibody to Skin
Pemphigus Vulgaris	Generalized vesiculobullous lesions; HLA-DW4; mouth lesions common; high morbidity	Suprabasilar, acantholytic	IC, *IgG*[b]; C3	IC, IgG
Vegetans	Lesions become papillomatous then heal	Suprabasilar, acantholytic	IC, *IgG*	IC, IgG
Foliaceous	Chronic superficial flaccid blisters	Subcorneal	IC, IgG subcorneal	IC, IgG
Erythematosus	Lesions on face, upper chest	Subcorneal	IC, IgG & BMZ	IC, ANA
Pemphigoid Bullous Pemphigoid	Tense vesiculobullous lesions; mouth lesions 30%; morbidity variable	Subepidermal	C3, IgG, IgM, IgA linear BMZ	Linear BMZ IgG (60%)
Herpes gestationis	Papulovesiculobullous lesions during pregnancy; postpartum remission	Subepidermal	C3, IgG linear BMZ	Linear BMZ IgG, uncommon
Cicatricial pemphigoid	Chronic, erosive scarring lesions; oral, eye, genital lesions common; remissions rare	Subepidermal	C3, *IgG*, IgA, IgM linear BMZ	Linear BMZ IgG (rare)
Epidermolysis bullosa acquisita	Bullae, atrophic scars, milia produced by mild trauma, dystrophic nails, adult onset, no family history	Subepidermal	C3, IgG, IgM, IgA linear BMZ	Linear BMZ IgG (rare)
IgA bullous dermatosis, childhood	Vesiculobullous lesions in childhood; central face, lower trunk, genitalia; self-limited course, spontaneous remission	Subepidermal	*IgA*, C3, linear BMZ	
IgA bullous dermatosis, adult	Vesiculobullous lesions; no typical distribution; no association with gluten sensitive enteropathy; response to sulfones variable	Subepidermal	*IgA*, C3, linear BMZ	

Disease	Clinical features	Histopathology	IMF	ANA
Dermatitis Herpetiformis	Papulovesicular lesions, extensor surfaces of extremities; severe pruritus chronic, recurrent course, HLA-B8, DW3 associated with gluten sensitive enteropathy	Subepidermal blister; dermal papillae microabscesses	Perilesional & normal skin; *IgA* & C3 in papillary tips	None
Erythema Multiforme Simplex	Recurrent episodes of maculopapulo-vesiculobullous and target-like skin lesions	Subepidermal blister; vasculitis	*C3*, *IgM* in dermal vessels	None
Stevens-Johnson syndrome	Vesiculobullous skin and mucous membrane lesions (oral, eye, genitalia, etc.)		Not determined	None
Toxic epidermal necrolysis	Generalized skin and mucous membrane bullous lesions with extensive areas of denuded skin	Necrosis of epidermis	Not determined	None

[a] The abbreviations used are BMZ, basement membrane zone; IMF, immunofluorescence; IC, intercellular area of epidermis; ANA, antinuclear antibody.
[b] Predominant immune reactant italic.

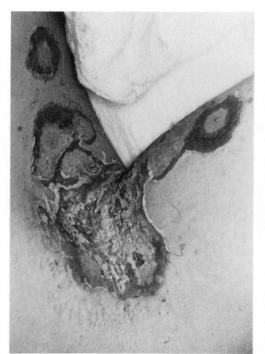

Fig. 16.1. Pemphigus vulgaris. Flaccid ruptured bullae and erosions of the skin of the axilla.

long clinical remission. Currently, there are a variety of therapeutic regimens available which must be individualized to the particular needs of the patient. Patients with early mild disease, especially limited to the oral cavity, may be managed by moderate (40 mg) single dose daily, or by alternate-day equivalent dose of prednisone. More extensive disease requires daily, high (80–160 mg) divided dosage of prednisone therapy or combination immunosuppressive therapy using azathioprine or cyclophosphamide. Plasmapheresis alone or in combination with immunosuppressive therapy is currently being evaluated in the management of difficult patients. Gold therapy is also useful to control some patients who have steroid-aggravated complications. Long-term complications of these therapeutic regimens have yet to be determined.

To achieve the best therapeutic results, it is important to adequately control the blistering phenomenon as soon as possible after the diagnosis is made. If the disease is extensive, combination prednisone and azathioprine or prednisone and cyclophosphamide therapy is

indicated, so that in 4–6 weeks the steroid dosage may be tapered. Drug toxicity, bone marrow suppression, and septicemia are the major life-threatening early complications. Both the skin exudate and blood should be cultured at frequent intervals to anticipate intercurrent infection. Isolation procedures are mandatory to protect these patients with impaired defense mechanisms.

The skin and oral cavity should be meticulously cleansed several times daily to remove the necrotic epidermis that clings tenaciously to the partially denuded epithelium. The continuous exudation provides an ideal substrate for bacterial growth. Debris is carefully removed from the oral cavity after each meal and washed with dilute hydrogen peroxide. To decrease the discomfort of eating, diluted Benadryl Elixer can be held in the mouth for a few minutes prior to eating a liquid or soft diet.

PEMPHIGUS VEGETANS

Pemphigus vegetans was first described by Neumann in 1869 to describe a very rare clinical varient of pemphigus in which the lesions, especially in the intertriginous areas, appear as an exuberant growth of granulation tissue at the site of a previous blister. The areas may become verrucous and form pink papillomas. Histologic sections show acanthosis, papillomatosis and, occasionally, an area of acantholytic blister formation. Immunofluorescence studies of biopsy material and serum are similar to pemphigus vulgaris.

PEMPHIGUS FOLIACEOUS

Pemphigus foliaceous was recognized as a clinical form of pemphigus by Cazenave in 1844. He reported that the "bullae flow together, break as soon as they have formed and cover large areas with small scales, resembling the flakes of fine pastry." The lesions of pemphigus foliaceous are very superficial and often appear as scaly, crusted, eczematoid plaques or as an exfoliative dermatitis. A characteristic musty odor is usually noted. The characteristic pathology of a very early

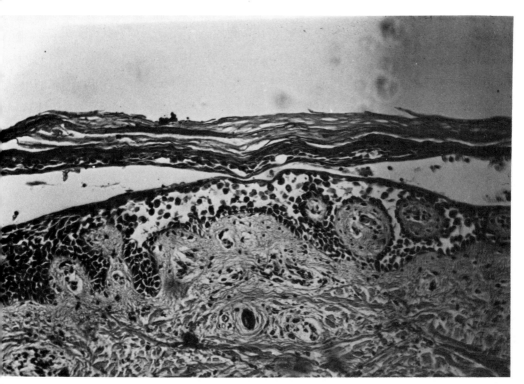

Fig. 16.2. Pemphigus vulgaris. Suprabasal bulla formation with acantholytic cells in the cavity (×210).

lesion is a subcorneal blister with acantholytic cells. The immunopathology of the lesions in most patients is similar to pemphigus vulgaris except that the antibody reacts specifically with antigens present in the intercellular spaces of the subcorneal layer, the site of the earliest histologic lesion. Indirect immunofluorescence findings are identical to pemphigus vulgaris. The course of pemphigus foliaceous is more benign than vulgaris and responds more readily to prednisone therapy. Occasionally, combined immunosuppressive therapy is needed.

PEMPHIGUS ERYTHEMATOSUS

In 1926, Senear and Usher described another rare varient of pemphigus in patients whose lesions appeared mainly in scalp, face, and upper trunk. This entity combines features of pemphigus and lupus erythematosus. Most clinicians believe pemphigus erythematosus represents a localized form of pemphigus foliaceous. The immunopathology has been reported to be similar to pemphigus vulgaris but, in addition, antinuclear antibody has been detected in the serum, and deposition of IgG along the basement membrane has been demonstrated. Several instances of pemphigus erythematosus and lupus erythematosus occurring in the same patient have been documented. Pemphigus erythematosus also has been associated with thymoma and myasthenia gravis.

PEMPHIGOID

The pemphigoid group of blistering disorders is the most difficult to classify. Pemphigoid is the term that has come into usage to indicate the subepidermal blistering disorders that also have deposition of immunoglobulin and/or complement along the basement membrane zone of the epidermis. Some of the

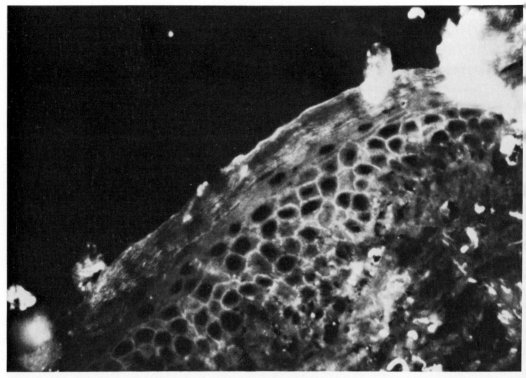

Fig. 16.3. Pemphigus vulgaris. Positive direct immunofluorescence staining (IgG) of the intercellular area of the epidermis of a pemphigus patient (×335).

disorders are also characterized by the presence of a serum antibody to the basement membrane zone of the skin.

Bullous pemphigoid and cicatricial pemphigoid are closely associated immunologically but differ clinically in that bullous pemphigoid generally spares mucous membranes and does not heal with scarring, while cicatricial pemphigoid has a predilection for mucous membranes and characteristically resolves with severe scarring. Herpes gestationis is clinically, pathologically, and immunologically similar to bullous pemphigoid but is unique in that it can be provoked by estrogens, is associated with pregnancy, and resolves completely after the last pregnancy. Epidermolysis bullosa acquista and cicatricial pemphigoid have many common features but are distinguished by the extensive cutaneous involvement of the former and different site of blister formation by electron microscopic examination. The inclusion of IgA bullous dermatosis in the child and the adult is based merely on similar clinical and immunologic features, but

the predominant class of immunoglobulin involved differs from bullous pemphigoid and may reflect the presence of a totally different pathogenetic mechanism. As they are further investigated, these patients may be classified quite differently. In all these varieties of "pemphigoid," the clinical presentation and laboratory findings vary sufficiently to suggest that either different pathogenetic mechanisms are operative or that the host's immunologic defenses are different when challenged by the same causative agent.

BULLOUS PEMPHIGOID

Clinical Manifestations. Bullous pemphigoid (BP) is a relatively benign, self-limited disease with a duration rarely exceeding 5 years. The disease is most common in the elderly but has been reported in children. There is no sex or ethnic predisposition. In the typical patient, the initial lesions are large tense bullae filled with clear serum. After 24 hours, the blister fluid becomes cloudy or hemorrhagic. The blisters arise in normal or erythematous skin (Fig. 16.4). Recurrent crops of lesions may remain localized for weeks but most often they become generalized. Oral lesions occur, but are less severe than pemphigus vulgaris and rarely occur initially. The blisters in the mouth often remain intact, unlike pemphigus in which the roof easily ruptures. Other mucous membranes including the esophagus and vagina may occasionally be involved. Pruritus may or may not be present.

The clinical presentation of bullous pemphigoid unfortunately can be highly variable, and a diagnosis based on clinical presentation and routine histologic findings is not reliable. Some patients present with erythematous plaques and urticarial lesions more suggestive of erythema multiforme. Other patients present with only small vesicles, sometimes even herpetiform, and are initially thought to have dermatitis herpetiformis. The clinical differentiation between dermatitis herpetiformis, bullous pemphigoid, and erythema multiforme is sometimes impossible and immunologic studies should be done so that the correct disease is recognized.

Pathology and Immunopathology. There are no histopathologic features unique to bullous pemphigoid to differentiate this disorder from dermatitis herpetiformis or erythema multiforme. Since all these disorders have a subepidermal blister (Fig. 16.5) and a variable inflammatory infiltrate, the definitive diagnosis of bullous pemphigoid should be based on direct immunofluorescence studies of a biopsy of skin taken adjacent to a blister. The third component of complement and IgG is found deposited in a linear pattern along the basement membrane zone. Frequently, only complement is found. Ultrastructural studies show that the deposits are in the lamina lucida, between the basal cell plasma membrane and the basal lamina.

A serum antibody to the basement membrane zone (BMZ) is detected in approximately 60% of patients (Fig. 16.6). Serial determinations during the course of the disease show that no correlation exists between the titer and the clinical activity. Some patients with generalized bullae have no detectible serum antibody. The bullous pemphigoid antibody, if detected, is usually of the IgG class and can fix complement. Immune complexes have been identified in the serum and in the

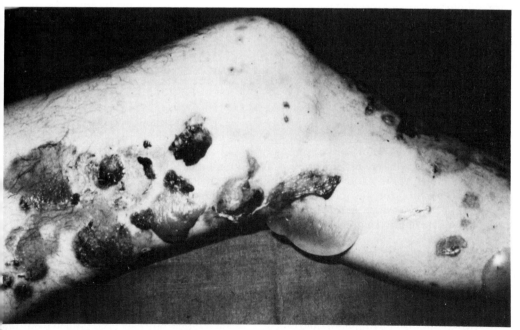

Fig. 16.4.   Bullous pemphigoid. Large, tense bullae: filled with clear or hemorrhagic serum.

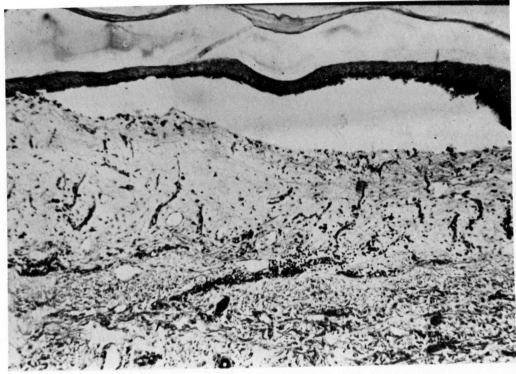

Fig. 16.5. Bullous pemphigoid. Subepidermal bulla formation (×84).

blister fluid in bullous pemphigoid but the significance of this finding has yet to be determined.

Therapy. Patients with localized bullous pemphigoid can be treated with topical steroids, intralesional triamcinolone injections, or alternate-day prednisone. If the lesions are generalized, moderate dosages of daily prednisone (40 mg) are usually needed initially, then, gradually alternate daily therapy can be introduced. If the eruption is severe and recalcitrant to steroids or if the patient has diabetes mellitus, combination therapy with cytoxan or azathioprine and prednisone can be used. The majority of patients with bullous pemphigoid will obtain complete remission of their disease.

The association of bullous pemphigoid and malignancy has been the subject of many case reports. Analysis of the data comparing age-matched controls fails to support this association. However, any patient who develops generalized bullous pemphigoid deserves a complete history and physical examination and appropriate laboratory studies to try to find a triggering factor. In any case, such an evaluation is needed before beginning daily steroid therapy to anticipate possible complications.

HERPES GESTATIONIS

Herpes gestationis is a rare vesiculobullous eruption in pregnancy. The incidence has been estimated to be 1 in 30,000 deliveries. The clinical manifestations, pathology, and immunologic features are similar to bullous pemphigoid and herpes gestationis and may simply represent a variant. Perhaps a better name would be gestational pemphigoid.

Clinical Manifestations. The clinical lesions are variable and include discrete vesicles, grouped vesicles, erosions, crusts, erythematous urticarial plaques, and large tense bullae. The eruption is usually very pruritic. The symptoms often begin during the fifth month of pregnancy but can occur during the first trimester and during the first few postpartum menstrual periods.

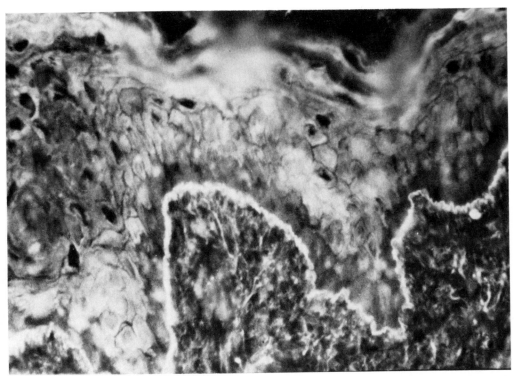

Fig. 16.6. Bullous pemphigoid. Positive indirect immunofluorescence staining (IgG) of the basement membrane zone of human skin (×335).

Pathology and Immunopathology. The immunopathology of perilesional skin is similar to bullous pemphigoid and shows deposition of C3 at the BMZ with concomitant IgG deposition in approximately 30% of patients. Occasionally IgA and IgM have been noted.

Newborns of mothers with herpes gestationis occasionally have a similar transient rash, and the immunopathology of these skin lesions have shown C3 along the basement membrane zone. The antibody readily crosses the placenta. This type of self-limited newborn syndrome has been described in other immunologic disorders such as myasthenia gravis. Fetal wastage is increased and there is an increased incidence of premature deliveries.

Although herpes gestationis is similar to bullous pemphigoid, clinically and immunologically there are several differences which must be resolved before the two entities are considered to be the same with identical pathogenetic mechanisms. Herpes gestationis is restricted to pregnancy, is provoked by estrogens or progesterones, and ultrastructural studies suggest that the blister in herpes gestationis may occur slightly higher, since the basal cell layer is usually destroyed.

Therapy. Systemic prednisone therapy is usually necessary to control the symptoms although there are some patients who can be managed with topical steroids and antihistamines. If daily dosages are needed for the mother during pregnancy, the newborn infant should be monitored for adrenal insufficiency.

CICATRICIAL PEMPHIGOID

The first case of cicatricial pemphigoid was probably reported by Wichmann in 1794 when he described a woman with chronic blisters of her eyes and mouth. The name, benign mucous membrane pemphigus, was proposed by Thost in 1917. He wished to emphasize that this type of blistering disorder was usually limited to mucous membranes and could lead to chronic scarring of the eyes and mouth but, unlike pemphigus, was not life-threatening. Pathologic studies by Civatte in 1949 showed that the blister was subepidermal like pemphigoid instead of suprabasilar like pemphigus. This observation led to the changing of the name to benign mucous membrane pemphigoid. Cicatricial pemphigoid has been preferred recently, since the disease is not totally benign since it can cause blindness nor is it limited to the mucous membranes.

Clinical Manifestations. Cicatricial pemphigoid usually occurs in elderly persons and occurs in women more frequently than in men (2:1). The most commonly involved mucosal surfaces are, in order of frequency, the mouth, eyes, larynx, genitalia, and esophagus. Oral blisters may be intact but may be eroded and desquamative gingivitis can occur. Cutaneous lesions are present in 25% of patients and consist of scattered tense bullae or areas of erythema with recurring blisters and erosions which heal with atrophic scarring.

The course is chronic and progressive, and the final outcome of ocular pemphigoid is often blindness (Fig. 16.7). Severe laryngeal or esophageal involvement is rare, but stenosis requiring tracheostomy and strictures needing dilatation have been reported.

Pathology and Immunopathology. Biopsy of a lesion shows a subepidermal blister that is indistinguishable from bullous pemphigoid. Immunofluorescence studies show that IgG, C3, and an admixture of IgA and IgM are deposited along the BMZ of skin and mucous membrane lesions identical to bullous pemphigoid (Fig. 16.8). Immunoelectronmicroscopy studies show deposition of immune reactants in the lamina lucida as in bullous pemphigoid. A serum antibody is not commonly detected.

In patients with erosive gingivitis, scarring alopecia, or conjunctival erosions, direct immunofluorescence studies of the involved tissue is essential to confirm the diagnosis. The disorders that can be clinically confused with cicatricial pemphigoid include oral pemphi-

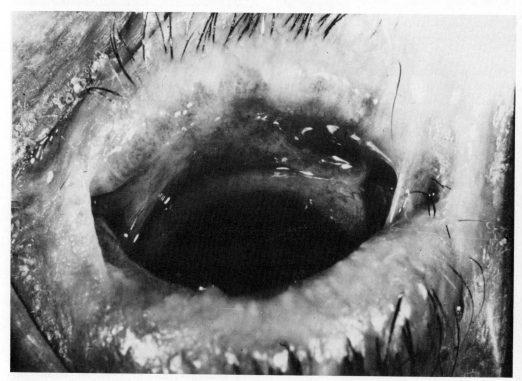

Fig. 16.7. Cicatricial pemphigoid. Conjunctival scarring with symblepharon formation and trichiasis.

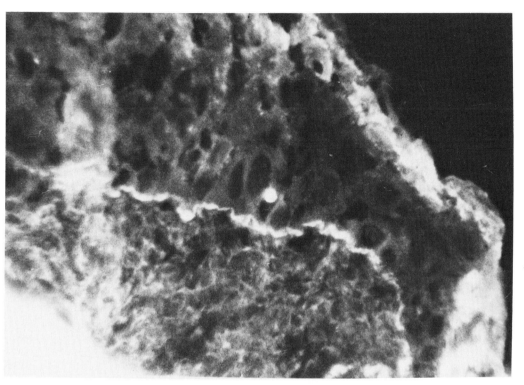

Fig. 16.8.   Cicatricial pemphigoid. Positive direct immunofluorescence staining (IgG) of the basement membrane zone of the conjunctiva of a patient with cicatricial pemphigoid (×335).

gus vulgaris, lichen planus, erythema multiforme, Behçet's disease, and nonspecific conjunctival erosions erroneously attributed to wearing contact lenses.

Therapy.   Since the course of the disease is protracted with little tendency for remission, continuous immunosuppressive and steroid therapy may not control the disease. Exceptions occur if there are esophageal or laryngeal strictures and if the disease is disabling. Eye complications, trichiasis, blepharitis, and dry eyes, should be carefully managed by an ophthalmologist. There are unconfirmed reports of milder forms of cutaneous cicatricial pemphigoid responding to sulfapyridine.

EPIDERMOLYSIS BULLOSA ACQUISITA

A nonhereditary form of epidermolysis bullosa was recognized by Elliot in 1895 and the word acquisita was added to emphasize this point by Kablitz in 1904. By definition epidermolysis bullosa acquista (EBA) is acquired, the onset usually occurs during adulthood and there is no family history. The bullae and erosions are produced by mild trauma especially over the joints of the hands, feet, elbows, and knees. The lesions heal with atrophic scars and milia. Nail dystrophy is common. Routine histology shows a subepidermal blister. Immunofluorescence studies of skin show deposition of IgG and/or C3 at the BMZ in all of the nine recently reported patients. One patient had detectable serum IgG and IgM BMZ antibody and had essential mixed (IgG-IgM) cryoglobulinemia.

The exact nosology of this entity is still uncertain. This disease has many features seen in cicatricial pemphigoid including scarring lesions, high incidence of oral lesions, and immunopathology studies compatible with the pemphigoid group of disorders. However, more widespread cutaneous lesions, the propensity to develop traumatic blisters over joints, and dystrophic nail lesions are characteristic of EBA. Preliminary immunoelectron microscopic studies show that the site of immunoglobulin deposition is below the basal lamina in contrast to cicatricial pemphigoid in which the immune reactants are in the lamina lucida. There is also a high incidence of associated autoimmune disorders, especially Crohn's disease. Many therapeutic agents, mostly steroids but also gold compounds, have been used with varying success in patients with EBA.

LINEAR IgA BULLOUS DERMATOSIS

A distinct group of patients have been described who have overlapping clinical, histologic, and immunologic features of both dermatitis herpetiformis and bullous pemphigoid. In adults, this entity has been called atypical dermatitis herpetiformis. In children, it has been known by a variety of descriptive terms including chronic bullous dermatosis of childhood, atypical dermatitis herpetiformis with linear IgA, juvenile dermatitis herpetiformis, mixed bullous pemphigoid, dermatitis herpetiformis, and juvenile pemphigoid.

LINEAR IgA BULLOUS DERMATOSIS IN ADULTS

Linear deposition of IgA along the basement membrane in the skin has been described in a group of patients with papulovesicular lesions like dermatitis herpetiformis or with larger blisters of the type associated with bullous pemphigoid. These linear deposits are present in the lamina lucida and just beneath the basal lamina of the basement membrane. Routine histologic examination shows a subepidermal blister and is not diagnostic. The response to sulfones is variable. These patients do not have a gluten-sensitive enteropathy and the intestinal biopsies in six patients have been normal. The incidence of HLA-B8 is not significantly different from the normal population in contrast to dermatitis herpetiformis in which 90% of patients are HLA-B8.

LINEAR IgA BULLOUS DERMATOSIS IN CHILDREN

A unique blistering disorder has been recognized for many years which, although uncommon, occurs more frequently in children than bullous pemphigoid, dermatitis herpetiformis, or pemphigus vulgaris. The disease is usually seen in children of preschool age. The eruption is characterized by tense, clear, or hemorrhagic bullae. There are often many rosette-shaped lesions consisting of a ruptured crusted central blister surrounded by new smaller blisters. Many patients also have dry erythematous plaques with polycyclic margins bordered by intact bullae. The eruption is generalized but most of the lesions occur on the lower trunk, genital-crural areas, and central part of the face, especially around the mouth (Fig. 16.9). Pruritus is variable and may be completely absent or may be intense. The course is characterized by periodic remissions and decreasing frequency of exacerbations with ultimate remission within 2 or 3 years. This feature contrasts sharply with dermatitis herpetiformis where the patient may have exacerbations throughout life.

Histologic examination of a blister shows a nondiagnostic subepidermal blister. Microabscesses are sometimes seen in the dermal papillae. IgA is the immunoglobulin most commonly detected at the basement membrane zone. Less commonly, IgG, IgM, and C3 are found.

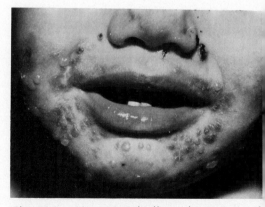

Fig. 16.9. Linear IgA bullous dermatosis of childhood. A preschool child with tense, clear, blisters around the mouth.

The immunofluorescence findings in IgA bullous dermatosis of childhood differ from the findings in dermatitis herpetiformis and bullous pemphigoid. The linear BMZ pattern is similar to bullous pemphigoid but IgA instead of IgG is found more consistently in bullous dermatosis of childhood. Circulating anti-BMZ antibody is rarely detected but in bullous pemphigoid approximately 60% of patients have serum IgG antibody. None of the children with large rosette-shaped lesions have had granular deposition of IgA in the dermal papillae, the characteristic finding in dermatitis herpetiformis. The incidence of intestinal mucosal changes in bullous dermatosis of childhood has not been determined.

The disease usually responds to sulfapyridine or sulfones, similar to dermatitis herpetiformis, but the response can be variable and, unlike dermatitis herpetiformis, corticosteroids are occasionally added to control the eruption.

DERMATITIS HERPETIFORMIS

In 1893, Duhring described a group of patients with a blistering disease of the skin characterized by a great variety of primary lesions of a herpetic nature and by severe itching and burning. Many entities other than dermatitis herpetiformis (DH) were probably included in this report. After sulfone therapy was found to dramatically suppress the eruption, it was widely used as a diagnostic test as well as a therapeutic agent. Recently, dermatitis herpetiformis has been found to have immunologic and genetic markers that have greatly helped in diagnosis, and sulfone responsiveness has been found to be an unreliable test.

Clinical Manifestations. The primary lesions of dermatitis herpetiformis are erythematous papules, urticarial plaques, or vesicles. If DH presents in its classic form, it is intensely pruritic and there are many grouped papulovesicular lesions that occur mostly on the extensor surfaces, elbows, knees, and buttocks, as well as the posterior nuchal area and scalp (Fig. 16.10, 16.11). It persists indefinitely, although for unknown reasons, the severity and treatment requirements vary from time to

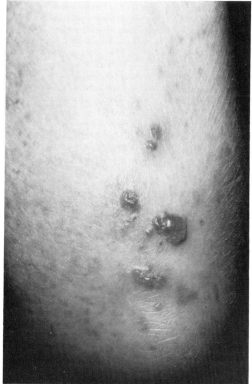

Fig. 16.10. Dermatitis herpetiformis. Grouped vesicular and bullous lesions on the elbow.

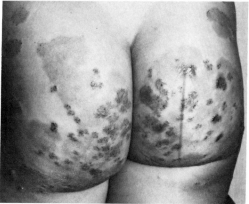

Fig. 16.11. Dermatitis herpetiformis. Grouped papulovesicular lesions on the buttocks.

time. The clinical presentation is highly variable and many patients with dermatitis herpetiformis present with only excoriations and crusted lesions with no primary intact lesions.

However, dry, excoriated skin is a common problem in office practice and most patients with severe pruritus and excoriations do not have DH.

Pathology and Immunopathology. Routine histologic study of a lesion shows a subepidermal blister with microabcesses in the dermal papillae (Fig. 16.12). However, the light microscopic findings are not sufficiently distinctive to differentiate dermatitis herpetiformis from bullous pemphigoid. Immunofluorescence studies of both perilesional and uninvolved skin of DH patients show IgA deposited in a granular pattern in the tips of the dermal papillae (Fig. 16.13). When repeated biopsies are done over a long period of time, even if the rash is in remission, IgA deposits are still detected. Immunoelectronmicroscopic studies have demonstrated that the IgA is localized in clumps closely associated with microfibrillar bundles within the dermal papillae.

DH patients do not have a detectable serum IgA antibody to microfibrillar structures. Serum IgA is elevated in less than 10% of patients. Low serum IgM levels have been reported in one-third of the patients with untreated DH and celiac disease. Complement components of both the alternate and the classic pathways are detected in DH skin. It has been postulated that activation of the alternate pathway of the complement system by IgA complexes is responsible for the skin lesions. However, it is difficult to reconcile this idea with the finding of complement in the skin of patients on a gluten-free diet, who have no active skin lesions.

The incidence of antireticulin antibody in DH is about 20%, in adult celiac disease 40%, and in childhood celiac disease 60%. It has been shown that the more severe the enteropathy is on biopsy of small intestine, the higher the incidence of antireticulin antibody. If the patient is treated with a gluten-free diet, the incidence is reduced, suggesting a cross-reactivity between gluten and reticulin. More than 90% of patients with celiac disease and patients with dermatitis herpetiformis (defined clinically and immunologically by the presence of IgA skin deposits) have HLA-B8-DW3, indicating there is a strong immunogenetic basis for the disease.

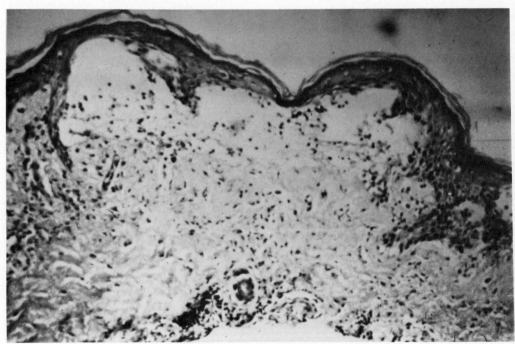

Figs. 16.12. Dermatitis herpetiformis. Subepidermal blister with microabscesses in the dermal papillae (×84).

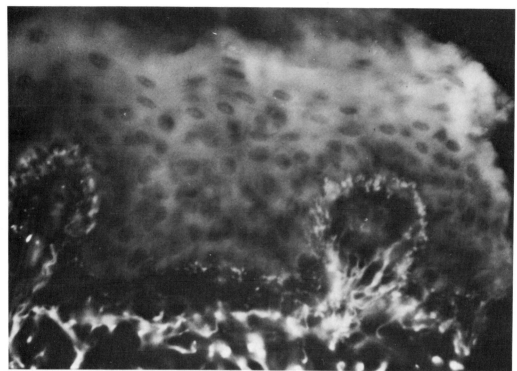

Fig. 16.13.   Dermatitis herpetiformis (DH). Positive direct immunofluorescence staining showing granular deposition of IgA in the dermal papillae of uninvolved skin of a patient with DH (×335).

Since skin lesions respond to gluten-free diet and relapse on introduction of gluten, gluten is responsible in a basic way for the disease. Antigliadin antibodies are thought to destroy epithelial cells of gut mucosa either by antibody mediated cytotoxicity or by immune complex deposition. Gliadin challenge causes an increase in local mucosal immunoglobulin synthesis with antigliadin specificity. Recent studies have demonstrated that a small, but significant amount of antigliadin antibodies forms stable immune complexes in vitro. Much effort has been expended to identify antibodies to wheat (gliadin) proteins and recently IgG antibodies to gliadin have been identified in 5 of 14 patients with DH. The triggering event in gluten-sensitive enteropathy may be the binding of gluten protein to lymphoid cells or to mucosal epithelial cells expressing HLA-B8, DW3 antigens. The binding of gluten may cause local production of gluten antibodies which could induce complement-mediated, antibody-induced cytotoxicity damaging intestinal epithelium.

In DH, the morphologic evidence of the enteropathy on gut biopsy is patchy. However, structural changes can be induced in a previously "normal looking" intestine by exposure to gluten suggesting gluten sensitivity may exist even if the intestine appears structurally normal. Essentially, all gut biopsies of DH patients show abnormal increased infiltration of lymphocytes in the lamina propria, even in the absence of flattened villae. Gluten-sensitive enteropathy has been found in over 90% of patients with DH but it is mild and rarely presents symptoms. Patients with DH can have increased fat excretion and deficient iron and folate levels similar to patients with celiac disease.

Therapy.   Both the enteropathy and skin lesions in DH are gluten dependent and most patients improve with a gluten-free diet. After elimination of gluten from the diet, sulfone therapy can be stopped or a significant reduction in the dose of dapsone is possible. If gluten is reintroduced, the skin lesions reappear within 1 week. In some patients, it may take a few years before dapsone can be totally discontinued. The most likely reason for failure of the rash to respond to the gluten-free diet, is that the diet is not strictly maintained.

ERYTHEMA MULTIFORME

In contrast to pemphigus, pemphigoid, and dermatitis herpetiformis, erythema multiforme is not a chronic bullous disorder but is acute and self-limited. It is often considered in the differential diagnosis at the onset of the other disorders, however, so it is important to recognize the specific clinical manifestations and immunologic features of erythema multiforme and its variants.

Bateman first described the target lesions in 1814 and Bazin recognized the prodromal symptoms and associated mucosal lesions in 1862. Hebra contributed the name when he described the multiform character of the eruption in 1866. The severe mucosal complications of the disorder were recognized by Stevens and Johnson in 1922.

ERYTHEMA MULTIFORME SIMPLEX

The distinctive clinical lesion of erythema multiforme simplex is the iris or target lesion (Fig. 16.14). This lesion is a dull red flat macule that can enlarge to about 2 cm over 48 hours. The periphery remains erythematous while the center either clears, becomes purpuric or, at times, becomes vesiculobullous and even necrotic. Target lesions usually de-

velop in an acral distribution on the extensor surfaces and on the palms and soles. Crops of lesions appear and recede over several weeks. Many patients also develop urticarial edematous wheals which persist for days but, unlike urticaria, are not pruritic and do not expand and disappear within hours. When vesicles and bullae occur (Fig. 16.15) the patient often develops mucosal lesions.

ERYTHEMA MULTIFORME MAJOR

Erythema multiforme major, or Stevens-Johnson syndrome as it is also known, is characterized by erosive bullae of the skin and mucous membranes as well as by significant constitutional symptoms. The prodrome consists of fever, malaise, and myalgia followed by the sudden appearance of erosive lesions of the oral mucosa, lips, and bulbar conjunctiva. The extent of the cutaneous lesions is variable. The eyes become coated with a gray-white exudative membrane and hemorrhagic crusts. The mucosal lesions can extend to involve the pharynx, larynx, esophagus, and genital mucosa. Ocular lesions can result in

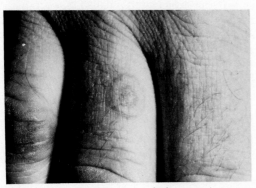

Fig. 16.14. Erythema multiforme. A target lesion on the finger.

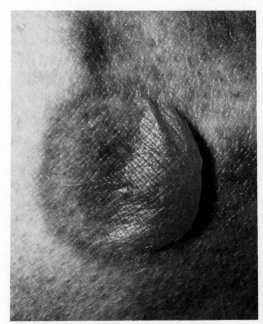

Fig. 16.15. Erythema multiforme. A bullous lesion.

corneal ulceration, panopthalmitis and even blindness. Less commonly, pneumonitis, diarrhea, polyarthritis, and otitis media are complications.

TOXIC EPIDERMAL NECROLYSIS

Toxic epidermal necrolysis (TEN) may in some instances represent the most severe form of erythema multiforme. The toxic epidermal necrolysis type of erythema multiforme is usually drug induced. Like erythema multiforme, the eruption is heralded by fever, malaise, and myalgia. A generalized painful violaceous erythema suddenly occurs and, within 24 hours, blisters and large areas of denuded skin appear. Characteristically, the erythematous areas are symmetrical and discrete with irregular borders. The bullae are flaccid and often not numerous. The striking findings are the large areas of denudation superimposed on an erythematous skin (Fig. 16.16). The Nikolsky sign is present. Erosive, desquamative oral lesions are common.

Differential Diagnosis. Erythema multiforme is a spectrum of disorders and does not represent a specific disease with a specific cause. Rather, it represents a hypersensitivity pattern of the epidermis and vasculature of the dermis and other organs to a variety of agents including drugs, viruses, bacteria, fungi, hormones, neoplasia, and a variety of miscellaneous conditions (Table 16.4). By far, drugs account for almost 50% of the episodes. Since this figure is based on circumstantial evidence, it may be high, for many drugs are given for prodromal symptoms. But Dilantin, barbiturates, and sulfonamides are well established precipitating agents.

In the patients with classic skin lesions of erythema multiforme, especially those who present with target lesions, the disorder is not easily confused with other problems. However, atypical cases may have lesions simulating chronic urticaria, necrotizing vasculitis, bullous pemphigoid, or toxic erythema from drugs or infection (secondary syphilis, chronic meningococcemia, subacute bacteria endocarditis, viral exanthems). If erythema multiforme is limited to the oral mucosa, the clinical presentation is not diagnostic but other possibilities are limited. These include cicatri-

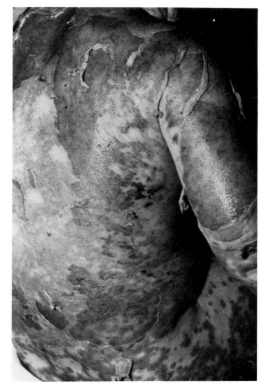

Fig. 16.16. Toxic epidermal necrolysis. Extensive denuded areas of skin with multiple discreet erythematous macular lesions.

cial pemphigus, pemphigus vulgaris, erosive lichen planus, Behçet's syndrome, and primary herpetic gingivostomatitis.

Pathology and Immunopathology. The pathology depends on the age and severity of the lesion biopsied. In early erythematous macules, only minimal dermal edema is present. There is a mixed lymphohistiocytic perivascular infiltrate and endothelial swelling. If the lesion is purpuric or bullous, the vascular changes are more striking, with pronounced papillary edema and spongiosis of the lower epidermis. As the papillary edema increases, a subepidermal cleft forms.

In bullous lesions, the epidermis is necrotic, and separates entirely from the dermis. The mononuclear infiltrate in the dermis is often sparse. These changes are similar to the findings in TEN. A frozen section of a peel of desquamated epidermis and a punch biopsy of skin can be done to confirm the diagnosis and to distinguish TEN from staphylococcal

Table 16.4
Some Factors Blamed for Causing Erythema Multiforme

Infections	Drugs
Viral	Antibiotics, especially penicillin
Adenovirus	Sulfonamides
Coxsackie virus	Anticonvulsants especially hydantoins
ECHO 9 virus	Barbiturates
Hepatitis	Antipyretics
Herpes simplex	Analgesics
Infectious mononucleosis	Gold salts
Influenza A	Hydralazine
Ornithosis	Nitrogen mustards
	Phenolphthalein
Mycoplasma pneumoniae	Phenylbutazone
Bacterial	
Gonorrhea	*Others*
Streptococcus hemolyticus	Physical factors
Staphylococcus	Cold
Tuberculosis	Sunlight
Vibrio parahaemolyticus	X-ray therapy
Trichomoniasis	Neoplasms
Fungus	Collagen-vascular disorders
Coccidioidomycosis	
Dermatophytosis	
Histoplasmosis	

scalded skin syndrome (SSSS). In TEN, the peel and the biopsy of skin shows full thickness of epidermis but in SSSS the biopsy shows a split high in the epidermis in the granular cell layer. However, to the experienced observer, the two entities are clinically quite dissimilar and histologic confirmation is rarely necessary.

Immunofluorescence studies of skin biopsies in early lesions of erythema multiforme may show deposits of IgM and complement in the dermal vessel walls. Direct immunofluorescence studies of skin biopsy material from drug-induced TEN have been inconclusive. Immune complexes and cryoprecipitins have been identified in the serum of a high percentage of patients with erythema multiforme. Current investigative evidence strongly suggests multiple agents (drugs, viruses, etc.) can trigger the formation of immune complexes. In selected individuals, perhaps those with immunologic incompetence manifested by depressed T cell function, complexes can be sequestered in the blood vessels of the superficial dermal plexus and activate the complement cascade and cause local tissue destruction.

Therapy. In mild cases of erythema multiforme, no specific treatment is necessary, the disease has a mild course and abates in 2–3 weeks. A search for the provocative agent should be made. Antihistamines are sometimes indicated but usually are not helpful.

The use of prednisone is still controversial. Prompt administration of corticosteroids may be helpful as an antiinflammatory agent. In moderately severe forms, when no provocative cause is found, corticosteroids, in tapering dosages, will abort recurrences and can be justified.

In the most severe forms, especially Stevens-Johnson type and also in toxic epidermal necrolysis, when large areas of skin are denuded, steroids may be harmful if administered late in the course of the disease because the patient's resistance to infection may be suppressed and wound healing can be delayed. Dedicated, skilled nursing care such as is found in a burn unit is essential for the survival of these patients who have lost large areas of full thickness epidermis. The main goal of therapy becomes the prevention of complications, to prevent secondary infection of denuded areas, and to maintain the patient's fluid and electrolyte balance.

References

1. Lever, W.F.: Pemphigus and pemphigoid, a review of the advances made since 1964. Am. Acad. Dermatol., *1:* 2, 1979.
2. O'Loughlin, S., Goldman, and G.C., Provost, T.T.: Fate of pemphigus antibody following successful therapy. Arch. Dermatol., *114:* 1769, 1978.
3. Judd, K.P., and Lever, W.F.: Correlation of antibodies in skin and serum with disease severity in pemphigus. Arch. Dermatol., *115:* 428, 1979.
4. Ruocco, V., Rossi, A., and Argenziano, G. et al.: Pathogenicity of the intercellular antibodies of pemphigus and their periodic removal from the circulation by plasmapheresis. Br. J. Dermatol. *98:* 237, 1979.
5. Chorzelski, T.P., Jablonska, S., and Beutner, E.H.: Pemphigoid. In E.H. Beutner et al. (Eds) *Immunopathology of the Skin*, p. 243. John Wiley & Sons, New York 1979.
6. Ahmed, A.R., Maize, J.C., and Provost, T.T.: Bullous pemphigoid, clinical and immunologic follow up after successful therapy. Arch. Dermatol., *113:* 1043, 1977.
7. Lawley, T.G., Stingl, G, and Katz, S.I.: Fetal and material risk factors in herpes gestationis. Arch. Dermatol., *114:* 552, 1978.
8. Katz, A., Minta, J.O., and Toole, J.W.P., et al.: Immunopathologic study of herpes gestationis in mother and infant. Arch. Dermatol., *113:* 1069, 1977.
9. Reunala, T., Karvonen, J., and Tiilikainen, et al.: Herpes gestationis. Br. J. Dermatol. *196:* 563, 1977.
10. Person, J.R., and Rogers, R.S., III: Bullous and cicatricial pemphigoid. Clinical, histopathologic and immunopathologic correlations. Mayo Clin. Proc., *52:* 54, 1977.
11. Bean, S.F., Furey, N., and West, C., et al.: Ocular cicatricial pemphigoid (immunologic studies) Trans. Am. Acad. Ophthalmol. Otolaryngol., *81:* 8067, 1976.
12. Krivo, J.M., and Miller, F.: Immunopathology of epidermolysis bullosa acquisita. Arch. Dermatol., *114:* 1218, 1978.
13. Chorzelski, T.P., Jablonska, S., and Beutner, E.H., et al.: Linear IgA bullous dermatosis. In E.H. Beutner et al. (Eds) *Immunopathology of the Skin*. p. 315 John Wiley & Sons, New York, 1979.
14. Esterly, N.B., Furey, N.L., and Kirschner, R.S., et al.: Chronic bullous dermatosis of childhood. Arch. Dermatol., *113:* 42, 1977.
15. Thune, P., Husby, G. and Fausa, O., et al.: Immunologic and gastrointestinal abnormalities in dermatitis herpetiformis. Int. J. Dermatol., *18:* 136, 1979.
16. Fry, L., and Seah, P.P.: Dermatitis herpetiformis: an evaluation of diagnostic criteria Br. J. Dermatol., *90:* 137, 1974.
17. Fry, L: Dermatitis herpetiformis: basic findings. In E.H. Beutner, et al. (Eds) *Immunopathology oof the Skin*, p. 283 John Wiley & Sons, New York, 1979.
18. Kazmierowski, J.A. and Wuepper, K.D.: Erythema multiforme: immune complex vasculitis of the superficial cutaneous microvasculature. J. Invest. Dermatol., *71:* 366, 1978.

CHAPTER **17**

BENIGN AND PREMALIGNANT TUMORS OF THE SKIN

MARK GORDON

Tumors of the skin can be classified according to their tissue of origins (1). Accordingly, we can classify tumors as arising from the epidermis, from the melanocyte system, and of mesodermal origin.

TUMORS ARISING FROM THE EPIDERMIS

Benign Tumors

SEBORRHEIC KERATOSIS

Seborrheic keratosis occur in the later decades of life and are the most common epidermal tumors of the elderly. They are seen with equal frequency in both sexes. No specific etiologic factors are known; however, some authors have emphasized their familial occurrence. They occur most commonly on the trunk (Fig. 17.1) and arms and occur with lesser frequency on the face (as shown in Fig. 17.2, see color Plate III), neck, and scalp (Fig. 17.3). Usually, the lesions are multiple. Once these lesions start developing, new lesions continue to appear without any of them spontaneously disappearing. Seborrheic keratosis are not considered premalignant and, even though basal cell carcinoma has been re-

ported, this complication is extremely rare. They usually begin as small, raised, light-yellow areas which enlarge and become more deeply pigmented, so that when they are fully developed they become deep bluish brown in color. They are covered with a thick greasy scale which has the appearance of being "stuck on." The scale is easily removed by light friction, adding to the feeling that the lesion was almost "stuck on or glued" to the skin. When the superficial scale is removed, a granular surface appears with small follicular plugs in it. Occasionally, especially on the face, the lesions become warty and dry. The lesions may become inflamed due to irritation, resulting in rapid growth and darkening of the lesions. This is one of the main reasons why patients consult physicians. Other reasons include unsightly appearance or just general concern about the lesions. Of special interest is the sudden appearance of multiple seborrheic keratosis in patients (2) which may be associated with an adenocarcinoma, usually of the gastrointestinal tract. The pathology of seborrheic keratosis consists basically of a benign proliferation of epidermal cells resulting in a superficial plaque rising above the epidermal surface. Most seborrheic keratosis can easily be diagnosed by their clinical appearance. However, in the differential diagnosis, we have to consider verruca vulgaris

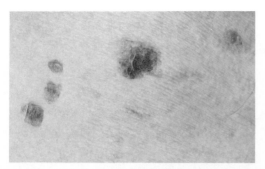

Fig. 17.1. Seborrheic keratosis. Irregular surface with different degrees of pigmentation.

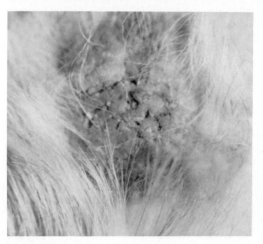

Fig. 17.3. Seborrheic keratosis. Large lesion on scalp.

and occasionally nevus cell nevi and actinic keratosis. Occasionally, because of the pigmentation of these lesions, pigmented basal cell carcinomas and malignant melanomas have to be considered. In the majority of these lesions, there is no need for any treatment. The reasons for treatment are cosmetic appearance of the lesions, discomfort caused by the lesions becoming inflamed or irritated or, occasionally, for diagnosis. The treatment of seborrheic keratosis should not leave a scar and excision is never recommended except when, on a rare occasion, one needs an excisional biopsy for diagnosis. Cryotherapy is a favorite treatment. The lesions can also be curetted with light electrodesiccation of the base. The curettings can be submitted as a biopsy.

KERATOACANTHOMA

Keratoacanthoma (3) is a rapidly growing skin tumor which bears a striking resemblance to squamous cell carcinoma, yet has a potential to regress and heal spontaneously. There are basically three types of keratoacanthomas: solitary, multiple (Ferguson-Smith), and eruptive. The latter two are extremely rare and in most discussions, when one refers to keratoacanthomas, one usually means the solitary form. Our discussion will be limited mainly to the solitary lesion. The lesion usually starts on normal skin with the nose and cheek being the most common areas of occurrence. However, it should be emphasized that keratoacanthomas can occur on any part of the body including, rarely, the mucous membranes. The etiology of keratoacanthomas is unknown, however, a few causal factors have been suggested; namely viral etiology, sunlight (since most keratoacanthomas occur on light-exposed areas), tar, oil products, and trauma. The pathogenesis of the lesions appears to be a growth of benign keratinocytes arising from the follicular epithelium. The possibility has been suggested that the growth of keratoacanthomas is under the influence of factors which normally regulate the hair cycle. As in the hair cycle, when a telogen hair is cast off with involution of the hair follicle, so in the keratoacanthoma there is an expulsion of the central cornified plug with a regression of the lesion. The tumor seems to predominate in males and Caucasians, the most common decade of onset being the sixth or seventh. The incidence appears to be 20–40% of all squamous cell carcinomas and keratoacanthomas together. Keratoacanthoma usually starts as a small maculopapule, which rapidly becomes a nodule and within 4–8 weeks becomes a raised hemispherical tumor with a large keratotic plug which is deeply imbedded (Fig. 17.4). The fully developed lesion can be up to 2 cm in diameter; however, larger lesions have been reported. It usually has gently sloping, smooth, shiny, nontranslucent borders which blend into the normal surrounding skin. The tumor is not fixed to the underlying structure and lacks induration of the base. After a stationary period, lasting 4–8 weeks, the lesion usually regresses spontaneously in another 6–8 weeks, usually leaving an irregularly shaped

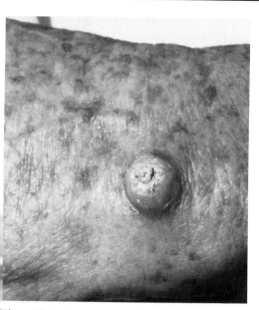

Fig. 17.4. Keratoacanthoma. Crateriform lesion with hyperkeratotic plug.

scar. While classical keratoacanthoma has a definite clinical appearance, variants occasionally arise. For example, lesions may simulate seborrheic keratosis, cutaneous horns, or verrucae. Occasionally, keratoacanthomas may obtain a huge size and become locally destructive. The pathology consists of an invaginated pseudoepitheliomatous hyperplasia of the epithelium overlying the central core of dense keratin. The cells appear normal but somewhat larger. Most important differential diagnosis is between keratoacanthoma and a rapid-growing squamous cell carcinoma. In the diagnosis, one has to consider the history of rapid growth of the keratoacanthoma with its classical clinical features versus the slow growing squamous cell carcinoma which occurs later in life, usually on abnormal skin, and which can ulcerate. However, the diagnosis can still be difficult, and then one has to turn to the pathologist. When a biopsy is done, one has to remember that the pathologist can only help us if he has an adequate specimen. In the case of a keratoacanthoma, it means excision of the whole lesion, or at least a central wedge of the lesion which includes the total breadth of the lesion and central core. Even then, with a complete history, physical appearance of the lesion, and

the pathology, occasionally one cannot differentiate except if one waits long enough for the keratoacanthoma to spontaneously regress. However, waiting for a lesion to resolve, when considering the possibility of the squamous cell carcinoma metastasizing, can be a very dangerous choice. Most keratoacanthomas should be treated for multiple reasons. First, and most important, if the lesion is treated early, one can prevent the lesion from becoming large and one can obtain a good pathologic specimen for interpretation. Secondly, the scar left from treating lesions is usually more cosmetically acceptable than the scars left from spontaneous involution of the lesions. Finally, most patients prefer therapy instead of waiting, because the lesions are on exposed areas. The treatment is simple and effective. The best treatment is simple surgical excision. One method is to remove the protruding portion, by shave excision to the level of the skin, followed by curettage and electrodesiccation of the base. However, it should be remembered that the pathologist may not be able to interpret this type of surgical specimen, as the depth of the lesion is missing, and this treatment probably should be reserved for lesions only where surgical excision is not feasible, either because of size or debilitation of the patient.

EPIDERMAL NEVI

The term nevus is used to designate a congenital localized area of any abnormal tissue. Epidermal nevi are due to the hyperplasia of epithelial cells present at birth or developing soon after. However, hereditary nevi always predominate. They affect both sexes equally. These lesions may be small or large, single or multiple, and of varied sizes. The surface is frequently verrucous (Fig. 17.5). They may appear on any part of the body but are especially seen on the extremities. They may be skin colored, light or dark brown, or grey depending upon the amount of pigment. Because of these different variations, the epidermal nevi are known under different names, i.e. linear nevi, which usually run in streaks or bands with a segmental distribution; systematized nevi, in which large areas of the body are involved; and other names such as

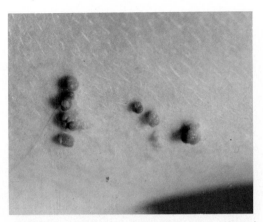

Fig. 17.5. Epidermal nevus. Pedunculated linear lesions.

ichthyosis hystrix, or nevus verrucosus. Of special interest is a report of Solomon et al. (4) in which they found a high association of extensive epidermal nevi with skeletal and central nervous system abnormalities. They strongly recommend extensive study of infants born or seen later in life with extensive epidermal nevi. The treatment of these lesions is very difficult. When presented with these lesions, one has to consider that they are harmless and that the patients usually are seeking reassurance and cosmetic improvement. When seen in small infants, it is important also to remember that these lesions grow for a while, then become stationary. Accordingly, one should not treat these lesions until such time. When one has established that the lesions are stationary, removal of lesions may be requested for cosmetic improvement. In all small or linear lesions, the best treatment is surgical excision. Careful curettage with electrodesiccation or the use of cryosurgery can be useful, but recurrences are common and, occasionally, the resulting scarring is not acceptable (Fig. 17.6). Dermabrasion of epidermal nevi has resulted in acceptable results with minimal scarring (see Chapter 30).

EPITHELIAL CYSTS

Under the term "epithelial cysts" we include the epidermal cysts, the pilar or sebaceous cysts, and milia.

Epidermal Cysts. Epidermal cysts comprise 80% of the epithelial cysts. Their genesis varies; most arise from obstructed or occluded follicles or, rarely, from a traumatic innoculation of epidermal cells (5). They have a wall composed of true epidermis, as seen on the skin surface, or the uppermost part of the hair follicle (6). Accordingly, they appear to result as proliferation of the cells of the surface epithelium and upper part of the follicle epithelium (7). Epidermal cysts usually occur on the face, scalp, neck, and trunk. They can occur any time in life, equally in both sexes, and usually are asymptomatic, unless they become secondarily infected. They are slow growing and, when fully developed, they may be up to 5 cm in diameter, elevated, freely movable, elastic, and usually raised. These lesions are usually benign with rare reports of malignant transformation. The pathology shows a lining of epidermis with horny material in laminated layers filling the sack.

Pilar Cysts. Pilar cysts are clinically indistinguishable from the epidermal cysts. However, they are almost exclusively limited to the scalp, comprise only 10–15% of all cysts, and their origin appears to be from the middle portion of the hair follicle and from the cells of the outer root sheath. The pilar cysts have a wall comprised of epithelial cells that do not have intercellular bridges. The cells close to the cavity are swollen, do not have a granular layer, and seem to float off into the lumen. The contents of the cyst consist of a homogenous, eosinophilic material. Treatment of epidermal and pilar cysts is by excision or by dissecting them through an incision in the overlying skin (see Chaper 27).

Milia. These are basically small, 1–2 mm epidermoid cysts. They have the appearance

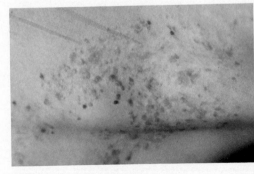

Fig. 17.6. Epidermal nevus. Some scarring visible due to treatments with electrodesiccation and cryotherapy. All lesions recurred.

of small, white firm lesions. One variety usually occurs de novo and probably represents a benign skin tumor; or they occur secondary to trauma and other dermatoses in which they represent retention cysts caused by occlusion of the pilar-sebaceous orifices. Milia are frequently a late complication of dermabrasion.

Premalignant Skin Tumors

ACTINIC KERATOSIS

Actinic keratosis (senile or solar keratosis) which usually occur on sun exposed areas, namely face, neck, back of hands, and forearms are the most common premalignant skin lesions. Their etiology is solar irradiation. They usually occur in the aged but may occur at a younger age in people who are exposed more to the sun, namely farmers, sailors, etc. They also may occur more commonly in people with certain predispositions, mostly in people of Celtic background or from the British Isles or of Anglo-Saxon ancestry.

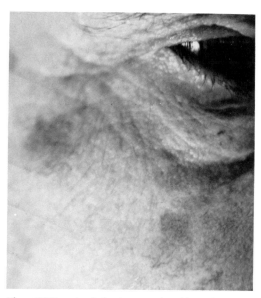

Fig. 17.7. Actinic keratosis. Sharply marginated, scaly area.

Fair complected people with a greater than average exposure to the sun are more prone to actinic keratosis. Males seem to be more affected. From a geographic standpoint, actinic keratosis are more prevalent in regions that receive a lot of sunshine, and in rural areas. They usually appear as sharply circumscribed, slightly raised or depressed, reddish, light, or dark brown lesions (Fig. 17.7) and are usually covered by an adherent scale (Fig. 17.8) and are usually multiple. Without treatment (8), 12–13% will go on to become squamous cell carcinomas. Metastases rarely, if ever, occur in squamous cell carcinoma arising from actinic keratosis. The signs that point to malignant transformation include rapid growth, ulceration and bleeding, induration, and surrounding inflammation. Treatment of actinic keratosis can easily be achieved by destructive methods, namely, cryosurgery with liquid nitrogen or curettage and electrodesiccation. Multiple lesions can be treated with 5-fluorouracil.

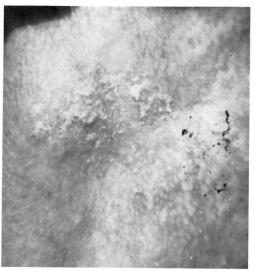

Fig. 17.8. Actinic keratosis. Large, scaly lesion.

BOWEN'S DISEASE

Bowen's disease can be defined as an intraepidermal squamous cell carcinoma. Thus, it represents biologically but not morphologically "a precancerous dermatosis" (9). Three causative theories for Bowen's disease have been proposed. First, as an actinic keratosis, solar radiation is an important factor on exposed skin. Secondly, it can be caused by ingestion of arsenic when it occurs on nonexposed skin (10). Thirdly, a virus etiology has been implicated. The lesions occur in the older age group, past age 55, and, like actinic keratosis, favor sun-sensitive individuals. Lesions seem to affect males more than females. They are evenly distributed on sun-exposed and covered areas such as palms, soles, scalp, and anogenital regions. Usually, the lesions are single. These lesions present themselves as slowly growing erythematous plaques which are crusted and sharply marginated from normal skin (Fig. 17.9). In the differential diagnosis, the following should be considered: superficial basal cell carcinoma, Paget's disease, actinic and seborrheic keratosis, lichens simplex chronicus, verrucae, and psoriasis. In Bowen's disease, at least 5% of these patients develop an invasive carcinoma in the primary plaque (8). Once the invasive carcinoma develops in Bowen's disease, up to 37% of the patients can show metastasis. Patients with Bowen's disease also have a much higher incidence of both cutaneous and mucocutaneous premalignant and malignant lesions (up to 42%), and they have a much higher incidence of primary extracutaneous cancers. Included in the tumors, are actinic keratosis, basal cell carcinoma, de novo squamous cell carcinomas, malignant melanomas, and internal malignancies involving the respiratory, gastrointestinal, genitourinary, and reticuloendothelial systems, breasts, endocrine system, soft tissues, and mucous membranes. The best treatment for Bowen's disease is local excision. However, in the areas in which this

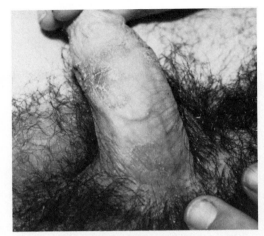

Fig. 17.10.   Bowenoid papules of penis.

is not possible, destruction with curettage and electrodesiccation or treatment with 5-fluorouracil can be tried. However, recurrences with the latter two modalities can occur. Of special interest are reports (11) about the so-called "bowenoid papulosis" of the genitalia. These are reddish brown or violaceous papules of the genitalia (Fig. 17.10). The lesions appear perfectly benign, but histopathologically they appear to be carcinomas in situ. Some precedent viral infection has been reported in many of these patients. At the present time, they are being treated conservatively but no one knows their biologic behavior.

TUMORS OF THE MELANOCYTE SYSTEM

Benign

NEVUS CELL NEVI

As stated previously, the term nevus can be used to designate any localized area of abnormal tissue. Here we will discuss nevi which basically consist of nevus cells.

Nevus cell nevi, which are the most common tumors in men, can be subdivided into three types, namely junctional nevi (Fig. 17.11), compound nevi (Fig. 17.12) and intradermal nevi (Fig. 17.13, 17.14). All three have certain clinical features that differentiate them, however the definition of the three types is based upon the anatomical location

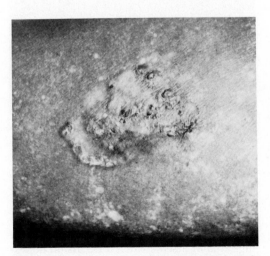

Fig. 17.9.   Bowen's disease. Irregular, scaly plaque with features of psoriasis.

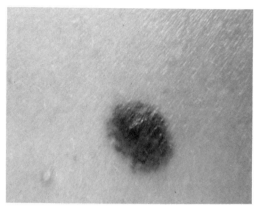

Fig. 17.11. Junctional nevus. Slightly raised pigmented lesion.

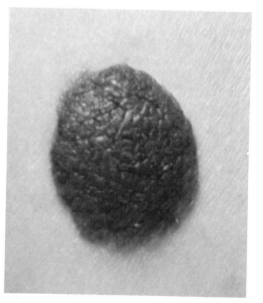

Fig. 17.12. Compound nevus. Raised, pigmented nodule.

will become malignant, usually the junctional component transforms into malignant melanomas. However, this transformation is rare. At birth, the nevi cannot usually be recognized. They start appearing soon after birth and slowly increase in number with some rapid growth during puberty and pregnancy. By the third decade, they seem to peak, and an average person will have about 40 nevi (13). Subsequently, they seem to start disappearing so that by age 50 the average number of nevi is four. Another important factor in the natural history of nevi is that (14) in the

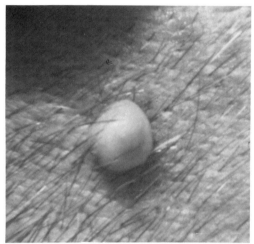

Fig. 17.13. Intradermal nevus. Pedunculated, lightly pigmented lesion.

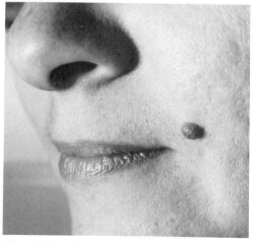

Fig. 17.14. Intradermal nevus. Pedunculated, flesh-colored lesion.

of the nevus cells. In the junctional nevus, the cells lie in nests in the epidermis or at the dermoepidermal junction. The compound nevus has an intermediate location, in which nevus cells lie both at the junction and in the dermis. The original definition of the intradermal nevus was that the cells lie entirely in the dermis. However, Kopf and Andrade (12) have shown that if biopsies of intradermal nevi are sectioned serially, in 80% of these biopsies a junctional component can be seen. Of great importance is the fact that if a nevus

prepubertal children, 98% have junctional elements while only 12% of nevi in adults have junctional activity. The common nevus in adults is the intradermal nevus. Nevi are so common that it is impossible to find a person without one. The clinical appearance of nevi varies according to type. The junctional nevus is usually flat, hairless, and light to dark brown in color. They may be a few millimeters in size to a few centimeters, and can occur on any part of the body. Most of the nevi on the palms, soles, and genitalia are of the junctional variety. Before, it used to be believed that nevi in the last three locations, because of their junctional component and frequent friction, were the most likely to transform into malignant melanoma. However, in the study done by Cullen (15), it was shown that the incidence of nevi of the palms, soles, and genitalia was 14.9% in 10,000 young people being examined for induction into the Armed Forces. Allyn et al. (16), in a study of 1,000 patients showed that every sixth person had one pigmented nevus on the palms or soles. These statistics show that removing all of these nevi in these areas becomes totally impossible and probably not necessary. Compound nevi are similar to junctional nevi, but are more raised. The intradermal nevus, the most common in adults, is usually up to 1 cm in size and may be brown or nonpigmented, can be hairy or dome shaped, and can be sessile or pedunculated (Fig. 17.15). Patients usually consult physicians because of two reasons: 1) cosmetic appearance, and 2) fear of malignancy. Change in nevi will bring the patients into the office for reassurance. The reason that most nevi change is usually due to trauma or infection. However, a change without explanation in an elderly person (such as in color, size of the lesion, spread of pigment into surrounding skin or symptoms of pain and itching) should be of concern to the clinician. Spontaneous bleeding and ulcerations are late findings. Especially of concern should be a new pigmented lesion in an elderly patient. In the differential diagnosis, besides malignant melanoma, consider pigmented basal cell carcinoma, seborrheic keratosis, and dermatofibromas. In the treatment of nevi, if malignant melanoma is considered, it should be totally excised for biopsy. If malignancy is not considered, the lesion should be removed only if the patient desires. One method is to remove the elevated part of the lesions, by cutting them flush with the surface of the skin (shave excision) and then the base can be lightly electrodesiccated. If the lesion is flat, then simple excision is the treatment of choice (see Chapter 27). In a study of 355 pigmented nevi that were treated by electrodesiccation, no evidence of malignant change was seen (17), but clinical diagnosis should always be checked histopathologically.

HALO NEVUS

Halo nevus (Leukoderma Aquisitum Centrifugum) (18) has a centrally placed cutaneous tumor which has become surrounded by a zone of acquired hypochromia (Fig. 17.16, and as shown in Fig. 17.17 on color

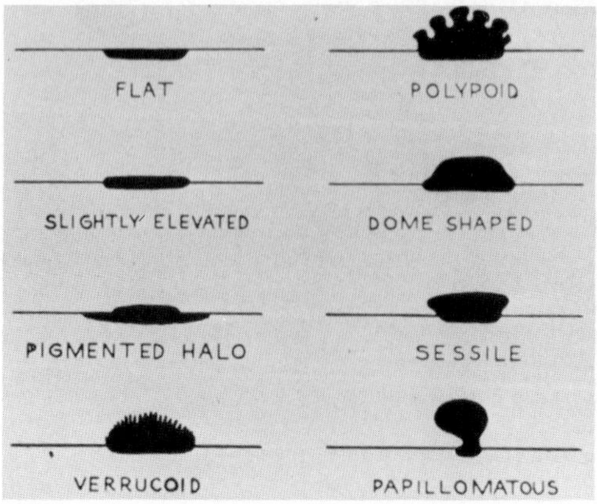

FLAT

POLYPOID

SLIGHTLY ELEVATED

DOME SHAPED

PIGMENTED HALO

SESSILE

VERRUCOID

PAPILLOMATOUS

Fig. 17.15.   Types of nevi.

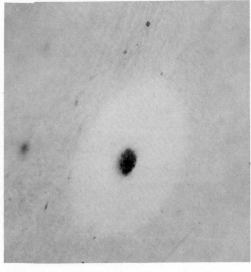

Fig. 17.16.   Halo nevus. Central lesion is a junctional nevus.

Plate III). The central tumor is usually a nevus but neural nevi, blue nevi, or malignant melanomas have been reported. The average age of occurrence is in the late teens. The lesions usually occur on the trunk in which a long standing lesion suddenly developes a white halo. The central nevus may occasionally disappear. The area of depigmentation may subsequently repigment. However, often the lesions are static. Since these lesions may regress spontaneously, no treatment is necessary. If the patient desires treatment for cosmetic reasons, excision is the treatment of choice. In a rare instance where malignant melanoma is considered, treatment of choice is excision (see Chapter 27).

CONGENITAL NEVOCYTIC NEVI

Congenital nevocytic nevi are present at birth and pose a different problem to the clinician since they seem to have a higher rate of transformation into malignant melanomas, especially before puberty. Congenital nevocytic nevi can be classified (19) according to size: small (1.4 cm or less), medium (1.5–19.9 cm), large or giant (20 cm or more). The incidence of all congenital nevi is between 1.3–2%. Out of these, a great majority fall into the first two categories. The small and medium nevi, when first seen at birth, resemble café au lait spots which are flat and tan colored.

With age, they darken, become raised or verrucous, and may develop hair (Fig. 17.18).

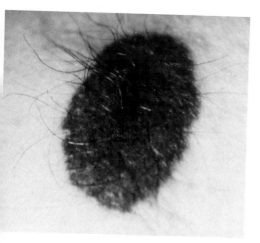

Fig. 17.18. Congenital nevocytic nevus.

The giant nevi may involve contiguous areas of the body, sometimes in dermatome distribution or, occasionally, multiple lesions are seen. These lesions are often verrucous, sometimes flat and hairy, and the pigmentation in them may vary. An additional problem with the giant variety is that they may be associated with leptomeningeal melanocytosis which, in turn, may produce seizures, mental changes, and hydrocephalus. This occurs especially with cervical lesions. The histopathology of these lesions is sometimes helpful and a biopsy will occasionally help in deciding the diagnosis. However, in most cases, the clinical appearance and the presence of the lesion at birth confirms the diagnosis. Congenital nevocytic lesions present two problems to the clinician: the patients, usually children, are seen because of the cosmetic appearance and, also, to determine whether these lesions will become malignant. From the cosmetic point of view, the clinician has to consider whether there will be an improvement in appearance and what psychological trauma these lesions will pose for the patient later. From the medical point of view, there is enough evidence to show that there is definitely an increased rate of malignant melanoma developing in the giant lesions to warrant their removal, if at all feasible. With the medium and small lesions, no good statistics are available at present. There are, however, reports of malignant melanoma developing in medium and small lesions. While opinions differ, our approach is to remove these lesions if they are easily accessible and if one can expect good cosmetic results. When dealing with lesions that are larger and not easily removable, one can explain the problem to the parents by stating that malignancy has been reported in these lesions but its incidence, while probably low, is unknown. A congenital nevocytic nevus registry has been established at the Skin and Cancer Hospital of New York University to which all lesions should be reported. This study eventually should help resolve this problem. Treatment of these lesions is surgical and, with the giant nevi, the surgery may be quite extensive.

SPINDLE CELL NEVUS

Spindle cell nevus (Benign Juvenile Melanoma) are benign nevus cell nevi with peculiar histologic features resembling malignant melanoma. These lesions occur primarily in the first two decades of life, but reports are available of an occurrence at birth and at age 56. The clinical appearance (20) is that of a smooth nodule, raised, round or oval, firm to hard, pink to red. There is an overlying telangiectasia and the lesions appear to be translucent. Of importance, they contain no pigment. The classical picture, as described above, may be varied, however, making the diagnosis more difficult. The size of the lesion varies from a few millimeters up to 3 cm. The most common area of occurrence is on the face. In the differential diagnosis, consider nevus cell nevi, pyogenic granulomas, fibromas, hemangiomas, verrucae, juvenile xanthogranuloma, solitary lesion of urticaria pigmentosa and keloids. Its spontaneous course is unknown; however, the following has been suggested: that they may remain stationary for life, they may involute, or that they may transform into ordinary nevi. The consensus is that it acts as a benign lesion and does not have a malignant potential. The treatment is conservative, but total excision is usually recommended, otherwise, recurrences may occur. In addition, since the diagnosis may be doubtful originally, and the pathologist may have difficulty interpreting it because of its resemblance to malignant melanoma, total excision provides the total lesion for pathological confirmation.

TUMORS OF MESODERMAL ORIGIN

DERMATOFIBROMA

Dermatofibroma usually occurs as a hard, fibrous nodule which is commonly situated on the legs and arms, but may occur almost anywhere on the body. Usually one lesion is found, but multiple lesions can occur. They start as pinhead lesions which slowly enlarge from a few millimeters up to a centimeter in size. Once they reach their full development, they become stationary. The lesions are usually flesh-colored, brown, tan or almost bluish black. They are attached to the overlying epidermis. Dermatofibromas represent a reactive process in which there is a proliferation of fibroblasts and histiocytes. Occasionally, there is also reactive hyperplasia of the epi-

dermis associated with this. In some cases, there is a precedent history of injury such as an insect bite or scrape, suggesting injury as a possible etiology. This may explain why the lesions are found commonly on the legs of women who shave. Dermatofibromas are most commonly found in the fourth or fifth decade, but people of any age may be affected. They are usually asymptomatic and the patient seeks help because of their cosmetic appearance or diagnosis of a dark lesion. In the differential diagnosis, consider scars, keloids, nevi, hemangiomas, or malignant melanomas. Treatment is simple excision (see Chapter 27).

SKIN TAGS

Skin tags (Achrochordons) usually occur as multiple filiform, soft papules, a few millimeters in size, that are seen mostly on the neck, upper chest, and axillae (Fig. 17.19). Occasionally, they present a solitary bag-like pedunculated growth on the trunk or extremities. These lesions are usually flesh-colored or brown, and are seen in middle-aged women and elderly men and women. The etiology is unknown; however, there seems to be an increase of these lesions during pregnancy or menopause. In many cases, the patients give a history of their parents having similar lesions. The lesions are harmless and persist indefinitely. Patients are usually seen because

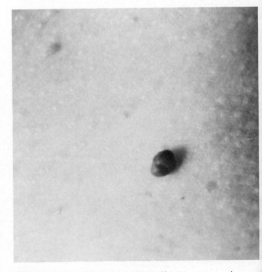

Fig. 17.19. Skin tag. Small pigmented papilloma.

of the cosmetic appearance of these lesions and, occasionally, these lesions become irritated in friction areas. Occasionally, a patient is seen with sudden development of a painful black lesion. Usually, this is due to, a skin tag on a long stalk becoming twisted, infarcted, and turning black. Treatment can be accomplished by clipping the lesions at the base with small scissors and electrodesiccating the base for hemostatis; or the small lesions can simply be electrodesiccated. Cryosurgery with liquid nitrogen also can be used, especially when the patient comes in for cosmetic reasons with many lesions.

KELOIDS

Keloids are peculiar hyperplastic responses, usually following injury, that show progressive growth often resulting in huge scars. In the cases where there is no obvious history of trauma (spontaneous keloids), most probably some minor trauma preceded the onset of the lesion. Usually, black and other deeply pigmented individuals are more susceptible to keloids. Occasionally, a familial history of keloids is obtained. There also seems to be a regional predilection for keloids, as the sternal area, ears (Fig. 17.20), face, shoulders, neck, and extremities are common locations. These lesions may be of any size or shape. They may be oval, round, or irregular with a claw shape, nodular, lobulated, sessile, or pedunculated. The early lesions are pink and rubbery, but older lesions are dark and firm. Sometimes, the lesions may distort the involved areas. Especially in young lesions, symptoms such as pain and itching are common. These lesions may begin within a few weeks following trauma and continue to grow for months and years. The pathology of these lesions consist, in the early stages, of proliferation of fibroblasts but older lesions show thick bundles of collagen. Prevention of keloids is an important function of the physician. In patients susceptible to keloids, surgical procedures should be avoided, if at all possible. Cosmetic surgery in these patients should be weighed very carefully, and susceptible patients should be examined carefully for other keloids. Always remember that electrodesiccation seems to predispose more to keloids than scalpel surgery, and lesions that become infected or inflamed are more prone to develop keloids. In the treatment of these lesions, remember that simple excision may lead to regrowth and sometimes result in larger keloids. However, excision followed by x-ray to the area sometimes prevents recurrence. Cryotherapy may improve some of these lesions. Injection of long-acting insoluble corticosteroids, such as triamcinolone acetonide, may produce regressions, but multiple injections over long periods of time may have to be used. Occasionally, in large lesions, excess tissue may have to be first removed and corticosteroids injected into the remaining tissue. This is especially true in the long-standing lesions seen on ear lobes. The pain and itching seen in early keloids can be alleviated by intralesional corticosteroids and in smaller lesions, by potent topical steroids.

PYOGENIC GRANULOMAS

Pyogenic granulomas are rapidly growing lesions that frequently occur at the site of injury. They occur at any age and at any place on the skin, but are found more commonly in areas more prone to trauma. They usually start as few millimeters in size, red papules that rapidly enlarge up to a centimeter (Fig. 17.21). As they enlarge, they become friable and bleed easily. They also fre-

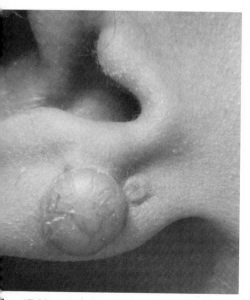

Fig. 17.20.   Keloid. Lesion ear, caused by ear piercings.

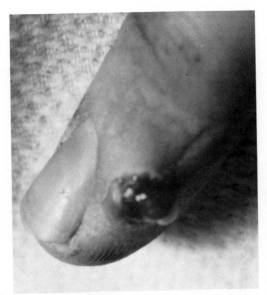

Fig. 17.21. Pyogenic granuloma. Friable vascular lesion.

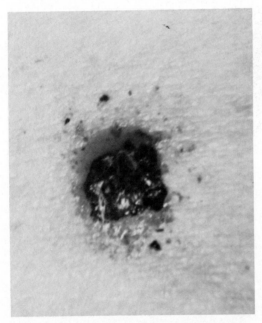

Fig. 17.22. Pyogenic granuloma. Note bleeding tendency.

quently become pedunculated and the surface lobulated. The color of the lesion is different shades of red and the surface has crusting ulcerations and necrosis (Fig. 17.22) and, occasionally, purulent discharge. In the differ-

ential diagnosis, hemangiomas and malignant melanomas are considered occasionally. The patients seen in the office are most commonly children, probably because they are more prone to injury. They are usually brought to the office because of the bleeding. When the physician makes the diagnosis, the lesion should be treated because, occasionally, the lesion can be double the size within a few days. Treatment consists of either excising the lesions or curetting them with electrodesiccation. The specimen should be sent for histopathological confirmation.

SENILE HEMANGIOMAS

Senile hemangiomas are small, few millimeters in size, red papules, usually found on the trunk and proximal extremities. They are commonly seen in the elderly, but occasionally younger people develop them. If these patients present themselves to the office for treatment, it is usually for cosmetic reasons and these lesions can easily be removed with electrodesiccation.

SENILE SEBACEOUS HYPERPLASIAS

Senile sebaceous hyperplasias usually occur on the face of the elderly as small yellow nodules (Fig. 17.23). They are multiple with a surface which is lobulated or umbilicated. Occasionally, they may occur in younger people. Some of these lesions occasionally enlarg

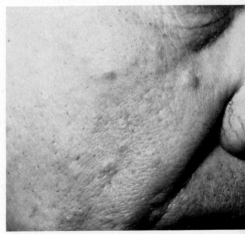

Fig. 17.23. Sebaceous hyperplasia. Sma yellow nodules.

so that differentiation from basal cell carcinoma becomes a problem. Histopathologically, they represent enlarged mature sebaceous glands. Treatment is not necessary but, if the patient desires it, they can be removed, for cosmetic reasons, electrosurgically.

LIPOMAS

These are the most common tumors of mesenchymal origin. They are usually 1–2 cm in size, soft, easily movable, subcutaneous tumors that can occur in almost any location of the body. However, they are seen more commonly on the posterior neck, trunk, and proximal extremities. They have to be differentiated from epidermoid cysts. Treatment is not necessary but, if desired by the patient, they can be excised.

References

1. Caro, W.A.: Tumors of the skin, In S.L. Moschella, D.M. Pillsbury, and H.J. Hurley (Eds) *Dermatology*, Vol. II, W.B. Saunders, Philadelphia, 1975, p. 1323.
2. Dantzig, P.I.: Sign of Leser-Trélat. Arch. Dermatol., *108:* 700, 1973.
3. Baer, R.L., and Kopf, A.W.: Keratoacanthoma. In *Yearbook of Dermatology, 1962–1963 Series.* Year Book Medical Publishers, Chicago, 1963.
4. Solomon, L.M., Fretzin, D.F., and DeWald, R.L.: The epidermal nevus syndrome. Arch. Dermatol., *97:* 273, 1968.
5. McGavran, M.H., and Binnington, B.: Keratinous cysts of the skin. Arch. Dermatol., *94:* 499, 1966.
6. Lever, W.F.: *Histopathology of the Skin*, Ed. 5, p. 460. J.B. Lippincott, Philadelphia, 1972.
7. Pincus, H.: "Sebaceous cysts" are tricholemmal cysts. Arch. Dermatol., *99:* 544, 1969.
8. Helwig, E.B., and Graham, J.H.: Precancerous skin lesions and systemic cancer, In *Tumors of the Skin. The University of Texas M.D. Anderson Hospital and Tumor Institute Seventh Annual Conference on Cancer*, p. 209. Year Book Medical Publishers, Chicago, 1964.
9. Lever, W.F.: *Histopathology of the Skin*, Ed. 5, p. 473. J.B. Lippincott, Philadelphia, 1972.
10. Peterka, E.S., Lynch, F.W., and Goltz, R.W.: An association between Bowen's disease and internal cancer. Arch. Dermatol., *84:* 623, 1961.
11. Wade, T.R., Kopf, A.W., and Ackerman, A.B.: Bowenoid papulosis of the genitalia. Arch. Dermatol., *115:* 306, 1979.
12. Kopf, A.W., and Andrade, R.: A histologic study of the dermoepidermal junction in clinically "intradermal" nevi, employing serial sections: 1. Junctional thèques. Ann. N.Y. Acad. Sci., *100:* 200, 1963.
13. Stegmaier, D.C., and Becker, S.W., Jr.: Incidence of melanocytic nevi in young adults. J. Invest. Dermatol., *24:* 125, 1960.
14. Sulzberger, M.B., Wolf, S., Witten, V.H., and Kopf, A.W.: *Dermatology, Diagnosis and Treatment*, Ed. 2, p. 401. Year Book Medical Publishers, Chicago, 1961.
15. Cullen, S.I.: Incidence of nevi. Arch. Dermatol., *86:* 40, 1962.
16. Allyn, B., Kopf, A.W., Kahn, M., and Witten, V.C.: Incidence of pigmented nevi. JAMA *186:* 890, 1963.
17. Walton, R.G., and Cox, A.J.: Electrodesiccation of pigmented nevi. Arch. Dermatol., *87:* 342, 1963.
18. Kopf, A.W., Morrille, J.D., and Silberberg, I.: Broad spectrum of leukoderma aquisitum centrifugum. Arch. Dermatol., *92:* 14, 1965.
19. Kopf, A.W., Bart, R.S., and Hennessey, P.: Congenital nevocytic nevi and malignant melanomas. J. Am. Acad. Dermatol., *1:* 123, 1979.
20. Kopf, A.W., and Andrade, R.: Benign Juvenile Melanoma, In *Yearbook of Dermatology, 1965–1966 Series.* Year Book Medical Publishers, Chicago, 1966.

CHAPTER **18**

MALIGNANT SKIN TUMORS

WILLIAM A. CARO

Although the vast majority of skin tumors are benign, a significant number of malignant tumors occur in this organ. These tumors range from the common basal cell epithelioma (basal cell carcinoma), with its usual low grade of malignancy, to the much less common malignant melanoma, usually a highly malignant tumor.

Environmental and genetic factors play an important role in the development of malignant skin tumors. Solar irradiation represents the most important recognized environmental carcinogen although, in the past, systemic administration of arsenic and improperly used superficial x-ray therapy also had the capacity of inducing malignant skin tumors, usually years later.

Fair-skinned, blue-eyed individuals have a genetic susceptibility to solar carcinogenesis, and this effect is heightened in patients with certain rare genetic disorders such as xeroderma pigmentosum.

BASAL CELL EPITHELIOMA (BASAL CELL CARCINOMA)

Basal cell epithelioma represents the most common malignancy of man, although the incidence has wide racial and geographic variations. Individuals with red to blond hair, blue eyes, and fair skin are especially susceptible to the development of basal cell epithe-

lioma, while the tumor is rare in blacks. These racial differences in the incidence of basal cell epithelioma are directly related to the presence or absence of protection against solar irradiation afforded by melanin pigmentation.

Patients of similar skin pigmentation are at greater risk in geographic areas with more intense sun exposure, and this risk is exemplified by the high incidence of basal cell epithelioma in such areas as Texas and Australia. Although no longer in therapeutic use today, systemic administration of arsenical medications in the past made individuals more susceptible to the development of basal cell epitheliomas as well as other premalignant and malignant skin tumors.

In most studies, the incidence of basal cell epithelioma is somewhat higher in men, although this may relate to greater exposure of men to solar irradiation. Most tumors arise after the age of 40, although younger individuals also may be affected. On rare occasions, basal cell epithelioma may occur in children as a solitary lesion, although children with multiple lesions must be studied for one of the genetic disorders leading to the early development of such tumors—the nevoid basal cell epithelioma syndrome and xeroderma pigmentosum.

Basal cell epithelioma tends to favor sun-exposed areas with relatively high numbers of pilosebaceous follicles, such as the face. The neck also represents a common site, although these tumors are uncommon over such sun-exposed areas as the dorsa of the hands and forearms.

Several clinical types of basal cell epithelioma may be recognized: 1) nodulo-ulcerative, 2) pigmented, 3) sclerosing, 4) superficial, and 5) the nevoid basal cell epithelioma syndrome. Nodulo-ulcerative basal cell epithelioma represents the most common type, and these lesions are especially common on the face and neck. The onset is heralded by a small papule which slowly enlarges. The fully developed lesion usually is flesh colored but may have an erythematous, bluish or tan shade. The tumor characteristically has a somewhat translucent or pearly hue and a smooth to slightly irregular surface (Fig. 18.1). Careful examination of the surface usually reveals a fine play of small telangiectatic blood vessels.

With enlargement, the center becomes umbilicated and eventually may ulcerate to be covered by a friable crust. In ulcerated lesions, the characteristic pearly or translucent nodular border usually provides the main diagnostic feature (Fig. 18.2). Untreated lesions continue to enlarge with destruction of contiguous tissue through local invasion. Such long neglected lesions may reach massive proportion and eventually may cause the death of the patient from invasion of a vital organ, infection, or massive hemorrhage from an eroded blood vessel.

Pigmented basal cell epithelioma represents a variant of the nodulo-ulcerative type with large amounts of melanin pigment within the tumor. Such lesions are light to dark brown in color and may resemble malignant melanoma clinically.

The sclerosing basal cell epithelioma is an uncommon form and also usually occurs on the face. This lesion usually has a flat and often somewhat depressed surface and poorly defined borders. The color usually is yellowish to white with a smooth surface and a firm consistency (Fig. 18.3). The appearance often suggests a scar or a small patch of scleroderma. Sclerosing basal cell epithelioma usually enlarges slowly, and deep invasion and ulceration are must less likely than with the more common nodulo-ulcerative types.

Superficial basal cell epithelioma falls between nodulo-ulcerative and sclerosing types in frequency and more commonly occurs on the trunk. This lesion has a somewhat greater tendency to be multiple than do the preceding two types.

Superficial basal epithelioma often will be misdiagnosed by the untrained eye, as the

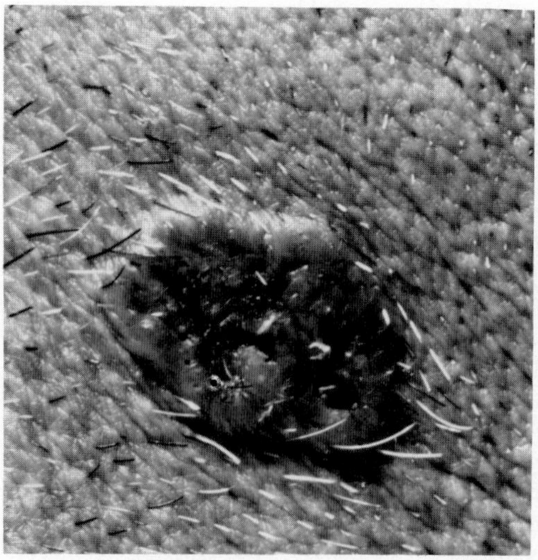

Fig. 18.1. Nodulo-ulcerative basal cell epithelioma. Lesion has a pearly appearance and irregular surface.

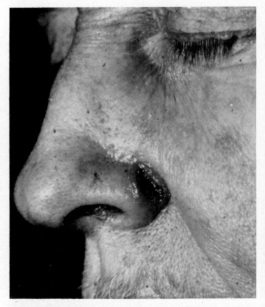

Fig. 18.2. Ulcerated basal cell epithelioma. Pearly nodular border.

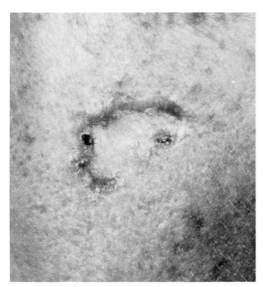

Fig. 18.3. Sclerosing basal cell epithelioma. Lesion depressed, has a smooth surface and pale color. The border is nodular in some areas and blends into normal skin in others.

clinical appearance may more closely resemble an inflammatory lesion than a tumor. The lesion presents as an erythematous, slightly scaly patch with an irregular thread-like border. There may be slight infiltration to palpation. The lesion expands slowly and may develop small superficial areas of ulceration as shown in Figure 18.4 (see color Plate III). These lesions usually remain superficial, although, rarely, they may develop a nodular component.

The nevoid basal cell epithelioma syndrome (basal cell nevus syndrome) represents a rare autosomal, dominantly inherited, disturbance characterized by 1) multiple basal cell epitheliomas with their onset in childhood and with a wide distribution, 2) small pits on the palms and soles, 3) characteristic bony abnormalities including jaw cysts and bifid ribs, 4) calcification of the falx cerebri, and 5) other connective tissue and endocrine abnormalities. The basal cell epitheliomas, although gradually increasing in number, usually remain indolent during childhood. After puberty, and into adult life, these lesions behave more aggressively with enlargement, ulceration, deep invasion and destruction of normal tissue. Such lesions may be consider-

ably more destructive than the ordinary basal cell epitheliomas arising on sun-exposed skin.

Although basal cell carcinomas of all types show progressive growth with the capacity of deep invasion, metastatic spread is a distinct rarity. This has been reported in approximately 100 cases, and frequently the original tumor was atypical or had recurred many times with apparently adequate treatment prior to the identification of metastatic spread.

The histopathologic picture of basal cell epithelioma shows a component of epithelial cells and a stromal component. Nodulo-ulcerative lesions most commonly are composed of solid masses of cells with deeply basopholic nuclei and scanty, poorly defined cytoplasm (Fig. 18.5). The cells bordering these masses show a tendency for palisading with their nuclei oriented perpendicularly to the surface of the masses (Fig. 18.6). The cells of the basal cell epithelioma bear some resemblence to cells of the epidermal basal layer and are called basaloid or basalioma cells. The stroma supporting the cellular masses characteristically shows a fibrous reaction (Fig. 18.6). Pigmented basal cell epitheliomas have melanin pigment within the tumor. Sclerosing basal cell epitheliomas have a much more pronounced fibrous stroma with irregular strands and small groups of basaloid cells interspersed within the stroma (Fig. 18.7). Superficial basal cell epitheliomas have broad masses of basaloid cells extending downward from the dermoepidermal junction into the upper dermis (Fig. 18.8). Nevoid basal cell epitheliomas cannot be distinguished microscopically from the more common forms.

Three methods of treatment are commonly employed in the initial management of basal cell epithelioma and, in experienced hands, each will give cure rates in excess of 95%. The selection of a method of treatment will depend upon the experience of the physician, the age and general health of the patient, and the type and site of the lesion. The three methods consist of surgical excision, curettage and electrodesiccation, and irradiation. Most basal cell epitheliomas can be excised without difficulty, although the surgeon must pay attention to the borders of the lesion. Sclerosing basal cell epitheliomas have poorly defined borders, and inadequate excisions with recur-

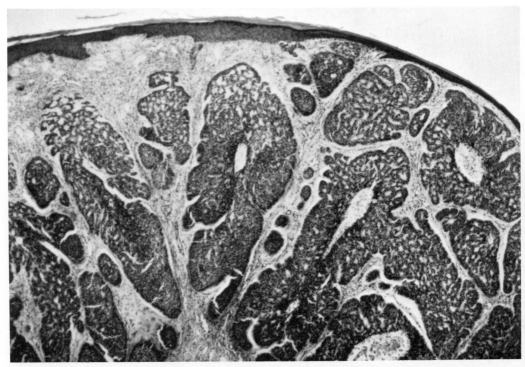

Fig. 18.5. Basal cell epithelioma. Irregular masses of small dark cells (basaloid cells).

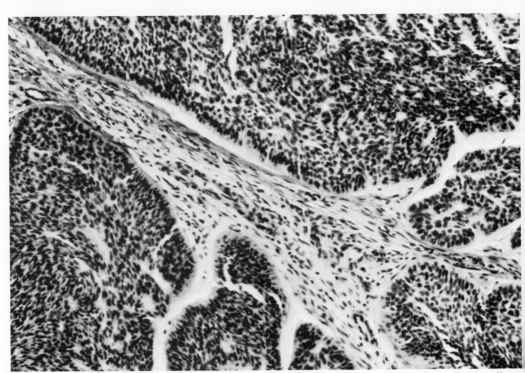

Fig. 18.6. Basal cell epithelioma. Higher power showing palisading of basaloid cells at borders of tumor masses and fibrotic stromal response.

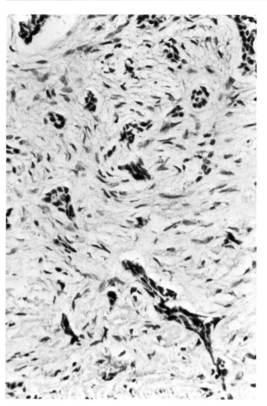

Fig. 18.7. Sclerosing basal cell epithelioma. Irregular strands and small groups of basaloid cells within a fibrous stroma.

rences may occur if the microscopic extent of the tumor is not appreciated.

Removal of the tumor with a dermal curette depends upon the contrast between the soft consistency of the most common tumors and the firm consistency of the underlying dermis. This removal is followed by the application of the electrodesiccating current until a dry eschar is produced. This procedure usually is repeated once or twice. The eschar separates within several weeks, and the resulting scar usually is quite acceptable cosmetically. Nodular lesions of less than 1 cm and superficial types lend themselves well to this treatment, while it should not be employed for sclerosing lesions or for larger or deeply infiltrating nodular lesions. This form of treatment is widely used by practicing dermatologists.

Irradiation in the form of superficial x-ray therapy has more limited application. X-rays are generated at 60–100 kVp with a half value layer (HVL) of 0.8–1.0 mm. Al. With appropriate lead shelding of surrounding tissues, the lesion is usually treated in five to eight fractional doses with a total of 3500–4500 rads over a 1- to 2-week period. Such treatment requires considerable technical skill and experience and should be undertaken only by those throughly familar with its use. X-ray therapy in general should be limited to patients over 40 years of age and is especially appropriate in older or debilitated individuals. Lesions of the eyelid margins, canthi, and areas of the nose are especially amenable to x-ray therapy, and this modality also has been used on occasion for incompletely excised lesions or lesions recurrent after some other mode of therapy.

Cryotherapy, a technique of destroying the lesion by controlled freezing with a liquid nitrogen-cooled probe, has been used by a limited number of clinicians and produces satisfactory results in carefully selected cases.

Mohs' surgery (Mohs' chemosurgery) was developed as a technique for excising tumors under microscopically controlled conditions. Although not as widely employed as excisional surgery, curettage or irradiation, Mohs' surgery occupies an important position in the management of basal cell epithelioma.

In the original technique, the tumor is fixed in situ by the application of zinc chloride paste and then excised and subjected to immediate microscopic examination using frozen sections cut horizontally. The various borders of the specimen are marked with ink of differing colors for orientation, and additional fixative is applied to areas of residual tumor. The area is then re-excised until a tumor-free plane of tissue is achieved. In the newer fresh-tissue technique, the chemical fixative is eliminated and a direct surgical approach is employed. The microscopic control remains the same. Because Mohs' surgery is tedious and time consuming, it is not employed for easily treated lesions. The technique is especially valuable in tumors with poorly defined borders and in recurrent lesions. Excellent results often have been achieved in complicated lesions where other treatment methods have failed.

Adequate patient follow-up forms an essential component in the management of basal cell epithelioma. Although adequate treatment produces an excellent cure rate, an occasional lesion may recur. Besides the usual

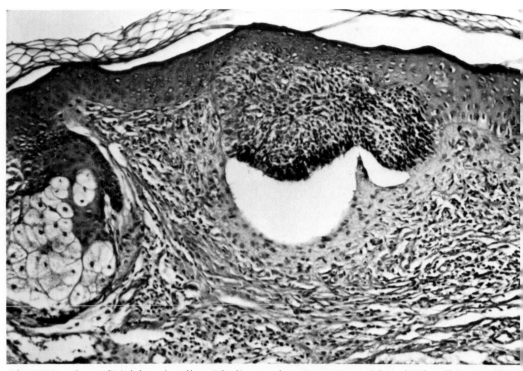

Fig. 18.8. Superficial basal cell epithelioma showing mass of basaloid cells extending from the dermoepidermal junction into the upper dermis. The open space represents retraction of the tumor mass during processing.

postoperative visits, we usually examine our patients 1 month following the completion of treatment and then at 3 months, 6 months, 1 year, and annually thereafter for 5 years. In addition, the patient is asked to contact us without delay if he develops symptoms in the treatment site or if the area changes in any suspicious way.

Although the cure rate for initial treatment of basal cell epithelioma approximates 95%, the cure rate for recurrent lesions is substantially lower. The new plan of treatment must take this into account, and treatment of recurrent lesions will have to be more aggressive than that used initially. More extensive surgery or Mohs' surgery often will be selected for these difficult lesions, and careful long-term follow-up remains essential.

SQUAMOUS CELL CARCINOMA

Squamous cell carcinoma represents a malignant tumor derived from surface epidermis.

Although skin is the most common site, lesions also occur on mucosal surfaces. Squamous cell carcinoma is the second most common malignant skin tumor after basal cell epithelioma. In comparison with basal cell epithelioma, squamous cell carcinoma tends to occur at an older age and has an even greater incidence in men.

The development of squamous cell carcinoma is influenced by the same environmental and genetic factors which influence the development of basal cell epithelioma. Most squamous cell carcinomas arise on sun-damaged skin, especially in individuals with fair skin. This relationship to solar irradiation appears to be more direct than with basal cell epithelioma, as squamous cell carcinoma also occurs commonly in such sun-exposed areas as the dorsa of the hands and forearms.

Prior exposure to high doses of therapeutic x-ray, arsenicals, and local exposure to certain tar compounds have been important environmental factors.

The clinical appearance and development

of squamous cell carcinoma vary considerably depending, in part, on where and how the lesion arises. Most squamous cell carcinomas arise from sun-damaged skin either de novo or from a pre-existing lesion. Of these pre-existing lesions, development of squamous cell carcinoma from actinic keratosis is most common, although cutaneous tumors also arise from Bowen's disease, erythroplasia of Queyrat and certain damaged skin areas such as chronic radiodermatitis, burn scars, and chronic sinusitis. On mucosal surfaces, squamous cell carcinoma may develop from leukoplakia and actinic cheilitis. A much smaller number of squamous cell carcinomas developed from clinically normal skin.

The lesion usually begins as a small, firm erythematous nodule with variably defined borders. In the patient with sun-damaged skin, more than one squamous cell carcinoma may be present. These lesions enlarge more rapidly than basal cell epitheliomas, although the rate of growth varies considerably. With enlargement, lesions frequently ulcerate revealing a friable to firm granulating, often hemorrhagic, surface (Fig. 18.9).

The clinical appearance of some lesions may resemble basal cell epithelioma, although squamous cell carcinoma usually has a much harder consistency. The developing lesion of squamous cell carcinoma also may resemble keratoacanthoma, although squamous carcinoma usually grows more slowly.

As it enlarges, squamous cell carcinoma invades deeper tissue, and this invasion is less confined and more irregular than in the usual basal cell epithelioma.

The biologic activity of a squamous cell carcinoma varies depending upon its origin. Squamous cell carcinomas arising from actinic keratoses usually grow slowly and seldom metastasize. At the other end of the spectrum, squamous cell carcinomas arising on mucosal surfaces such as the lip usually grow rapidly and have a distinct tendency to metastasize. Squamous cell carcinomas arising from Bowen's disease, erythroplasia of Queyrat, chronic radiodermatitis, and burn scars tend to be more aggressive than those arising from actinic keratoses, and squamous cell carcinomas arising from normal skin also may be quite aggressive. Metastatic spread occurs through lymphatic channels to regional lymph nodes, and either the original tumor or its metastatic spread may lead to the death of the patient.

Microscopically, squamous cell carcinoma shows a disorganized proliferation of squamous cells with varying degrees of differentiation. Well differentiated tumors have keratinizing cells, but this keratinization usually is irregular and disordered (Fig. 18.10). Some well differentiated tumors may be almost impossible to distinguish from keratoacanthoma. Poorly differentiated tumors have no appreciable keratinization and may appear as atypical spindle cell tumors difficult to differentiate from other malignant spindle cell tumors. Intermediate degrees of differentiation also occur.

Treatment of squamous cell carcinoma usually employs the same modalities as used for basal cell carcinoma: surgical excision, curettage and electrodesiccation, x-ray therapy, and Mohs' surgery. The choice of technique, again, will depend upon the age and health of the patient, and the nature, size, and location of the tumor. The physician must always bear in mind that squamous cell carcinoma is basically a more aggressive tumor than basal cell epithelioma and should plan his therapy accordingly. With metastatic disease, systemic chemotherapy may be employed, and the ad-

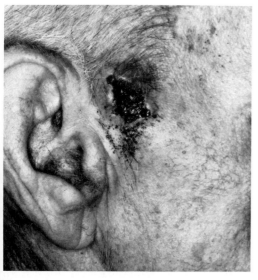

Fig. 18.9. Ulcerated squamous cell carcinoma arising in sun-damaged skin. The lesion was firm to palpation.

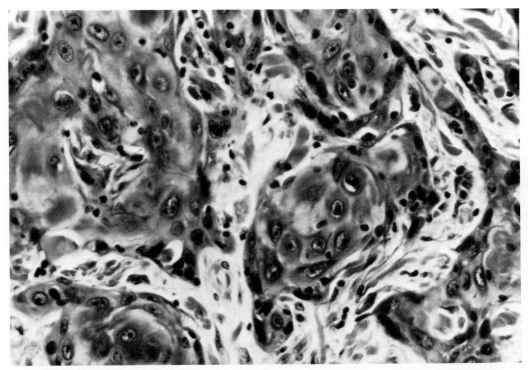

Fig. 18.10. Squamous cell carcinoma showing small irregular masses of abnormal, keratinizing cells.

ministration of bleomycin has been of some value.

Follow-up of the treated squamous cell carcinoma follows the same principles as those for basal cell epithelioma, but the physician must remain alert to the more serious nature of squamous cell carcinoma and the greater likelihood of recurrence.

MALIGNANT LYMPHOMAS

With the exception of mycosis fungoides, a primary malignant lymphoma of the skin, malignant lymphomas ordinarily do not originate in this organ. When lymphomatous infiltrates involve the skin, they usually do so late in the course of the disease and represent spread beyond the lymph nodes of origin. On rare occasions, such a lymphoma will originate in the skin and may not show later involvement of lymph nodes.

In comparison with the small number of patients who develop lymphomatous infiltrations in the skin, a larger number of patients

with malignant lymphomas develop nonspecific skin lesions thought to be on a toxic or hypersensitivity basis. Such lesions usually mimic a spectrum of benign dermatoses and do not resemble lymphoma lesions clinically or microscopically.

Mycosis fungoides represents the most important malignant lymphoma seen by the dermatologist. This disease begins in the skin and usually remains confined to the skin throughout its course. Extracutaneous dissemination to lymph nodes and visera may occur later in the course of the disease, however. Classical mycosis fungoides consists of three sequential clinical stages: 1) erythematous or premycotic stage, 2) infiltrative or plaque stage, and 3) tumor stage, and the disease usually progresses at a slow rate. Transition from one stage to the next usually is gradual. Although patients in the erythematous stage may live 15–20 years with their disease, when the tumor stage has occurred survival rarely exceeds 2 years.

In the erythematous stage the lesions often are not diagnostic and consist of erythematous patches of variable distribution (Fig. 18.11). There may be mild scaling and the contours of the lesion may be irregular. Lesions may have an eczematous or psoriasiform appearance, and itching often is severe.

With progression to the infiltrative stage the lesions become somewhat elevated and have an infiltrated feel on palpation (Fig. 18.12 & 18.13). They may be smooth to somewhat rough or scaling, and the color often will be a dusky hue of reddish blue or reddish brown. In patients with the fully developed infiltrative stage, lesions may involve large areas of the skin surface but usually will be sharply marginated from uninvolved skin (Fig. 18.14).

With progression to the tumor stage, the patient develops tumors and nodules of varying size and thickness. These usually increase in size and number and commonly ulcerate (Fig. 18.15). The patient at this stage often will have a grotesque appearance and short survival. Death usually results from inanition or sepsis. In the late stage of mycosis fungoides, the disease often spreads to lymph nodes and internal organs, especially lung, spleen, liver, and kidney.

Occasional patients with mycosis fungoides may develop cutaneous tumors from the on-

set, and such lesions may be difficult to distinguish from other forms of malignant lymphoma.

The Sézary syndrome consists of generalized erythroderma (Fig. 18.16) with severe pruritus, generalized lymphadenopathy, hepatomegaly, and a markedly elevated white blood count characterized by atypical lymphocytes having hyperconvoluted nuclei

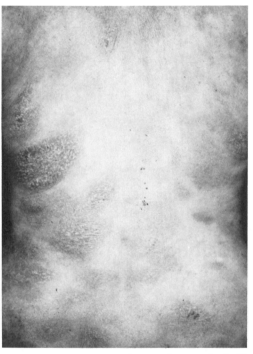

Fig. 18.12. Mycosis fungoides, early infiltrative stage. Some lesions are elevated, others are not.

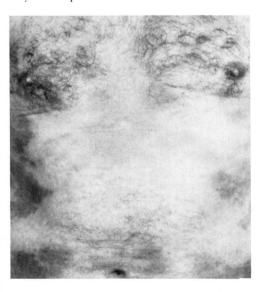

Fig. 18.11. Mycosis fungoides, erythematous stage. These patches resemble a dermatitis and are not diagnostic of mycosis fungoides.

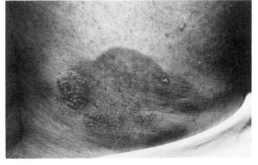

Fig. 18.13. Mycosis fungoides, infiltrative stage. This plaque is elevated and palpable, and has an irregular contour.

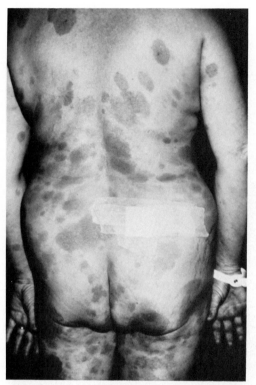

Fig. 18.14. Mycosis fungoides, infiltrative stage: extensive involvement but sharply marginated from normal skin.

Treatment of mycosis fungoides rarely is curative, although prolonged periods of remission following therapy have been reported in some patients treated in early stages. Management should be multidisciplinary utilizing the skills of the dermatologist, medical oncologist, and radiotherapist. Erythematous and early infiltrative stage disease are treated with topical nitrogen mustard, radiotherapy using the electron beam, and photochemotherapy using oral psoralens and long wave ultraviolet light (PUVA).

In more advanced disease, systemic chemotherapy will be employed, although no single drug or combination of drugs has proved entirely satisfactory. Treatment at this stage of disease is usually considered palliative.

Other malignant lymphomas, including Hodgkin's disease and lymphomas of undifferentiated, lymphocytic and histiocytic types, produce nodules and tumors which require microscopic examination for identification as to type (Fig. 18.17). These lesions often have a bluish or brownish hue and may ulcerate (Fig. 18.18). They may be single or multiple and are almost always radiosensitive. Treatment will be directed toward the underlying lymphoma.

(Sézary cells). The atypical cells are also found in skin and in many clinically enlarged lymph nodes. Most investigators believe the Sézary syndrome to represent a form of mycosis fungoides, and the histopathologic picture is indistinguishable from mycosis fungoides.

Microscopically, the hallmark of mycosis fungoides is a proliferation of the same atypical lymphocytes as seen in the Sézary syndrome. These cells have been identified as T lymphocytes and characteristically invade the epidermis. Such epidermal invasion may produce small microabscesses (Pautrier's microabscesses), although more diffuse epidermal infiltration also occurs. In some cases, the epidermis is spared.

The degree of dermal involvement usually parallels the clinical stage of the disease. Early lesions have few atypical cells in the dermis, while late infiltrative and tumor-stage lesions show extensive infiltration by atypical cells.

OTHER MALIGNANT TUMORS

Other components of skin may produce malignant tumors, although such tumors are uncommon. Examples include dermatofibrosarcoma protuberans, a malignant fibrohistiocytic tumor, and Kaposi's sarcoma, a malignant vascular tumor.

Malignant tumors originating elsewhere may metastasize to the skin, although such spread is not common. The female breast represents the most common primary source followed by gastrointestinal tract, genitourinary tract, and lung. Cutaneous metastases are usually present as discrete nodules, often in the general region of the primary tumor. Less commonly, the skin lesions will present as infiltrative plaques. Although the clinical appearance of the lesion often will suggest its metastatic nature, microscopic examination will be essential for accurate diagnosis.

Such lesions can be effectively excised, al-

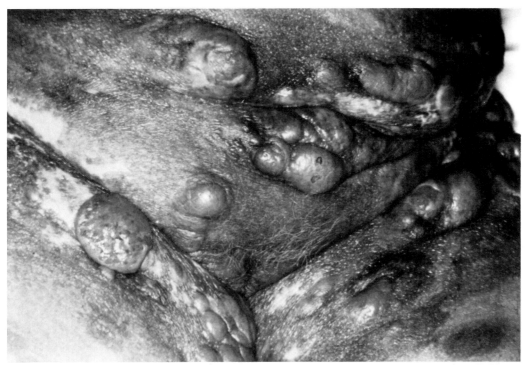

Fig. 18.15.   Mycosis fungoides, tumor stage. Large tumor nodules with ulceration.

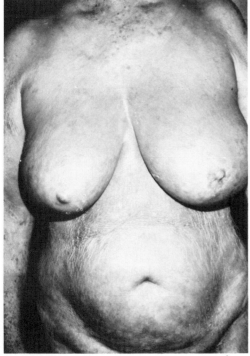

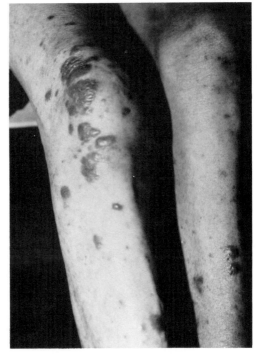

Fig. 18.16.   Sézary syndrome. Generalized erythroderma.

Fig. 18.17.   Malignant lymphoma, lymphocytic type. Discrete erythematous nodules.

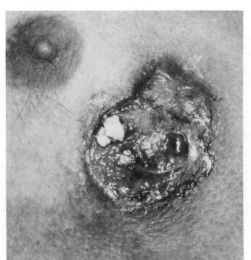

Fig. 18.18. Hodgkin's disease, ulcerated nodule.

though the major attention must be directed toward the primary disease and the possibility of spread elsewhere.

References

1. Andrade, R., Gumport, S.L., Popkin, G.L., and Reese, T.D.: *Cancer of the Skin.* W.B. Saunders, Philadelphia, 1976.

2. Bluefarb, S.M.: *Cutaneous Manifestations of the Malignant Lymphomas.* Charles C Thomas, Springfield, Ill. 1959.

3. Brownstein, M.H., and Helwig, E.B.: Patterns of cutaneous metastasis. Arch. Dermatol., *105:* 862, 1972.

4. Costanza, M.E., Dayal, Y., and Binder, S. et al.: Metastasizing basal cell carcinoma. Cancer, *34:* 230, 1974.

5. Epstein, E., Epstein, N.N., and Bragg, K. et al.: Metastases from squamous cell carcinoma of the skin. Arch. Dermatol., *97:* 245, 1968.

6. Freeman, E.G., and Duncan, C.D.: Recurrent skin cancer. Arch. Dermatol., *107:* 395, 1973.

7. Freeman, R.G., Knox, J., and Heaton, C.L.: The treatment of skin cancer. Cancer, *17:* 535, 1964.

8. Gellin, G.A., Kopf, A.W., and Garfinkel, L.: Basal cell epithelioma. A controlled study of associated factors. Arch. Dermatol. *91:* 38, 1965.

9. Helm, F.: *Cancer Dermatology.* Lea & Febiger, Philadelphia, 1979.

10. Lutzner, M.A., Edelson, R., and Shein, P., et al.: Cutaneous T-cell lymphomas: the Sézary syndrome, mycosis fungoides and related disorders. Ann. Intern. Med., *83:* 534, 1975.

11. Rebuck, J.W., and Berard, C.W. *The Reticuloendothelial System.* International Academy of Pathology Monograph. Williams & Wilkins, Baltimore, 1975.

12. Reingold, I.M.: Cutaneous metastases from internal carcinoma. Cancer, *19:* 162, 1966.

13. Winkelmann, R.K., Caro, W.A. Current problems in mycosis fungoides and Sézary syndrome. Ann. Rev. Med., *28:* 251, 1977.

CHAPTER 19

MALIGNANT MELANOMA

HENRY H. ROENIGK, JR.

Malignant melanoma is one of the most dangerous tumors that arise on the skin. The lesion may begin from a benign nevus which has been present for years or may arise de novo and metastasize quickly. There appears to be an increased incidence of melanoma in the past decade despite earlier clinical diagnosis and new approaches to therapy.

Incidence

The Third National Cancer Survey (1975) indicated an annual incidence of malignant melanoma for the United States is 4.2/100,000 population. Blacks have a much lower incidence than whites and males slightly more than females. There is a higher incidence in the South than in the North leading to some implication of sunlight precipitating some lesions. The incidence of melanoma is constantly rising in various parts of the world. The age standardized incidence for females in Connecticut is rising by 11.8% per year and for males by 8.3%. Recent data from Los Angeles County for the decade 1970–1979 reveal an annual increase of 30% for native born Californians.

CLASSIFICATION OF MELANOMA

Primary cutaneous melanomas fall into four categories that can be recognized clinically and microscopically.

Lentigo Maligna Melanoma (LMN).
This growth pattern is the rarest of the four forms and accounts for about 10% of all cases. LMN develops at a median age of close to 70 years and is two to three times more common in females than in males. These large, variably pigmented, freckle-like lesions are often located on the cheek or temple but can occur on any exposed body surface (Fig. 19.1).

The lesion gradually increases in size and margins become very irregular. The color may be tan and brown with areas of deep black being suspicious of melanoma. The surface is very smooth and, when a noticeable thickening or elevated nodule develops, then malignant transformation must be suspected.

McGovern reported 33 cases of LMN that took from 15 months to 40 years to develop, with an average developmental period of 9 years. The prognosis of LMN is excellent because the tumor is very slow to invade deeply.

Superficial Spreading Melanoma (SSM).
These lesions are the most common type of melanoma, comprising approximately 75% of all cases. This variety usually occurs at an earlier age (40–50 years) than does LMN.

The major clinical feature of an SSM is the variety of colors ranging from tan-black, brown, blue-grey, to violaceous pink (Figs. 19.2, 19.3). These lesions are characteristically flat to slightly elevated with pigmentation ranging from 0.5 to 3.0 cm in diameter and they frequently have notched borders.

The lesions are most common on the upper back in both sexes and on the legs in women. When this evolves into the vertical-growth phase, papules and nodules appear clinically.

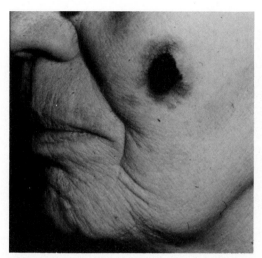

Fig. 19.1. Lentigo malignant melanoma which usually develops within a lentigo maligna (Hutchinson's freckle), usual location is face.

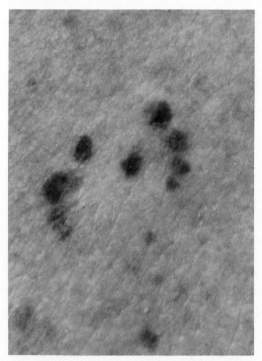

Fig. 19.2. Superficial spreading malignant melanoma with irregular borders and colors of blue-black, red, and white.

Nodular Melanoma (NM). This malignant pattern comprises 10–15% of all melanomas, occurs twice as frequently in males as in females, can occur in any location, and usually develops in patients who are around 50 years of age.

The color of a nodular melanoma is characteristically a shade of blue, e.g. blue-black, blue-grey, or reddish blue (Fig. 19.4, Fig. 19.5). An unpigmented (amelanotic) form of NM can be extremely difficult to diagnose by color, but occasionally there are small, dark specks at the base of the lesion.

Nodular melanoma can develop in a preexisting melanoma or de nova. There is usually an absence of lateral spread but, instead, a more dangerous vertical spread.

Acral-lentiginous melanomas. These lesions occur on the palms, soles, and terminal phalanges. There may be hyperpigmentation or distortion of the nail bed. Serial biopsies are often necessary to establish the diagnosis of melanoma since some areas may show only benign melanocytic hyperplasia. There is frequently a variety of colors similar to lentigo maligna melanoma.

CLINICAL DIAGNOSIS

The diagnosis of melanoma is usually based on the clinical appearance of a pigmented lesion in addition to a history of recent change, the latter being the most important clue. The following clinical criteria suggest the possibility of melanoma:

A change in the surface area of a nevus. Sudden enlargement.
A change in elevation of a lesion, with a flat mole becoming raised, palpable, nodular, or thickened.
A change in color, especially when brownish pigmentation becomes black.
A change in surface characteristics whereby a previously smooth cutaneous surface may become brown and scaly, with or without the occurrence of serous discharge or bleeding after minor trauma.
A change in sensation, e.g. the development of itching or tingling in an area of pigmentation.
A change in surrounding skin with signs of inflammation or appearance of satellite pigmentations.

Regardless of these considerations, it is not until the specimen has been removed and examined histologically that a definitive diagnosis of melanoma can be made.

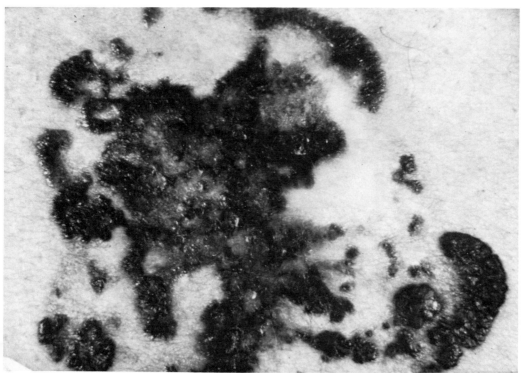

Fig. 19.3. Superficial spreading malignant melanoma—more extensive and larger lesions but still showing clinical features.

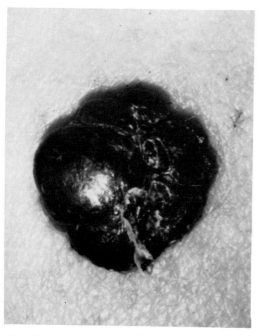

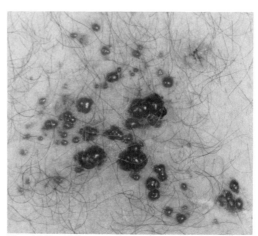

Fig. 19.5. Metastatic melanoma presenting with multiple nodules on the skin.

Clinical Staging

Clinical staging of melanoma relates to clinical spread of the tumor (Table 19.1). This type of staging is useful in planning further therapy or evaluating statistics on results of therapy.

Fig. 19.4. Nodular melanoma which has a smooth border with firm raised tumor.

Table 19.1
Clinical Setting

Stage 1
  Localized melanoma without metastasis to
  distant or regional lymph nodes
    1. Primary melanoma untreated or
       removed by excisional biopsy.
    2. Locally recurrent melanoma within 4 cm
       of primary site
    3. Multiple primary melanomas

Stage II
  Metastasis limited to regional lymph nodes
    1. Primary melanoma present or removed
       with simultaneous metastasis
    2. Primary melanoma controlled with
       subsequent metastasis.
    3. Locally recurrent melanoma with
       metastasis
    4. In-transit metastasis beyond 4 cm from
       primary site
    5. Unknown primary melanoma with
       metastasis

Stage III
  Disseminated melanoma
    1. Visceral and/or multiple lymphatic
       metastases
    2. Multiple cutaneous and/or
       subcutaneous metastases

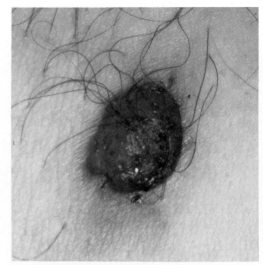

Fig. 19.7. Pigmented basal cell carcinoma which clinically resembles melanoma.

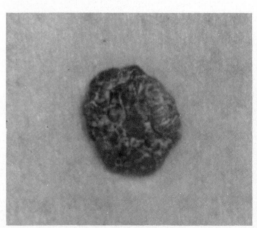

Fig. 19.8. Pigmented seborrheic keratosis with a halo surrounding the lesions. Resembles a melanoma.

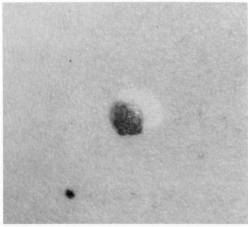

Fig. 19.6. Halo nevus—pigmented benign nevus with surrounding area of depigmentation.

Differential Diagnosis

The following clinical lesion must be considered in the differential diagnosis of malignant melanoma. If the diagnosis is uncertain, then a 4-mm diagnostic punch biopsy should be done to determine the correct diagnosis before embarking on a definitive procedure.

1. Nevi—Junctional nevi, compound nevi, and intradermal nevi. Benign juvenile melanoma (Spitz nevus), halo nevus (Fig. 19.6), and blue nevus often present deeply pigmented like a melanoma.
2. Pigmented basal cell carcinoma (Fig. 19.7).
3. Pigmented seborrheic keratosis (Fig. 19.8), and actinic keratosis rarely.
4. Granuloma pyogenicum.

5. Capillary hemangiomas, and hemorrhage into cyst or under nail plate.
6. Dermatofibroma.
7. Pigmented Bowen's disease.

Histopathologic Staging

Clark has determined five levels of histological invasion of malignant melanoma (Fig. 19.9). Clark's (1) microstaging classification has become widely adopted as the method for classifying melanoma. Based on the level of penetration of the melanoma through the skin, this system lends itself to objective verification. Clark's five levels of cutaneous invasion and clinical staging are shown in Table 19.2. Breslow (2) further refined Clark's classification, relating the prognosis of melanoma to the actual measured depth (thickness) of invasion as determined by a hand optical micrometer. It is generally accepted that a melanoma that has extended to a depth of 0.65 mm in Breslow's classification is comparable to Clark's level II and that a melanotic lesion that is 1.5 mm or thicker is comparable to Clark's levels IV and V, respectively. Clark's level III falls roughly between 0.65 mm and 1.5 mm in thickness.

In general, lentigo maligna melanoma has a better prognosis, level for level, than do the other types of malignant melanomas. The deeper the histologic invasion of melanoma (Clark's level IV and V) the worse the prognosis.

TREATMENT

Excision of Primary Melanoma

Adequate treatment requires a wide excision of the cutaneous tumor with the removal of a cuff of skin surrounding the lesion that should ideally be 4–5 cm in all directions. A critically located melanoma, such as one on the face, is not suitable for an excision of this magnitude, and clinical experience must dictate the extent of the excision.

The excision should include removal of the underlying deep fascia. Some surgeons believe that leaving the deep fascia intact at the time of melanoma removal improves survival statistics.

In some cases primary closure may be possible, but in other instances, a split-thickness skin graft is required to cover the area of

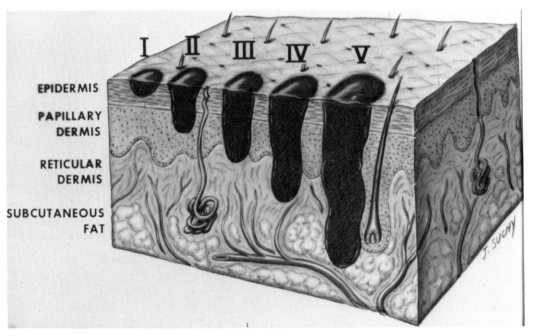

Fig. 19.9.   Clark's histological classification of malignant melanoma, showing levels *I–V*.

Table 19.2
Clark's Five Levels of Cutaneous Invasion (Histopathologic)

Level I
  Melanoma located above the basement membrane (basal lamina) of the epidermis. These lesions are essentially in situ, are extremely rare, and present no danger.
Level II
  Melanoma invades through the basement membrane down to the papillary dermis.
Level III
  Melanoma at this level is characterized by filling and widening by melanoma cells of the papillary dermis at its interface with the reticular dermis. Characteristically, there is no invasion of the underlying reticular layer.
Level IV
  These lesions show melanoma penetration into the reticular dermis.
Level V
  Melanoma at this level is evident by its presence in the subcutaneous tissue.

excision or rotation, or an advancement flap can be mobilized to cover the skin defect.

Breslow has shown that melanomas of the skin measuring less than 0.76 mm in thickness were excised with margins of as little as 1 mm up to 3 cm or more. All survived over 5 years, disease free.

Regional Lymph Node Dissection

If regional lymph nodes are palpable, then biopsy and possible therapeutic lymph node dissection is necessary for malignant melanoma.

There is controversy as to whether nonpalpable regional lymph nodes should be routinely excised. Surgeons are relying more on the histological depth of the melanoma in making this decision.

Clark levels I and II, or less than 0.76 mm in thickness, usually do not require lymph node removal. Melanomas of Clark level IV and V, or thicker than 1.5 mm, have a high incidence of lymph node metastasis and, therefore, probably should have a prophylactic lymph node dissection. There is controversy over the need for lymph node dissection

of Clark level III, or 0.76- to 1.5-mm thick lesions.

Other Modalities

Regional perfusion of an extremity for treatment of melanoma with large amounts of chemotherapeutic agents such as phenylalanine mustard and hyperthermic perfusion may reduce metatastasis in extremities. Elective lymph node dissection may not be necessary when isolation perfusion is performed.

Chemotherapy has mainly been used for widespread metastasis of melanoma. The agent with the best effect has been dimethyltriazeno-imidazole carboxamide (DTIC). Duration of remissions however last only 16–20 weeks.

Immunotherapy has been popular in the past 15 years because melanoma are known to have tumor antigens which produce antibodies against the tumor. Stimulation of a patient's immune system to produce more effective antibodies is the goal of immunotherapy. Bacillus Calmette-Guérin (BCG) is the most common agent being used for immunotherapy. Although initial trials with immunotherapy were encouraging, long-term complete remission of over 10 years are rare and late metastasis especially to the brain or other internal organs frequently occurs.

References

1. Clark, W.H., Jr., et al.: The histogenesis and biologic behavior of primary human malignant melanomas of the skin. Canc. Res., *29:* 705, 1969.
2. Breslow, A.: Thickness, cross-sectional areas and depth of invasion in the prognosis of cutaneous melanoma. Ann. Surg., *172:* 902, 1970.
3. Kopf, A.W., Bart, R.S., Rodriguez-Sains, R.S., and Ackerman, A.B.: *Malignant Melanoma.* Masson Publishing, U.S.A., New York, 1979.
4. Goldsmith, H.S.: Melanoma: an overview. CA - a Cancer J. Clin. *29:* 194, 1979.
5. Clark, W.H., Goldman, L.I., and Mastrangelo, M.J. (Eds.): *Human Malignant Melanoma,* Grune & Stratton, New York, 1979.
6. Veronesi, V. et al.: Inefficacy of immediate node dissection in Stage I melanoma of the limbs. New Engl. J. Med., *297:* 621, 1977.
7. McBride, C.M., Sugarbaker, E.V., and Hickey, R.C.: Prophylactic isolation-perfusion as the primary therapy for invasive malignant melanoma of the limbs. Ann. Surg., *182:* 316, 1975.
8. Krementz, E.T., Carter, R.D., Sutherland, C.M., and Ryan, R.F.: Malignant Melanoma of the Limbs: an

evaluation of chemotherapy by regional perfusion, in *Proceedings of the 20th Annual Clinical Conference on Cancer*, p. 375. M D Anderson Hospital and Tumor Institute, 1975, Houston, Texas.

9. Carter, S.K.: Decarbazine, Int. J. Dermatol. *15:* 59, 1976.

10. Roenigk, H.H., Jr., Doedhar, D.S., Krebs, J.A., and Barna, B.: Microcytotoxicity and serum blocking factors in malignant melanoma and halo nevus. Arch. Dermatol., *111:* 720, 1975.

11. Morton, D.L., Eilber, F., Malmgren, R. A., and Wood, W.C.: Immunological factors which influence response to immunotherapy in malignant melanoma. Surgery *68:* 158, 1970.

CHAPTER 20

LEG ULCERS

HENRY H. ROENIGK, JR.

Ulceration of the lower extremities is fairly common, and can present both diagnostic and therapeutic problems. Rare diseases such as tuberculosis, blastomycosis, and vasculitis can be mistaken for the more common chronic venous statis ulcers and ulcerations from arteriosclerosis obliterans. Thus, differential diagnosis is important, and a thorough history, physical examination, and certain laboratory tests are necessary.

DIAGNOSIS

History

Since many leg ulcers have certain characteristic features, a comprehensive history should include the following questions:

1. What did the ulcer look like when it first appeared?

   The appearance of leg ulcers often changes after secondary infection or after application of local medicine that the patient may have used in an attempt to heal the ulcer.

2. What started the ulcer?

   Local injury, strong medication, infection, thrombophlebitis, cold, and factitial (self-induced) injury may precipitate ulceration.

3. What is the family history?

   The family history is particularly helpful in cer-

tain hematologic disorders (sickle cell anemia or thalassemia) and connective tissue disorders (systemic lupus erythematosus or rheumatoid arthritis).

4. How quickly did the ulcer develop?

   Rapidly developing ulcers suggest venous insufficiency, while those that develop slowly suggest arterial insufficiency or malignancy.

5. How painful is the ulcer?

   Stasis ulcerations are often painless, whereas arterial ulcers are very painful. The patient with ischemic ulceration due to arterial insufficiency often finds that sitting in a chair all night and not elevating the legs relieves pain; the dependent position provides the best possible blood supply to painful ulcers. Venous ulceration, on the other hand, often improves with elevation, as this relieves the edema of the surrounding tissues.

6. What drug has the patient been on?

   It is important to obtain a complete list of all medications taken by the patient. Specific questions concerning nonprescriptive medications such as sedatives, sleeping pills, analgesics, and antacids should be included, since these drugs are often the cause of leg ulcers.

7. Is there a history of other systemic disorders?

   A current or past history of anemia, rheumatoid arthritis, collagen disorders, and other diseases often gives a clue to the cause of an unusual leg ulcer.

PHYSICAL EXAMINATION

The location of the ulcer is important in the differential diagnosis. Ulcers due to stasis dermatitis often occur over the internal malleolus, because this area is drained by the saphenous venous system. Ischemic ulcers occur in areas farthest from the occluded vessel. Those resulting from arteriosclerosis usually develop on the toes or dorsum of the foot, while those caused by hypertension occur on the lateral malleolus.

The skin surrounding the ulcer should be closely examined for such signs as stasis pigmentation, edema, presence or absence of arterial pulsations, evidence of scleroderma, petechiae, and hemorrhage. The color of the skin is also important. Pale skin indicates poor arterial blood supply, as in ischemic ulcers.

The patient should be examined for signs of systemic disease. A heart murmur caused by advanced cardiovascular syphilis, arthritis resulting from systemic lupus erythematosus, or other signs of diabetes mellitus (i.e. eyeground changes) may indicate the cause of the leg ulcer.

LABORATORY TESTS

Routine laboratory tests, including hemogram, blood chemistries, serologic test for

Table 20.1
Causes of leg ulcers

Vascular disorders	Tuberculosis
Arterial	Erythema induratum
Thromboangiitis obliterans	Lupus vulgaris
Arteriosclerosis obliterans	Papulonecrotic tuberculid
Livedo reticularis	
Hypertension	Metabolic disorders
Chronic pernio (chilblains)	Diabetic ulcer
Venous (chronic venous insufficiency)	Necrobiosis lipoidica diabeticorum
Lymphatic (elephantiasis nostras,	Pyoderma gangrenosum
lymphedema)	Gaucher's disease
	Gout
Vasculitis	Porphyria cutanea tarda
Atrophie blanche	
Allergic vasculitis	Tumors
Lupus erythematosus	Basal cell carcinoma
Necrotizing angiitis	Squamous cell carcinoma
Periarteritis nodosa	Kaposi's hemorrhagic sarcoma
Rheumatoid arthritis	Lymphoma
Degos' disease	Lymphosarcoma
	Mycosis fungoides
Hematologic disorders	Malignant melanoma
Sickle cell anemia	
Spherocytic anemia	Miscellaneous
Thalassemia	Drugs
Polycythemia vera	Halogens
Leukemia	Ergot
Dysproteinemia	Methotrexate
	Chemical burns
Infections	Trophic disorder
Fungal	Thermal injury
Blastomycosis	Lichen planus
Coccidioidomycosis	Weber-Christian disease
Histoplasmosis	Acrodermatitis chronica atrophicans
Sporotrichosis	Insect bite
Maduromycosis	Radiation
Syphilis	Frostbite
Bacterial infections	Factitial (self-induced) injury

syphilis, and bacterial cultures should be done in all leg ulcer patients, since other medical problems such as diabetes mellitus, electrolyte imbalance, and congestive heart failure can complicate the healing of the ulcer. Special procedures, such as skin biopsy, skin tests, and antinuclear antibody, should be ordered only when underlying systemic disease is strongly suspected.

Vascular Leg Ulcers

ARTERIOSCLEROSIS OBLITERANS

A history of intermittent claudication or severe pain in a leg ulcer suggests the presence of arteriosclerosis obliterans. Arterial insufficiency usually causes pallor, cyanosis, and coolness of the skin of the involved extremity. The loss of peripheral pulses is important in the diagnosis; however, the presence of pulses does not preclude a diagnosis of arterial insufficiency. When a partial or complete occlusion involves only a short segment of the terminal aorta or iliac arteries, the distal pulses may be present but dampened.

Postural color changes indicate the degree of ischemia in an extremity. An ischemic limb blanches when elevated and becomes excessively red or cyanotic when dependent. Failure of the color to return within 15 seconds after an extremity is changed from an elevated to a dependent position indicates moderate to severe ischemia.

Ischemic ulcers usually occur first at the tips of the digits (Fig. 20.1), around and under the nails, on the interdigital surfaces, or on the heels. They may also occur on the lateral and medial sides of the foot overlying the metatarsal heads. Usually small and shallow initially, these ulcers gradually increase in size, have a pale base devoid of granulation tissue, and are covered with necrotic debris, as shown in Figure 20.2 (see color Plate IV).

Noninvasive diagnostic procedures, such as use of Doppler ultrasound instrumentations and ultrasonic arteriography (1) are helpful in documenting arteriosclerosis obliterans; however, complete angiography (aortography and femoral arteriography) is the only diagnostic method available that will precisely locate the site of the arterial occlusions, the extent of the disease, and the amount of collateral circulation present. This information is essential in order to evaluate potential surgical repair of arterial insufficiency.

VENOUS INSUFFICIENCY LEG ULCERS

The cardinal features of ulceration from venous insufficiency are edema, superficial varicose veins, pigmentation, and eczematous dermatitis of the surrounding skin (Fig. 20.3). The pigmentation results from rupture of venules caused by excessive venous pressure and the subsequent extravasation of hemoglobin (hemosiderin) into the tissues. Stasis dermatitis causes erythema, weeping, scaling, and pruritus (Fig. 20.4), which may become generalized.

Ulcerations usually occur in the region of the ankle near the internal malleolus and may develop spontaneously or secondary to trauma. Aseptic cellulitis may develop in surrounding skin. The base of the ulcer is usually moist, with extensive granulation tissue, and is often secondarily infected. The ulcers may be painful but, in contrast to ulcers caused by arteriosclerosis obliterans, are often relieved by rest and elevation of the extremity.

Diagnostic tests are usually not necessary in ulcers due to venous insufficiency. Compe-

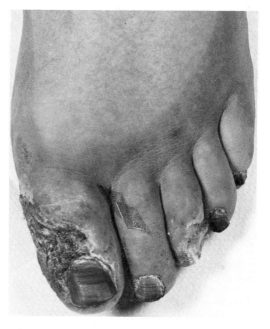

Fig. 20.1. Arteriosclerosis obliterans with ulceration of the tip of distal digits.

tency of the valves in the superficial veins can be tested by applying a rubber tourniquet to the leg with the leg in different positions, as outlined in the Trendelenburg test or the multiple-tourniquet test.

HYPERTENSIVE LEG ULCERS

Characteristically ischemic ulcers of the lower extremities may develop in patients who have had essential hypertension for a long time. Women in their fifth or sixth decades are most commonly affected, although ulcers occur in men. The ulcer usually starts as a painful, reddish-blue plaque over the lateral malleolus; the plaque ulcerates and is surrounded by a cyanotic or purpuric halo. The ulcer usually has little granulation tissue and is very painful. Diagnostic tests are not nec-

essary, except to exclude larger arterial insufficiency by arteriography. Control of essential hypertension is vital in the treatment of these ulcers.

Vasculitis

Many different terms have been applied to the entity of vasculitis, ranging from polyarteritis nodosa, hypersensitivity angiitis, Wegener's granulomatosis, allergic granulomatosis, to necrotizing vasculitis. Leg ulcers resulting from a vasculitis may be associated with other generalized disorders such as systemic lupus erythematosus or rheumatoid arthritis. The term vasculitis is often referred to as a hypersensitivity or allergic vasculitis. The hypersensitivity may often be due to an infection or an allergic reaction to drugs. The

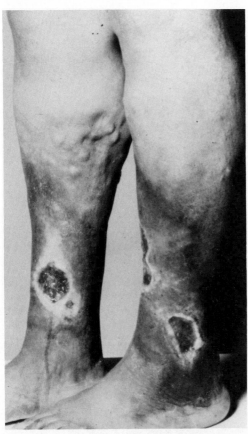

Fig. 20.3. Chronic venous insufficiency with ulceration usually over medial malleoleus. There is edema, pigmentation, and varicose veins.

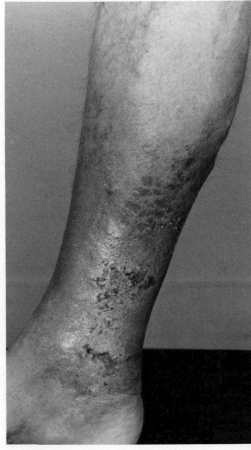

Fig. 20.4. Stasis dermatitis with early ulceration.

reaction is primarily in small blood vessels of the skin.

Cutaneous lesions of vasculitis vary from erythematous macules, purpura, hemorrhagic vesicles, urticarial lesions, nodular, and eventually necrotic lesions, and ulceration (Fig. 20.5, Fig. 20.6, and as shown in Figure 20.7 on color Plate IV). The skin is easily accessible for biopsy and this often will confirm the diagnosis of vasculitis. The histopathologic changes seen in skin biopsy specimens reveal swelling and degeneration of the endothelial cells of the small blood vessels, thickening of the vessel walls, and a fibrinoid degeneration of the perivascular tissue. A severe inflammatory infiltrate composed mostly of polymorphic neutrophils and eosinophils with some lymphocytes is often seen. The most common finding in acute vasculitis of the skin is leukocytoclasis or nuclear dust. This classic feature of vasculitis is the result of fragmentation of nuclear material from surrounding inflammatory cells. Other laboratory studies that may help to confirm a more generalized type of vasculitis include: blood hemoglobin, leukocyte count, erythrocyte sedimentation rate, lupus erythematosus (LE) test, antinuclear factor, renal function studies, and direct immunofluorescences of lesions.

The treatment of vasculitis ulcerations of the lower extremities involves treatment of the systemic disease producing the vasculitis. This may include antibiotics for an underlying infection, stopping a course of medications (hypersensitivity reaction), or administering systemic steroid, as in systemic lupus erythematosus. Stronger immunosuppressive agents, such as cytoxin and azathioprine, are sometimes needed to control the vasculitis.

Hematologic Ulcers

Various types of hematologic disorders will

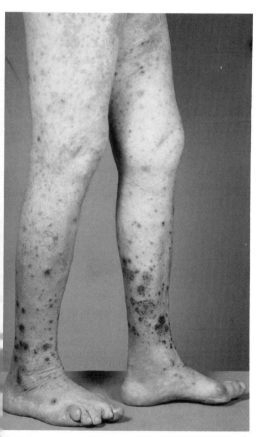

Fig. 20.5. Acute necrotizing vasculitis with purpura, hemorrhagic vesicles, urticaria, and ulceration of lower extremities.

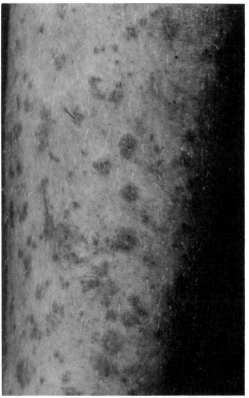

Fig. 20.6. Vasculitis with palpable purpura.

result in ulceration of the lower extremities. Sickle cell anemia, a genetically transmitted abnormality that results in an abnormal hemoglobin molecule in homozygous persons, is found almost entirely in the black race. The cutaneous manifestations of sickle cell anemia are indolent ulcers or scars on the lower parts of the legs (Fig. 20.8), which develop in about 75% of the older children or adults with the disease (Fig. 20.9). The ulcers which have sharply defined edges, are usually single, but may be multiple and bilateral. There is no distinctive feature of this ulcer, but in a young black with no other obvious cause of the ulcer, sickle cell anemia should be considered. Laboratory studies will show a normocytic and normochromic anemia, and the sickling phenomenon can be demonstrated in a moist, sealed, coverslip preparation.

Hereditary spherocytosis may produce ulceration of the lower extremities. Chronic ulcers of the leg in the region of the malleoli are reported to occur in 6% of patients. The ulcers are usually several centimeters in diameter and are surrounded by an area of hyperpigmentation. Increased fragility of erythrocytes in hypotonic saline solution has been recognized as a characteristic feature of hereditary spherocytosis.

Other hematologic disorders that rarely produce leg ulcers, but must be considered in the differential diagnosis are: thalassemia, polycythemia vera, leukemia, and the dysproteinemias. Macroglobulinemia, which occurs chiefly in persons between 50 and 70 years of age, will often have a presenting symptom of leg edema, and occasionally necrosis and ulceration. Cryoglobulinemia is characterized by the formation of immunoglobulins, or other proteins that precipitate on exposure to cold and redissolve on warming to body temperature.

Many patients with cryoglobulinemia also have multiple myelomas, macroglobulinemia, Hodgkin's disease, lymphosarcoma or other lymphomas, lupus erythematosus, polyarteritis nodosa, polycythemia vera, cirrhosis or, in endemic areas, kala azar. These patients may have the following presenting symptoms: Raynaud's phenomenon, purpura, necrosis ulceration, or gangrene of the upper or lower extremities especially at the tips of the fingers or toes.

Infectious Diseases

DEEP FUNGUS INFECTIONS

The deep fungus infections of the skin are produced as two distinct types. The rarer form, the chancriform syndrome, is an example of primary cutaneous inoculation. This form of the disease most commonly follows trauma to the skin, with an introduction of the pathogenic organisms into the tissues. An area of erythema and induration develops at the site of inoculation. In from 1 to 2 weeks, a chancre appears with subsequent lymphangitis and lymphedema of the involved limb.

The common form of the deep fungus infections are those associated with systemic involvement. The appearance of the lesion is usually a papular pustular nodule that enlarges peripherally to form an elevated ulcerated verrucous granuloma. The greatest activity of the infection occurs at the periphery

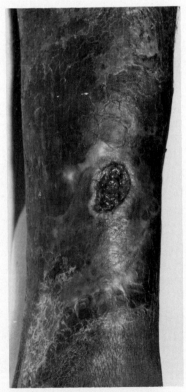

Fig. 20.8.   Leg ulcers associated with sickle cell anemia.

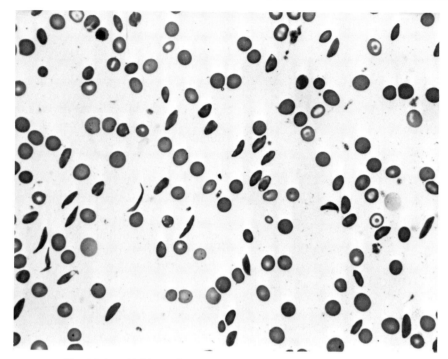

Fig. 20.9.   Sickle cell preparation from peripheral blood.

which is clearly demarcated from normal skin.

The deep fungi that could most commonly produce a lower extremity ulceration are: blastomycosis, coccidioidomycosis, histoplasmosis, and sporotrichosis. These can be differentiated by direct examination (smear), culture characteristics, and identification of the organism in tissue sections with periodic acid-Schiff (PAS) stain.

North American Blastomycosis is caused by *Blastomyces dermatitidis*. This organism most commonly produces a small papular pustule with an eventual verrucal plaque and advancing borders (Fig. 20.10). Direct examination of the exudate shows a large thick-walled blastospore or single budding yeast Fig. 20.11).

Coccidioidomycosis is caused by *Coccidioides immitis*. It is generally thought to be mainly a pulmonary infection that is commonly seen in natives of the San Joaquin Valley in California. This infection, however, does have a cutaneous form as usually seen on the exposed surfaces of the skin, e.g. the leg. It, too, has two forms of the disease, the typical chancres that in the late stages can become papillomatous and verrucal, or a systemic disease with resultant hematologic spread or fistula formation from an internal abscess that eventuates in the typical verrucal plaque, or draining abscess, respectively.

Histoplasmosis, a disease caused by *Histoplasma capsulatum*, is also usually a pulmonary disease. It also may produce the cutaneous form, but less frequently.

Sporotrichosis is a chronic fungus infection caused by *Sporotrichum schenkii*. The organism lives mainly on vegetation; therefore, most primary inoculations are made in gardeners or horticulturists who injure themselves while working. At the site of injury, a typical primary chancriform lymphoglandular type of eruption occurs with the development of many small abscesses and subsequent ulcerations. The verrucal plaque-like lesion occurs less frequently.

SYPHILIS

Syphilitic gumma, a late benign form of syphilis, develops as a deep subcutaneous fixed nodule or plaque that may be singular or multiple in number. Clinically, it appears as a firm, well defined painless indolent nod-

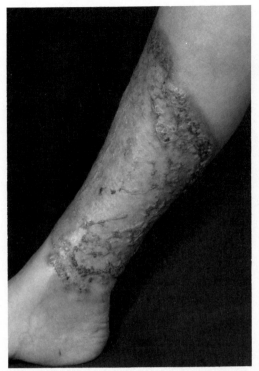

Fig. 20.10. North American blastomycosis with large plaque and advancing verrucal border.

ule or plaque. The lesions often ulcerate and extrude a thick sanguinous secretion (Fig. 20.12). The ulcers are clearly demarcated, deep, and have a purulent base. The ulcer heals from the base and leaves a contracted scar.

The causative organism, *Treponema pallidum*, is not identified on direct examination of the tissue. Serologic tests usually show high titers. The fluorescent treponema antibody (FTA) adsorption test is positive. A tissue biopsy of the nodule or ulcer shows a granulomatous process that extends from the dermis into the subcutaneous tissue. Epithelial and giant cells are numerous.

BACTERIAL-INFECTED ULCERS

Peripheral vascular ulcers of the leg often become secondarily infected and produce an increased inflammation of the ulcer and surrounding tissue. The clinical signs are those of erythema, edema, and purulent exudate or a heavy eschar (Fig. 20.13) with pronounced peripheral inflammation. In a study of the bacterial flora of the vascular ulcers, the most common significant bacteria in the inflammed leg ulcer were those of *Staphylococcus aureus* and *Enterobacter coli*. These ulcers respond to local antiseptic agents and topical or systemic antibiotics depending on the degree of inflammation and size of the ulcer. Appropriate cultures and antibiotic sensitivity testing are indicated.

TUBERCULOSIS

Lupus vulgaris of the lower extremities appears as a well demarcated reddish brown patch or patches containing small papules. The papules show positive diascopy (a yellow-brown color when the glass slide is pressed against them). These yellow lesions gradually become atrophic and show multiple areas of ulceration; occasionally, the borders develop a verrucal growth. It has been noted by some authors that squamous cell carcinomas can occur in these chronic lesions. A biopsy shows a typical tubercle with moderate caseation in the upper dermis. Acid-fast stains reveal the presence of small numbers of tubercle bacilli.

Tuberculid. In the past, tuberculids were thought to represent hematogenous dissemination of tubercle bacilli from a visceral focus into the skin. Over the years, four disorders have been classified as tuberculids: erythema induratum, (Fig. 20.14) papulonecrotic tuberculid, lichen scrofulosorum, lupus miliaris disseminatus faciei. These disorders are quite rare today and may not be related to tuberculosis.

Metabolic Disorders

NECROBIOSIS LIPOIDICA DIABETICORUM

Plaque-like lesions that occur over the anterior surface of the leg and are reddish yellow with a smooth glistening surface and numerous telandiectasia are often a clue to underlying diabetes mellitus, as shown in Figure 20.15 (see color Plate IV). Necrobiosis lipoidica diabeticorum (NLD) presents these distinctive clinical features, which can be confirmed by skin biopsy.

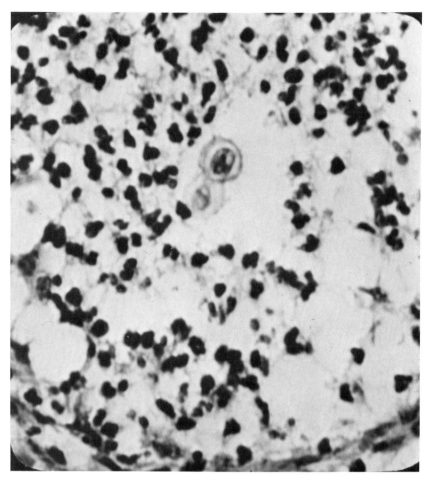

Fig. 20.11. Blastomycosis—direct smear of lesion showing yeast-like organisms.

Occasionally, as a result of minor trauma, the lesions of NLD will become ulcerated. Treatment with topical antibiotics and Unna boot will often result in re-epithelialization of the lesions. When the ulceration is extensive, then split-thickness skin grafting is indicated.

PYODERMA GANGRENOSUM

Acute necrotizing ulcerations of the lower extremity with a rolled vegetating border are suggestive of pyoderma gangrenosum and investigation for possible gastrointestinal disease will often disclose chronic ulcerative colitis.

The skin lesions usually begin as erythematous papulonodules that enlarge rapidly into plaques up to 12 cm or more in diameter. The active border is deeply violaceous red and the central portion is necrotic and ulcerated. A halo of erythema surrounds the lesion. Lesions of pyoderma gangrenosum are often extremely painful and, although they usually occur on the lower part of the leg, they may occur anywhere on the skin. Bacteriologic cultures of the ulceration often are sterile or grow contaminant organisms. Skin biopsy from the edge of the ulcer shows considerable proliferation of the epidermis (pseudocarcinomatous hyperplasia), and necrosis with chronic inflammatory cells in the dermis. The biopsy is not diagnostic of pyoderma gangrenosum, but helps to exclude other etiologic factors.

Although pyoderma gangrenosum at one time was considered pathognomonic of an underlying chronic ulcerative colitis, today

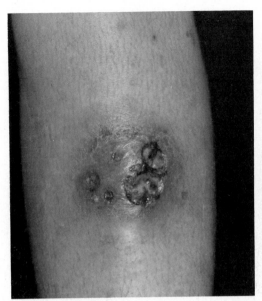

Fig. 20.12. Syphilitic gumma with nodule and ulceration.

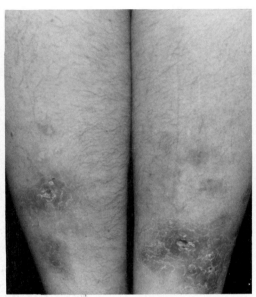

Fig. 20.14. Erythema induratum which is a tuberculid. There is induration and then ulceration on posterior portion of leg.

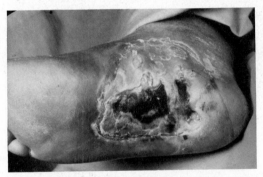

Fig. 20.13. Bacterial infected ulcer with purulent exudate and heavy eschar.

other conditions such as regional enteritis, gastric ulcer, empyema, and chronic debilitating infections may be associated with it. Therapy is directed primarily at the underlying systemic disorder. When the chronic ulcerative colitis is active, then treatment with salicylazosulfapyridine, adrenocorticotropic hormones, or corticosteroids will usually result in prompt healing of the ulceration.

PORPHYRIA CUTANEA TARDA

Porphyria cutanea tarda (PCT) is an acquired abnormality of porphyrin metabolism

which results in cutaneous lesions and increased urinary excretion of uroporphyrins and coproporphyrins. The majority of patients have abnormal liver function because of excessive use of alcohol, toxins, or drugs.

The clinical features include fragility of the skin and bulla formation of the sun-exposed areas, especially the hands. Healing of bullae results in scar formation and milia. Hyperpigmentation, hypertrichosis, and morphea-like plaques are other features.

Ulcerations of the lower extremity are not a common feature of PCT, but do occur.

Tumors

Benign and malignant tumors frequently will have presenting signs as ulcerations of the lower extremities. In each case, the diagnostic skin biopsy is essential to the correct diagnosis and thus early appropriate treatment. The following examples are tumors that more commonly will present as ulcers of the lower extremities: Kaposi's hemorrhagic sarcoma, lymphosarcoma, mycosis fungoides, (Fig. 20.16) and malignant melanoma (Fig. 20.17).

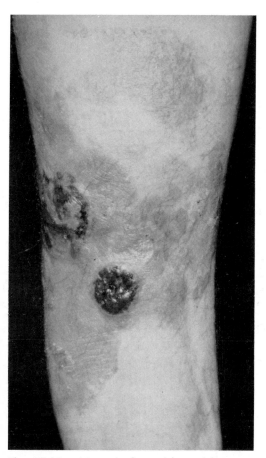

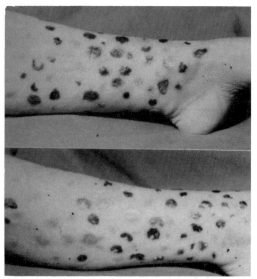

Fig. 20.18. Factitial ulceration produced by cigarette burns to leg.

nating are factitial or self-induced ulcerations. They are not confined to the lower extremity but are in areas easily accessible to the patient. Bizarre ulcers are produced by chemicals, cigarettes, syringes, and other devices used by psychotic patients (Fig. 20.18).

Fig. 20.16. Mycosis fungoides with eczematous plaque and ulcerative tumor lesions of the leg.

MANAGEMENT OF LEG ULCERS

The goal of treatment of all leg ulcers is to stimulate good granulation tissue and restore epithelial regrowth. General measures include clearing the surrounding skin (stasis eczema) with use of compresses, topical corticosteroids and, occasionally, topical antibiotics. Bed rest and reduction of edema speed healing. In ulcers caused by arteriosclerosis obliterans, bed rest is helpful, but the head of the bed should be elevated.

Local treatment of the ulcer is important in clearing the infection and stimulating granulation tissue that can accept either an entire skin graft or epithelial regrowth from the borders of the ulcer.

BENZOYL PEROXIDE

Benzoyl peroxide, a potent oxidizing agent widely used in treating acne vulgaris, recently

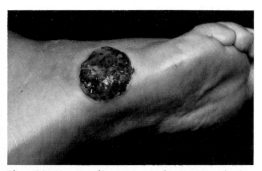

Fig. 20.17. Malignant melanoma of the foot.

Miscellaneous

Among the large group of miscellaneous causes of leg ulcers, probably the most fasci-

has been reported to give excellent results in promoting granulation tissue in ulcers.

A piece of terry cloth cut in the exact shape of the ulcer is moistened with normal saline solution, impregnated with 20% benzoyl peroxide lotion, and applied to the ulcer. The normal skin margins of the ulcer are protected with petrolatum jelly, and the padded ulcer is then occulated with plastic wrap. The dressings are changed every 8–12 hours. Excessive granulation tissue at epithelial borders may be cauterized with 10% silver nitrate solution. Benzoyl peroxide probably acts by providing bactericidal action, stimulating granulation tissue, and producing hyperbaric oxygen and debridement (Figs. 20.19–20.21).

DEXTRAN POLYMER BEADS

The treatment consists of applying a thick layer of a three-dimensional network of po-

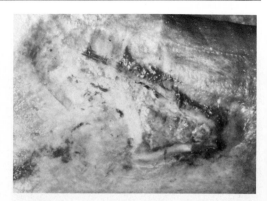

Fig. 20.21. Leg ulcer healed after 4 weeks of Benoxyl Lotion therapy.

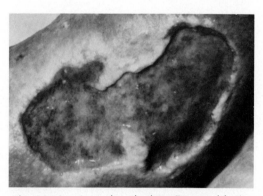

Fig. 20.19. Leg ulcer before Benoxyl lotion therapy.

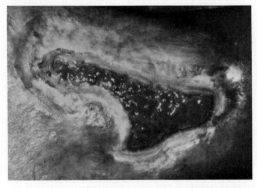

Fig. 20.20. Leg ulcer healing during Benoxyl Lotion therapy.

rous Dextran polymer beads 0.1–0.3 mm in diameter, to the ulcer. The beads are highly hydrophilic and absorb fluid until saturated, swelling in the process. When placed on a discharging ulcer surface, the beads promptly absorb the exudate, bacteria, and tissue degradation residues from the ulcer surface. The Dextran polymer beads are pharmacologically inert, and their action is entirely physical. By absorbing the protein-rich fluid from the ulcer surface, they prevent crust formation, greatly reduce the bacterial load on the ulcer surface, and remove inflammation mediators and toxins produced by bacteria, allowing more vigorous cell metabolism in the ulcer base.

Another excellent method of local debridement is to apply topical viscous lidocaine (Xylocaine 5% Ointment) and use a small sharp curette to remove the moist eschar that often inhibits re-epithelialization.

UNNA'S BOOT

The Unna paste boot is a flesh-colored roll bandage impregnated with a uniformly spread paste of zinc oxide, calamine, glycerin, and gelatin. Before the boot is applied, the leg is cleansed with lukewarm water or mineral oil to remove debris and any previous medication. Gentian violet 1%, Terra-Cortril Topical Ointment, fluocinolone acetonide ointment, or a topical antibiotic is then applied. The Unna boot is applied from an area just below the popliteal space. The foot should be kept at a right angle to minimize chafing

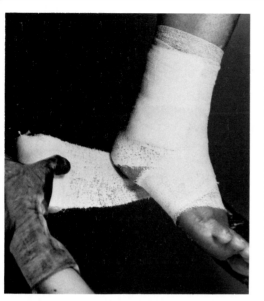

Fig. 20.22. Application of Unna boot.

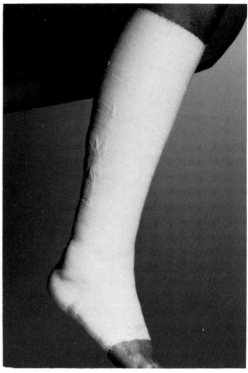

Fig. 20.24. Completed application of unna boot. Reproduced with permission from H.H. Roenigk, Jr. and J.R. Young: *Leg Ulcers—Medical and Surgical Management* Harper & Row, Publishers, Hagerstown, Md., 1975.

(Figs. 20.22). The bandage is placed around the foot and then directly obliquely over the heel and up the calf, in much the same manner as an elastic bandage is applied (Figs. 20.23, 20.24). It should be applied in a "pressure gradient manner," with the greatest pressure at the ankle and lower third of the leg. A double layer of Tubegauze is placed over the Unna boot (Fig. 20.25) and secured at the upper and lower limits with tape. The boot is changed weekly or more often if there is excessive drainage through the boot or if the boot becomes loose due to reduction of edema.

The Unna boot is ideal for stasis ulcers and stasis eczema but it also can be used in a variety of other ulcers, since it helps remove edema and protects the ulcer from external trauma. The patient may be ambulatory while wearing the Unna boot.

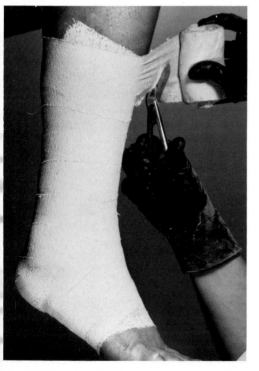

Fig. 20.23. Application of Unna boot. Reproduced with permission from H.H. Roenigk, Jr. and J.R. Young: *Leg Ulcers—Medical and Surgical Management* Harper & Row, Publishers, Hagerstown, Md., 1975.

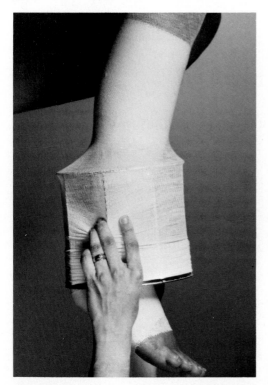

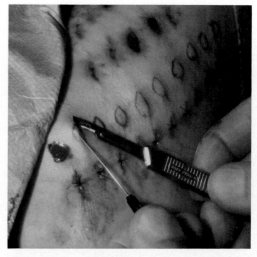

Fig. 20.26. Donor site for pinch grafts are from upper thigh. Taken with scalpel or razor blade. Reproduced with permission from H.H. Roenigk, Jr. and J.R. Young: *Leg Ulcers—Medical and Surgical Management* Harper & Row, Publishers, Hagerstown, Md., 1975.

Fig. 20.25. Double layer of Tubegauze placed over the Unna boot. Reproduced with permission from H.H. Roenigk, Jr. and J.R. Young: *Leg Ulcers—Medical and Surgical Management* Harper & Row, Publishers, Hagerstown, Md., 1975.

SKIN GRAFTS

The final goal in the treatment of all leg ulcers is to provide adequate skin coverage of the ulcer. Conservative methods may stimulate granulation tissue, with regrowth of epithelial tissue from the borders of the healing ulcer but healing by this method is not always satisfactory, since the epithelium may be fragile and ulceration can reoccur.

The underlying etiologic factors such as venous or arterial insufficiency and hypertension must be determined because, in general, skin grafting will not take well if arterial blood supply is poor. Venous stasis ulcers usually respond well to skin grafts. Porcine xenografting as a bedside procedure has proved to a be a reliable guide to definitive autografting. Adherence or loss of the porcine xenograft

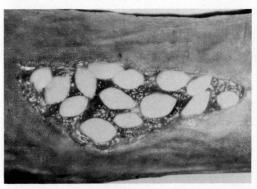

Fig. 20.27. Pinch grafts placed on the clean granulation tissue of ulcer base. Reproduced with permission from H.H. Roenigk, Jr. and J.R. Young: *Leg Ulcers—Medical and Surgical Management* Harper & Row, Publishers, Hagerstown, Md., 1975.

will be obvious on clinical inspection of the wound at 24 hours. Adherence may be allowed to continue for 24–72 hours, after which an immune rejection process begins. Split-thickness skin graft, applied in the routine fashion, probably will take successfully.

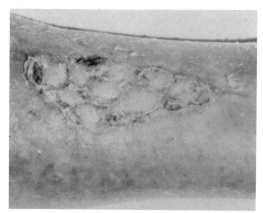

Fig. 20.28. Healed skin grafts several weeks later.

If bone or tendon is exposed, fully vascularized, full-thickness skin and subcutaneous tissue must be applied. Cross-leg pedicle flap or the application of distant tissue in the form of free-flap transfer revascularized by microvascular techniques is indicated over exposed bone or tendon. Small pinch grafts (4 mm) taken from the thigh and placed in on a clean ulcer with good granulation tissue will often give a good epithelial surface. This procedure can be done under local anesthesia and the rate of success is high (Figs. 20.26–20.28).

References

1. Bergan, J.J., Darling, R.C., and deWolfe, V.G., et al.: Report of the Inter-Society Commission for Heart Disease Resources: medical instrumentation in peripheral vascular disease. Circulation *54:* A-1, 1976.
2. Roenigk, H.H., Jr., and Young, J.R.: *Leg Ulcers—Medical and Surgical Management.* Harper & Row Publishers, Hagerstown, Md., 1975.
3. Fairburn, J.F., Juergens, J.L., and Spittell, J.A., Jr.: In E.V. Allen (Ed) *Peripheral Vascular Diseases,* Ed 4. W.B. Saunders Company, Philadelphia, 1972.
4. Pace, W.E.: Treatment of cutaneous ulcers with benzoyl peroxide. Can. Med. Assoc. J., *115:* 1101, 1976.
5. Coleman, G.J., and Roenigk, H.H., Jr.: Topical therapy of leg ulcers with 20 percent benzoyl peroxide lotion. Cutis, *21:* 491, 1978.
6. Jacobsson, S., Rothman, U., and Arturson, G., et al.: A new principle for the cleaning of infected wounds. Scand. J. Plast. Reconstr. Surg., *10:* 65, 1976.
7. Pace, W.E.: Dextran polymer beads in the local treatment of cutaneous ulcers. J. Dermatol. Surg. Oncol., *4:* 678, 1978.
8. Dinner, M.I., Peters, C.R.: Aids in management of vascular ulcer of the lower limbs. J. Dermatol. Surg. Oncol., *4:* 696, 1978.

CHAPTER 21

TOPICAL TREATMENT OF DISEASED SKIN

JAMES E. RASMUSSEN

THEORY AND GOALS

Successful topical therapy depends on much more than the selection of active ingredients for specific diseases. The best results occur when an equal amount of attention is given to the choice of a vehicle. To do otherwise may prevent the active ingredient from penetrating to the damaged areas, exacerbate the basic disease or induce a new problem such as secondary infection.

This chapter will discuss a variety of topical "active agents" and appropriate choices for vehicles.

VEHICLES

Choice of a vehicle (Fig. 21.1) should depend on 1) state of the skin (dry or wet), 2) location and amount of surface area to be treated, and 3) environment. The general goal for a vehicle is best explained as "if it's wet, dry it; if it's dry, wet it." Wet lesions—those that feature pus, exudate, vesicles, blisters, or maceration—should be treated with vehicles that promote drying. Dry lesions—rough, scaly, hyperkeratotic—need vehicles that provide lubrication.

State of the Skin

There are two ways to "dry" wet diseases or "wet" dry ones.

Wet diseases (Fig. 21.2) can be dried with either frequent application of absorbent powders (starch, zinc oxide, talc, bentonite) or with the intermittent use of vehicles, such as water, that evaporate. Powders can absorb small quantities of moisture but in doing so may form a hard coating on the surface of the skin. Water or other volatile liquids are very effective drying agents when used for 2–10 minute intervals three to five times a day. The water can be applied in the form of a compress, wet dressing, soak, bath, lotion, or spray.

Dry diseases (Figs. 21.3–21.5) can be softened with either water or with lubricants. Unfortunately, while water softens dry diseased skin it evaporates, rapidly producing an even drier situation. Lubricants, however, provide either physical occlusion which prevents the natural evaporation of water or act chemically to bind water to the skin. The oldest lubricants are either "pure" greases such as (petrolatum, lanolin, and mineral oil) or emulsions. Simply stated, emulsions are suspensions of oil in water (o/w) (producing a white cream) or water in oil (w/o). The percentage of water determines the lubricating potential and the ability to "vanish" or rub into the skin—high concentrations of water provide less lubrication, but rub in very well.

Cutaneous pharmacologists have fortunately progressed far beyond simple emulsions of o/w or w/o. Most vehicles are now complex mixtures of wetting agents, preservatives, solvents, and buffers with much greater bioavailability of active ingredients such as corticosteroids.

During the past 5 years, there have been considerable advances in the production of lubricating, but not "greasy," vehicles for topical steroids, many of which contain solutions of the active drug instead of the previous emulsion. The "new generation" of topicals is usually designated by the brand name followed by a hyphenated list of capital letters—

Aristocort A Topical Cream & Ointment, Cordran-SP Cream, Lidex-E Cream 0.05%.

These advances in pharmacology have blurred the once clear distinction between ointments, creams, and lotions, making it easier to treat patients, but more difficult to

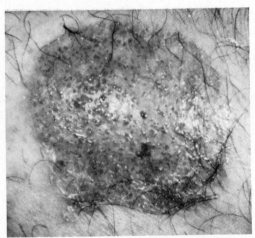

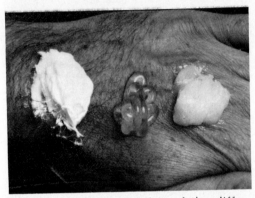

Fig. 21.1.   A demonstration of the differences in color of creams (white), gels (clear, usually) and pure ointments (grey).

Fig. 21.2.   A "wet" disease—exudative nummular eczema. Wet diseases should be treated with compresses; this disease could be treated with a steroid lotion or a cream followed by a wet compress.

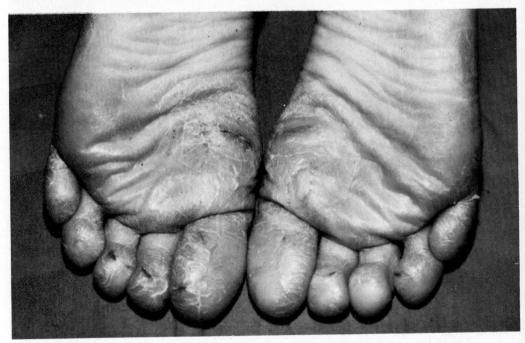

Fig. 21.3.   Atopic winter foot, a "dry" disease; treat with lubricating base.

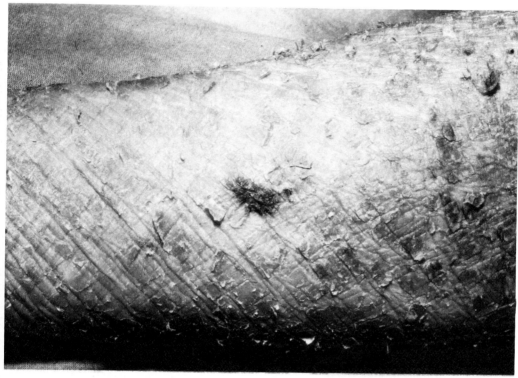

Fig. 21.4. Ichthyosis, a "dry" disease; treat with lubricating base.

explain the range of effects of the newer vehicles.

Vehicles for special situations. *Paints*—solutions of volatile solvents usually alcohol or acetone which rapidly leave a thin film of active ingredients. Paints are little used today, but a few are still worth mentioning.

Castellani's paint—a red/purple combination of phenol, boric acid, resorcinol, acetone, alcohol, and magneta. It is used as a drying, antibacterial-antifungal compound in chronic infection of the toe webs and groin. The relatively high concentration of phenol, boric acid, and resorcinol when applied over large areas can be toxic, especially in children.

Wart paint—varying concentrations of salicylic acid, lactic acid, benzoic acid and/or podophyllin in collodion and acetone which dries rapidly leaving a thin adherent membrane over the wart.

Cantharidin wart paint (Cantharone)—cantharidin (a blistering chemical derived from the Spanish fly of college folklore) in acetone and collodion. It is best used for periungual warts, occasionally (approximately 5%) producing a "ring around the wart" (recurrence of verrucae in a ring peripheral to the original lesion) (see Chapter 13).

Area of the Body

The body area to be treated is one of the most critical factors involved in the choice of a vehicle. Far from a homogeneous unit, the skin surface has oil on the face and scalp; moisture in the flexures, palms, and soles; and dry deserts on the extremities as well as substantial differences in the thickness from eyelids to feet. The cosmetic and functional aspects of the face, hands, and feet must also be considered.

Environment and Season

While dry diseases need lubrication, lubricants such as the "ointments" are poorly tolerated during the warm, humid months. Patients with atopic dermatitis are particularly

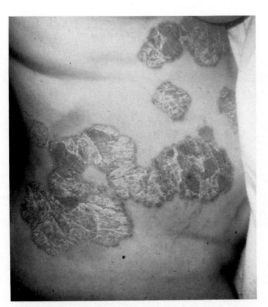

Fig. 21.5. Psoriasis, a "dry" disease; treat with lubricating base.

sensitive to occlusive vehicles at this time of the year and it is best to switch from ointments to creams during the summer. Conversely, many naturally dry lesions (psoriasis, atopic eczema) have a tendency toward *exacerbation* in the colder months; a time when *ointment* and the more lubricating creams are best used.

Failure to tailor the vehicles to suit the terrain and disease can result in poor compliance, decreased efficacy and adverse reactions.

Finally, remember that the quantity supplied should be enough to last until the next visit. An adult with widespread dermatitis needs a minimum of 30–60 g a day so do not write a prescription for 15-g tubes unless the area to be treated is small, such as the hands. Small quantities frequently refilled are much more costly than a few larger sizes, although availability is greater for 15- to 30-g trade packages.

Gels—Newer Vehicles

Gels are elegant, semisolid mixtures of alcohols, glycols, and water which are usually clear. They are not greasy, and they dry without leaving much of a residue on the skin. They are a good solvent system for many topical drugs and provide excellent bioavailability. Because of these cosmetic and pharmacological properties they are extensively used in over-the-counter (OTC) and prescription dermatologicals. Most are rather neutral in their direct effects on the skin although some are drying and may sting when applied. They are also somewhat more expensive than conventional vehicles.

The gels' greatest appeal is cosmetic and consequently one should restrict their routine use to face and scalp problems or to more generalized disease in fastidious patients.

CLINICAL PROBLEMS IN THE APPLICATION OF VEHICLES

Problem I. An adult presents with widespread dermatitis venenata (poison ivy) which is inflamed and weeping. Prescribe a regimen of therapy using only one vehicle.

Solutions
1. Frequent baths or showers (three to four times a day) for 5 or 10 minutes.
2. Shake-lotions which contain powders in a liquid vehicle (calamine lotion).
3. Widespread use of wet dressings is not practical and can result in a tremendous caloric loss.

Problem II. A 6-year-old girl has widespread chronic atopic eczema and visits your office in Buffalo, N.Y. on Christmas Eve. Treat her with a vehicle only.

Solutions
1. Atopic eczema is usually a dry, scaling dermatitis, especially during the cold winters in the northeast. Suggest a heavy cream (Eucerin, Nivea Creme is basically Eucerin plus perfume and a substantial price increase) or an ointment vehicle (Aquaphor will accept water so that it can be "thinned" but will not wash off). Suggest large quantities since the eczema is widespread and is usually a chronic problem. Avoid drying agents such as harsh soaps and gels.

Problem III. A 27-year-old woman has severe seborrheic dermatitis of her scalp which is best treated with a topical steroid. Suggest a vehicle.

Solutions

1. Aerosol, gel or lotion—not a cream or ointment since these are too greasy to use routinely on the scalp.
2. If the scale is very thick, apply cream or oils (mineral oil) at night and shampoo the following morning. Then use an aerosol, gel, or lotion vehicle for the topical steroid.

Problem IV. An 18-year-old man has a few small patches of psoriasis on the face, the axillae, and the gluteal cleft. Topical steroids will produce the best result; suggest a vehicle.

Solutions

1. Ointments are too occlusive for the moist axillae and gluteal cleft while gels may be irritating here; use light creams or lotions but watch out for acne on the face and intertriginous atrophy!

Problem V. A 38-year-old bus driver has severe hand eczema featuring xerosis and fissuring. Help him lubricate his skin using a topical steroid.

Solutions

1. Ointments are too greasy for most people who work with their hands. Use lubricating creams (such as Eucerin) or the special steroid emollients (Cordran-SP Cream, Aristocort-A, Topical Cream & Ointment, Lidex-E Cream).
2. Use ointment and cotton gloves, day and night.
3. Use cream which contains urea, lactic, or acetic acid (Alphaderm, LactiCare). These small molecules increase the emolliency of most vehicles but they can be slightly irritating.

ACTIVE INGREDIENTS

The following discussion is organized into either indication (such as acne), type of action (such as antiseptics) or type of drug (corticosteroids). The discussion is not all inclusive and directly reflects the authors preferences and bias.

Antiseptics

Halogenated phenolics are commonly used in "deodorant" soaps such as Dial and Safeguard.

Iodine (iodophor)—excellent degerming agent available in a wide range of soaps, scrubs, and ointments (Betadine, Efodine, etc.).

Alcohols—fair to poor skin degermers because they are irritating when the skin is damaged.

Silver nitrate—0.1–0.5% is an excellent broad spectrum germicide but the intense brown stain that it leaves severely limits its use.

Aluminum acetate (Burow's solution)—a 5% stock solution is usually diluted 1:40 with water and used as a soak and wet dressing. It is a *very* mild astrigent and antiseptic.

Hexachlorophene—(No longer available OTC) hexachlorophene is a good degerming agent which requires multiple applications over 1–2 days to be effective. Use with caution in babies and in anyone with widespread dermatitis because of the problems of percutaneous absorption.

Antifungals

Salicylic acid and *benzoic acid*—used alone or in Whitfield's ointment (6% benzoic acid, 3% salicylic acid).

Tolnaftate (Tinactin, Aftate; both OTC)—the *best* OTC antifungal drug currently available.

Undecylenic acid (Desenex)—can be used alone or in combinations.

Proprionates and Caprylates (Sopronol Ointment, Powder, and Solution and with other antifungals in Verdefam Cream, or Solution, OTC).

Haloprin (Halotex Cream and Solution, prescription required (Rx))—broad spectrum against bacteria, fungi and yeasts (*Candida albicans*).

Miconazole (MicaTin Brand Miconazole Nitrate Cream and Lotion 2%)—broad spectrum against bacteria, fungi and yeast (*C. albicans*).

Clotrimazole (Lotrimin, Cream, or Solution, 1%)—broad spectrum against bacteria, fungi and yeast (*C. albicans*).

Anticandidal

In addition to haloprogin, miconazole, and clotrimazole, consider:

Nystatin (Mycostatin Cream and Ointment, and others, Rx)—useful topically, on mucous membranes and orally.

Amphotericin B (Fungizone, Cream, Lotion and Ointment, Rx)—good anticandidal drug with slight orange color which can be used to check compliance.

Corticosteroids

Arranged in three groups according to decreasing potency (after Stoughton (1)). No substantial differences among the members of each group:

1. *High potency*—no substantial differences among the group
   Fluocinonide (Lidex) 0.05%
   Betamethasone dipropionate (Diprosone aerosol) 0.1%
   Halcinonide (Halog) 0.1%

2. *Middle potency*
   Fluocinolone acetonide (Synalar Creams, Fluonid) 0.025%
   Fluorandrenolide (Cordran) 0.05%
   Betamethasone Valerate (Valisone) 0.1%—may be somewhat more potent than other members of this group.
   Triamcinolone Acetonide (Aristocort A, Kenalog) 0.1%

3. *Low potency*
   Hydrocortisone (Cort-Dome Creme, Nutracort Cream, Hytone Cream) 1%
   Methylprednisolone (Medrol Acetate Topical) 1%

Remember that most of these products are available in ointment, cream, lotion and aerosol vehicle which directly affect potency. Most are also available at higher and lower concentration than the "standard" listed above.

Topical steroids of high potency (group 1) should be reserved for steroid-resistant diseases such as psoriasis or for areas where considerable hyperkeratosis is a problem (lichen simplex chronicus, dyshidrotic eczema of the palms and soles). They should not be used for more than 4–6 weeks or on large areas of the body (<20% surface area).

Group 2 steroids can be used over larger areas and for longer time periods with a greater margin of safety. They can cause an acne-like rash on the face and atrophy in intertriginous folds such as the groin. Wide-spread use of Valisone Cream, or Lotion, may cause adrenal suppression in children and any group II steroid may interrupt the adrenal-pituitary (HPA) axis in infants.

Group 3 steroids are usually free of local and systemic side effects unless used under occlusive dressing for long periods of time (<3 months). Also remember that each steroid listed above is available in a variety of vehicles and concentrations. Cost per gram decrease considerably when large sizes are prescribed.

Keratolytics and Keratin Modifiers

Salicylic acid—with benzoic acid in Whitfield's ointment or used alone in concentrations of 3–6% (Keralyt Gel and others) for the superficial removal of scale in diseases such as ichthyosis, psoriasis, seborrheic dermatitis, and fungal infections. Use with caution in children or when applying over greater than 20% of the body surface.

Urea—at concentrations of 10–40% (Carmol-10 and others). Urea probably acts as a humectant to bind water in the stratum corneum. Higher concentrations (20–40%) may be keratolytic. Lower concentrations are commonly added to steroids and appear to increase their potency, although the mechanism is not completely understood.

α-Hydroxic acids (lactic, pyruvic, or citric acids)—5% can be used alone for effective topical management of ichthyosis vulgaris. May also act as a humectant similar to urea.

Coal Tar

Byproducts of coking ovens; used as crude coal tar (CCT) or liquor carbonis detergens (LCD—an alcohol extract of CCT). CCT may be compounded at 2–5% concentrations in cream or ointment bases (Eucerin or petrolatum). It is also available commercially as Zetar or DOAK tar in the form of ointments, shampoos and bath additives and as a gel (Estar Emulsion and Psorigel).

Tars are best used in psoriasis, severe seborrheic dermatitis, and lichenified eczema. Tars are messy, smelly, and stain everything. Use them only at night and only after thorough patient education. Tar gels are much more cosmetically acceptable but some question their efficacy.

Antiseborrheic Dermatitis/Dandruff Preparations

Sulfur—with or without salicylic acid in creams or shampoos (Sebulex, Vanseb-T Tar Shampoo, and others, mainly OTC)

Selenium—in shampoos (Selsun and Excel, Rx; Selsun Blue, OTC)

Chloroxine—in shampoo (Capitrol Cream Shampoo, Rx) it yellows grey hair

Tar shampoos—Sebutone, Ionil-T, Vanseb-T Tar Shampoo, and others (all Rx)

Antiperspirants

Axillary—usually aluminum salts (Drysol, Rx; and many OTCs)

Palms and soles—aluminum salts (Drysol) formalin, gluteraldehyde (brown stain), and tannic acid (all Rx compounds)

Wart Remedies

Cantharidin—Cantharone (Rx) produces an intraepidermal blister which is variably painful. Five to seven percent of lesions develop ring-shaped warts at the periphery of the blister.

Wart paints (Duofilm, Rx or Compound W, OTC)—mixtures of salicylic acid ± lactic acid ± benzoic acid in flexible collodion. These require repeated daily applications but rarely scar.

Plasters—40% salicylic or a "corn plasters" (OTC) can be applied on palms and soles where grossly hyperkeratotic warts are most likely to form. Tape a closely trimmed piece in place for 2–3 days, remove, vigorously pare away the macerated keratin, and reapply the plaster. Repeat for a 3-week maximum or until the warts are gone. Do not use in patients with impaired circulation or sensation.

Podophyllin—a toxic extract from the rhizome of the mayapple or mandrake, podophyllin is usually applied in tincture of benzoin as a 20–25% solution. Apply *only* to moist warts (genital or perirectal) and do not use: 1) over large areas, 2) completely around any orifice or 3) during pregnancy without first consulting the obstetrician.

Antineoplastic

5-Fluorourocil (5-FU), 5% concentration (Efudex Topical Solutions and Cream Fluoroplex, both Rx) produces brisk inflammation of actinically damaged skin (solar keratosis). Treatment takes 2–4 weeks and works best on the head and neck. Unfortunately, the inflammation produced is quite annoying and places substantial limitation on the use of these products; others have questioned the long-term efficacy of 5-FU, noting that many actinic keratoses regrow in 3–12 months after therapy.

Antiviral (Other than Warts)

Idoxuridine—(Stoxil, Rx) available only as an ophthalmic ointment for the treatment of herpes simplex keratitis

Adenine arabinoside—(Videaraobine, Rx) only for the treatment of herpes keratitis

Sunscreens

Sunscreens (2) are now "rated" using the sun protective factor (SPF) which is the product of the minimal erythema dose (MED) of ultraviolet light using the sunscreen divided by the MED without the sunscreen. The larger the SPF, the more the protection from sunburning. Listed in order of rating, some SPFs are:

SPF Rating

10–15—SuperShade 15, Total Eclipse, PizBuin Exclusive

6–10—PreSun, Eclipse, Pabanol and others

4–6—ProTan, Pabafilm, Pagagel, A-Fil, Maxafil Cream, Solbar, Uval Sunscreen Lotion

2–4—Coppertone 2, Sundown Brand Sunscreen, RVP (red veteriary petrolatum)

References

1. Stoughton, R.B.: Perspectives on topical glucocorticosteroids. Prog Dermatol., *9:* 10, 1975.
2. Sunscreens, Med. Lett. Drugs Ther., *21:* 46, 1979.
3. Arndt, K.A.: *Manual of Dermatologic Therapeutics.* Little, Brown & Co. Boston, 1974.
4. Schmidt L.M.: Topical therapy for the pediatrician, In A. Jacob (Ed) *Pediatric Clinics of North America: Pediatric Dermatology,* p 191. 1978.
5. Rasmussen, J.E.: Percutaneous absorption in infants and children, In R.L. Dobson (ed) *Yearbook of Dermatology.* 1979.

CHAPTER 22

TOPICAL CORTICOSTEROIDS

RUTH K. FREINKEL

The introduction of the topical application of synthetic glucocorticoids almost a generation ago profoundly changed the treatment of cutaneous disease. The corticosteroids proved to be remarkably effective in relieving the signs and symptoms of so much skin distress that they have almost completely replaced the unpleasant but often effective paints, salves, and lotions of earlier times. Moreover, the commercially available, easily applied creams, ointments, and lotions obviated the need to compound complicated medications consisting of exotic materials in mysterious combinations and thus made it possible for nondermatologists to deal effectively with a great many skin complaints. It is necessary, however, to remember that in almost every instance, topical corticosteroids exert their effects in suppressing inflammatory reactions and that their panacea-like quality is due to the fact that inflammation is a major component in a vast variety of skin disease irrespective of etiology and pathogenesis.

Thus, corticosteroids do not "cure" disease but simply suppress reactions. In many instances, such as in allergic or irritant contact dermatitis, it is possible to alleviate the symptoms while the dermatitis runs its course. In other instances, suppression of inflammation prevents secondary effects such as bacterial infection or lichenification and thus mitigates complications. However, in many chronic disorders, such as psoriasis, the symptoms tend to recur when medication is discontinued. In others, such as fungal infections or scabetic infestations, suppression of inflammation actually invites propagation of the disease. Finally, topical steroids may produce a variety of undesirable and sometimes permanent side effects.

The indications for the use of topical corticosteroids can be found in other chapters of this volume. In general, they are most useful in those conditions where inflammation is the primary and/or major pathological manifestation and where the etiological factors are dealt with concurrently (e.g. removal of an allergen or irritant, suppression of a microbial infection, etc.).

PHARMACOLOGY

The anti-inflammatory activity of corticosteroids is expressed by vasoconstriction, suppression of inflammatory cells, and inhibition of the connective tissue response as well as of reactive epidermal hyperplasia. The hormones thus affect fundamental processes in virtually all of the cells in the skin. Synthesis of collagen and mucopolysaccharides is reduced while degradation is accelerated. Mitosis of epidermal cells is inhibited but keratinization is accelerated. More importantly, corticosteroids appear to directly interfere with responses of the mononuclear cells that mediate immune reactions and to inhibit the elaboration of mediators of cutaneous inflammation.

Such pharmacological effects produce the desired therapeutic effects. They also produce some of the undesired adverse responses. Thus, suppression of the connective tissue components can result in atrophy, poor wound healing and vascular changes such as telangectasia. Altered keratinization can lead to acne. Suppressed immune responses can permit bacterial, viral, and fungal infection.

The effectiveness of topical corticosteroids is determined by several factors which include 1) ability to penetrate the stratum corneum, 2) relative antiinflammation potency, and 3) metabolism of the compound in the skin.

PENETRATION OR PERCUTANEOUS ABSORPTION

Since corticosteroids are lipids, they penetrate stratum corneum more effectively than many other compounds that are applied to the skin. The rate at which corticosteroids penetrate is, to a large extent, determined by concentration and it is much less dependent on frequency of application.

Thus, less hydrocortisone is absorbed when a given concentration is applied four times a day than when four times the concentration is applied once a day. Moreover, absorption is dependent on body area and occurs in declining order from genital skin, face, scalp, trunk, extremities, and palmar or plantar skin. To some extent, percutaneous absorption can be enhanced or retarded by the vehicle in which they are presented. Physical laws governing partition coefficients between vehicle and stratum corneum dictate that penetration should be greatest from a lotion (low lipid content) and least from an ointment (high lipid content). However, other factors related to vehicles are of greater influence. Corticosteroids penetrate best through a well hydrated stratum corneum. Hydration is greater with an occlusive ointment than with a cream or a lotion but is enhanced even more by occlusion (as much as 10-fold) with a plastic film. Thus, the choice of vehicle is dictated by the degree of occlusion that is desired as well as cosmetic considerations.

Table 22.1
Common Topical Corticosteroids

Nonfluorinated
  Hydrocortisone (Hytone, Cort-Dome Cortef Acetate ointment)
  Prednisolone (Meti-Derm)
  Hydroxyprednisolone acetonide (Tridesilon)
Fluorinated
  Betamethasone benzoate (Fluorobate)
  Betamethasone valerate (Valisone)
  Betamethasone dipropionate (Diprosone)
  Triamcinolone acetonide (Kenalog Aristocort A)
  Fluocinolone acetonide (Synalar Lidex, Topsyn)
  Flurandrenolide (Cordran)
  Fluocinolone acetonide (Fluonid)
  Halcinonide (Halog)

In practice, chronic inflammation accompanied by scaling and thickening of the epidermis responds best to ointments while acute exudative responses are better treated with creams or lotions having less occlusive effects. Similarly, intertriginous areas are readily macerated by too occlusive a preparation and respond better to creams or lotions.

EFFECT OF STRUCTURE ON STEROID ACTION

The almost bewildering array of topical synthetic corticosteroids all represent structural modification of the natural hormone cortisol. Most of the modifications are designed to enhance antiinflammatory effects for which a hydroxy group on carbon 11 (C-11) and a ketone group on the side chain are essential (Fig. 22.1). Currently, most topical steroids are based on either prednisolone or prednisone and substituted at C-16 to minimize salt retention.

Penetration, and hence effectiveness, can be somewhat increased by substitution of a short chain acyl group on the side chain. However, enhancement of potency has been accomplished by addition of fluorine at C-9 or at both C-9 and C-6; however, the acetonide derivatives of flourinated corticosteroids are much more active. Addition of short chain acyl group at C-17 has provided even greater increases in potency.

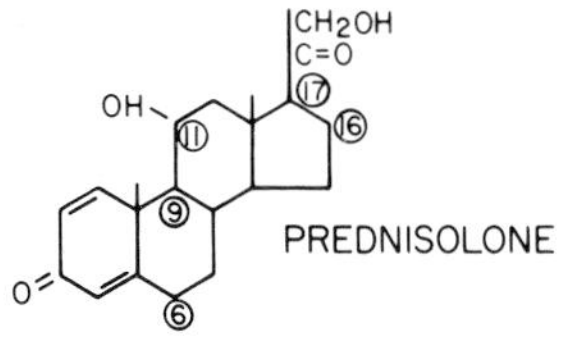

	CARBON	SUBSTITUTION
TRIAMCINOLONE	9	α fluorine
	16	α OH
FLUONCINOLONE	9,6	α fluorine
	16	α OH
BETAMETHASONE	9	α fluorine
	16	β CH₃

Fig. 22.1. Structure of common synthetic corticosteroids.

Biotransformation of corticosteroids in the skin is an important component of pharmacological effectiveness, since skin is an active site of steroid metabolism. The extent to which synthetic corticosteroids are metabolized determines the duration of their actions and thus their effectiveness. In this respect, prednisolone and prednisone are less rapidly metabolized than hydrocortisone. Thus, hydrocortisone can be oxidized to cortisone which has virtually no antiinflammatory effects.

THERAPEUTIC REGIMENS

Topical corticosteroids, while immensely useful, are not always indicated as the first or only therapeutic agent in treating even primarily inflammatory reactions. In acute exudative dermatitis, simple compresses and soaks should be used until swelling and exudation subsides. When bacterial cellulitis is present corticosteroids should be avoided until the infection has subsided. In chronic dermatitis, a combination of corticosteroids with less specific agents such as tar, sulfur, and salicylic acid may provide added inflammatory effects and reduce the requirement for corticosteroid.

Combinations of hydrocortisone and fluorinated corticosteroids with antibiotics and antifungal agents are commercially available and are used much too frequently. The rationale has been advanced that presence of antimycotic or bacterial agents will prevent superinfections which may occur especially when the corticosteroid is applied under wrap. There is little evidence to support this concept. The converse view, that secondary infection which often supervenes in acute dermatitis, justifies a combined therapy is equally untenable. Infection, if significant, responds best to simple compresses and specific antimicrobial agents. Topical antibiotics may promote emergence of resistant organisms and are helped in this regard by topical corticosteroids. A possible exception to this negative view is atopic eczema secondarily infected with *Staphylococcus aureus* where combinations of neomycin and steroids have been shown to be effective agents. If this therapeutic approach is chosen, cultures should be taken to verify the presence of specific microorganisms.

The choice of vehicle and type of corticosteroid (e.g. hydrocortisone, fluorinated, etc.) should be guided by the location of the disease, age of the patient, and degree of potency needed as well as the responsiveness of the particular disease.

Thus, nonfluorinated compounds such as hydrocortisone, should be selected for face, intertriginous, and genital areas, and the skin of infants and young children to avoid adverse local effects. If fluorinated compounds are required for such areas, they should be at low strength (e.g. 0.025% triamcinolone acetonide rather than 0.1%), and for short periods.

None of the available corticosteroids are specifically more effective for one disease or another except in terms of greater or lesser potency or absorption. Most are available as creams, ointments, and lotions and some are available in low concentrations while others are available in especially high concentrations. Choice is usually based on familiarity with the product. However, in chronic conditions such as psoriasis or atopic eczema, patients may become refractory to a given corticosteroid but will respond to another.

The choice of vehicle is extremely important both for effectiveness and patient acceptance. Lotions are more useful for scalp disorders where creams and ointments are frequently unacceptable to the patient. They are desirable for use in intertriginous areas where occlusive effects of ointments may be detrimental and in conditions where a drying effect is sought (e.g. rosacea). While creams are more cosmetically acceptable than ointments, for example on the hands, they are generally less effective in chronic conditions where there is hyperkeratosis (e.g. psoriasis or lichenified eczema). Alternation of creams during the day and ointments at night sometimes achieves an acceptable compromise. Formulations of corticosteroid in gels provides greater absorption plus a drying effect; unfortunately, the gels are frequently irritating to acutely inflamed skin. The use of occlusive plastic film wraps overnight or adhesive films impregnated with corticosteroid provides greater concentrations for longer periods of time, but must be used judiciously to avoid local adverse effects including candidal and bacterial infections.

One question that has not been fully resolved is that of frequency of application. Theoretically, it would be desirable to maintain constant levels of drug in the skin. For this reason, patients are usually instructed to apply the preparation three to four times per day. However, recent work has suggested that tachyphylaxis (acute tolerance) may occur with such frequent applications and could account for emergence of refractoriness. At present, recommendations are quite empiric. The physician should be flexible in instructing the patient and attempt to achieve the minimum effective frequency. In treating chronic skin disease, topical corticosteroid, like systemic drug, should not be discontinued abruptly but removed gradually. Maintenance therapy can sometimes be achieved with one or two applications a day or with occasional periods of treatment when disease becomes active. Healed skin should not be treated indefinitely to prevent recurrences.

ADVERSE EFFECTS

Two types of adverse effects occur with topical use of corticosteroids: systemic and local.

Systemic Effects

That topically applied steroids are absorbed is self-evident. The extent to which they become available through the circulation depends not only on how much is absorbed into the skin but also on how much is retained and degraded in the skin.

Despite their wide spread use, there have been few reports in recent years of manifestations of marked excess of systemic corticosteroids such as cushingoid facies, hypertension, diabetes, salt retention, etc. Exceptions to this are reports of iatrogenic Cushing's disease in infants treated over large body surfaces, in patients with liver disease, and in patients with exclusive skin disease using exceptionally potent corticosteroids (e.g. clobetasol proprionate and desoximetasone).

While manifestations of excessive glucocorticoids are rare, some degree of suppression of adrenal function due to absorption of the hormone is not. Many studies have demonstrated that endogenous corticosteroid levels are suppressed by administration of potent topical agents to as little as 20% of normal skin under occlusion, or to large areas of diseased skin without occlusion. Fortunately, the adrenal usually recovers rapidly when the treatment is discontinued. However, it is not really known whether prolonged suppression of the pituitary may permanently limit its ability to respond maximally in times of stress. The author has seen several cases with low levels of glucocorticoids requiring replacement therapy for several months after discontinuance of topical corticosteroids that had been used for long periods on large areas.

It is not known how frequently mild excesses of corticosteroids are achieved in patients treated over large areas and/or with occlusion. Abnormal carbohydrate tolerance has been reported without clinically evident Cushing's syndrome. The possible side effects are similar to those that occur with chronic low doses of oral corticosteroids. Further work is needed to resolve this question. For the present, the physician should be conscious of potential adverse effects especially in patients with concurrent diseases that might be exaserbated by corticosteroids.

A more practical consideration concerns the patient who undergoes surgery or some other physiologically stressful event during treatment with topical corticosteroids over large body areas. Such patients are like those on low maintenance doses of systemic corticosteroid and may require additional systemic corticosteroids during the acute stress. In such situations, measurements of A.M. and P.M. plasma cortisol is useful to determine if endogenous adrenal function is adequate.

Local effects of topical corticosteroids are much more common and relate to the potency, the method of administration and the site of application. Local atrophy of skin and subcutaneous tissue is not uncommon especially in intertriginous areas and on the face but is usually reversible.

Striae, however, may occur, especially in intertriginous areas, and are permanent. Telangectasia are especially common on the face. Such complications are rarely seen with hydrocortisone which makes it the compound of choice in these areas. The acnegenic effects of corticosteroids can occur with topical preparations and perioral dermatitis is often precipitated by fluorinated corticosteroids.

Another side effect occurs not infrequently when topical steroids are used under occlusive wrap. Occlusion with plastic film, per se, promotes candidal infection. Together with corticosteroid, candidal or bacterial infections (particularly folliculitis) is common. This also may occur in intertriginous areas without occlusion. When this complication arises, occlusion must be stopped and the area treated with appropriate antimicrobial agents and drying lotions.

One area where topical corticosteroids provide a potentially severe hazard is the eye. It is well recognized that instillation of corticosteroid into the conjunctival sac raises intraocular pressure significantly in 6–10% of patients. Excess application around the eyes can lead to glaucoma and to cataracts. Patients with elevated intraocular pressure are at particular risk. For this reason the use of corticosteroids on the eyelids should be minimal and limited to low potency preparations.

References

1. Feiwall, M., James V., and Barnett, E.: Effect of potent topical steroids on plasma cortisol levels of infants and children with eczema. Lancet, 2: 485, 1969.
2. Feldman, R.J., and Maibach, H.I.: Regional variation in percutaneous penetration of ^{14}C cortisol in man. J. Invest. Dermatol., 48: 181, 1967.
3. Gomez, E. C., and Frost, P.: Induction of glycosuria and hyperglycemia by topical corticosteroid therapy. Arch. Dermatol., 112: 1559, 1976.
4. Goodman, L.S., and Gilman, A.: The Pharmacological Basis of Therapeutics, Ed. 4, p. 1627. Macmillan, New York, 1970.
5. Leyden, J.J., and Kligman, A.M.: The case for steroid antibiotic combinations. Br. J. Dermatol., 96: 179, 1977.
6. McKenzie, A.S.: Percutaneous absorption of steroids. Arch Dermatol., 86: 911, 1962.
7. Munroe, D., and Clift, D.: Pituitary adrenal function after prolonged use of topical steroids. Br. J. Dermatol., 88: 381, 1973.
8. Plewig, G., and Kligman, A.M.: Induction of acne by topical steroids. Arch. Dermatol. Forsch. 247: 29, 1973.
9. du Vivier, A., and Stoughton, R.B.: Tachyphylaxis to the action of topically applied steroids. Arch. Dermatol., 111: 581, 1975.

CHAPTER 23

SYSTEMIC DRUGS IN DERMATOLOGY

CHARLES ZUGERMAN

The general principles of therapy are the same in dermatology as in other disciplines. In other words, the physician must successfully treat the patient's disease without damaging other organ systems. In pursuing this goal, the dermatologist has employed a variety of topical soaks, ointments, creams, and dressings. Traditionally, he has not relied heavily on systemically administered drugs. Recently, however, the systemically administered medication has begun to achieve an increasingly important place in the dermatologist's therapeutic arsenal. The following is a short description of some of the systemic drugs employed in the treatment of cutaneous disease.

CORTICOSTEROIDS

Indications and Counterindications in Dermatology

Indication for the use of corticosteroids (1) in dermatology varies with the prescribing physician. In general, two classes of dermatologic disease warrant the use of these potent medications. First, acute, severe, extensive eczematous processes which are of known etiology and which are self-limited may be treated with a short course of systemic corticosteroids. For instance, corticosteroids given early in the course of an acute allergic contact dermatitis to poison ivy serve to decrease the morbidity of the process *without* shortening its course.

Corticosteroids also are indicated in the treatment of certain dermatologic emergencies including bullous pemphigoid, pemphigus vulgaris, systemic lupus erythematosus and, in some instances, erythema multiforme, toxic epidermal necrolysis, and exfoliative dermatitis. Chronic idiopathic diseases such as psoriasis, atopic dermatitis, chronic hand eczema and seborrheic dermatitis are usually not treated with systemic steroids because long-term treatment is required and because the patient often becomes dependent upon the drug, exhibiting flares of the disease when the steroid is tapered.

Complications of Systemic Steroids

Corticosteroids, even used correctly, cause numerous significant and occasionally life-threatening side effects including fluid and electrolyte imbalances, ulcers, neurologic and psychiatric changes, increased tendency to develop infection and, perhaps, delayed healing of myocardial infarcts and birth defects, although the latter associations are controversial. Obvious hypothalamic-pituitary-adrenal (HPA) suppression occurs commonly in those who are on significant chronic steroid therapy. In addition, there are individuals who are prone to the development of cataracts and glaucoma while taking systemic corticosteroids. Many of these side effects can be minimized by varying the type of steroid given as well as its dosage and schedule of administration. In addition, if the use of steroids is minimized in those patients with a history of glaucoma, diabetes, osteoporosis, and hypertension, these problems may be partially avoided. Finally, there are a number of cutaneous side effects associated with the systemic use of corticosteroids including acneiform eruptions, easy bruisability, striae, obesity, and delayed wound healing.

Oral Corticosteroids

TYPES

Systemic corticosteroids are classified into three groups (Table 23.1) according to the duration of their suppression of the HPA axis. Long-acting corticosteroids suppress the HPA axis for over 48 hours and, although they do not have to be administered as often, their use is associated with a higher incidence of side effects. Short-acting corticosteroids suppress the HPA axis for 24–36 hours and produce fewer side effects because of their shorter duration of action. Intermediate-acting corticosteroids suppress the HPA axis for 48 hours and are ideal for instituting an alternate-day steroid regimen.

DOSAGE SCHEDULES

Administering a corticosteroid in a single daily dose is apparently as effective in controlling most skin disease as are daily divided dosage schedules. Giving the corticosteroid dose before 8 A.M. most closely approximates the normal diurnal variation and may minimize the development of iatrogenic Cushing's disease. Although the point is controversial, many physicians believe that it is unnecessary to slowly taper the steroid dosage if it has been administered for shorter than 2–4 weeks using a single 8 A.M. daily dose schedule.

Alternate-day corticosteroid therapeutic programs utilizing a relatively short-acting corticosteroid such as prednisone may minimize but not eliminate side effects associated with these drugs. This dosage regimen is best utilized in less severe dermatoses lasting for greater than a month. Unfortunately, many of the more severe dermatologic diseases cannot be controlled adequately in this manner.

Injectible Corticosteroids

Like the oral drugs, parenteral corticosteroids are classified according to their duration of action with long-acting preparations being effective for 3–4 weeks, intermediate ones for 1–2 weeks and short-acting steroids for hours or days (Table 23.2).

The advantages of these preparations often relate to ease of administration. It is unnecessary for the patient to be able to comprehend complex instructions or to be capable of accepting medication by mouth. Therefore, in individuals who are unreliable or who are vomiting, this route of administration seems ideal. In addition, the physician does not have to worry about withdrawing the drug or having the patient return routinely for follow-up.

Table 23.1
Oral Corticosteroids

Activity	Generic Name	Form	Dosage
Short acting	Prednisone	Tablets	1, 2.5, 5, 10, 20 and 50 mg
	Prednisolone	Tablets	5 mg
	Methylprednisolone	Tablets	2, 4, 8, 16, 24 and 32 mg
Intermediate acting	Triamcinalone	Tablets	1, 2, 4, 8 and 16 mg
		Syrup	2 mg/cc
Long acting	Dexamethasone	Tablets	0.75, 4, 5, 20 and 25 mg
		Elixir	0.5 mg/5 cc
	Betamethasone	Tablets	0.6 mg
		Syrup	0.6 mg/5 cc

Table 23.2
Injectable Steroids

Activity	Generic Name	Brand Name	Dosage
Long acting	Triamcinolone acetonide	Kenalog	10 mg/ cc
			40 mg/ cc
	Triamcinolone hexacetonide	Aristospan	5 mg/ cc
			40 mg/ cc
Intermediate acting	Triamcinolone diacetonide	Aristocort	25 mg/ cc
			40 mg/ cc
	Dexamethasone acetate	Decadron-La	8 mg/ cc
	Betamethasone sodium phosphate	Celestone Phosphate Celestone Soluspan	6 mg/ cc
	Methylprednisolone acetate	Depo-Medrol	20 mg/ cc
			40 mg/ cc
			80 mg/ cc
Short acting	Dexamethasone sodium phosphate	Decadron	4 mg/ cc

On the other hand, there are serious disadvantages to using injectible steroids. For instance, it is impossible to discontinue the medication if a serious side effect develops. In addition, the medication is absorbed unreliably with no regard to normal diurnal variation. Consequently, one expects and actually obtains considerably more suppression of the HPA axis than with oral preparations of comparable dosage. Finally, atrophy and striae may develop at the administration site.

Withdrawal from Corticosteroids

It is best in most cases to employ as short a course of corticosteroids as possible and to withdraw the drug at the earliest opportunity. There are many methods for withdrawing corticosteroids. These include gradually tapering the dosage on a daily basis or converting to an alternate-day regimen by gradually dropping the dosage on the "off" day. For more detailed information, the reader is directed to the review articles at the end of this chapter.

GRISEOFULVIN

Indications

Griseofulvin (2) is effective against all dermatophytes but is inactive against bacteria,

deep fungi, candida, viruses, and rickettsiae. It is strongly indicated for the treatment of dermatophyte infections of the hair and nails but it is also effective to various degrees against infections in other areas.

Pharmacodynamics

Griseofulvin is well absorbed orally, but older preparations are better absorbed with a fatty meal. It is ineffective topically and is not administered parenterally. After the drug is absorbed, it is deposited in the stratum corneum where it exerts a fungicidal effect on growing mycelia, probably by binding to lipids within the cell. Peak serum levels of the drug occur at about 4 hours after administration.

Dosage

Griseofulvin is available in both microsized and ultramicrosized preparations. Using the former, doses in adults range from 0.5 to 2 g daily, taken with a fatty meal. In children, 10 mg/kg/day can be given. Utilizing the ultramicrosized form of griseofulvin allows the dose to be cut in half. Treatment periods range from 2 to 4 weeks in treating tinea corporis to 4 or 6 months when tinea unguium is being treated.

Side Effects

Griseofulvin is derived from a species of *Penicillium* so that the possibility of cross-sensitivity to penicillin exists. Serious adverse reactions to this drug are rare. Commonly, patients who take griseofulvin develop a mild headache which can be minimized if the drug is taken at night. Griseofulvin interacts with Coumadin and with barbiturates, occasionally necessitating dosage adjustment. In addition, griseofulvin has been known to activate both acute intermittent porphyria and porphyria cutanea tarda. The drug should not be administered to individuals with severe liver disease or to pregnant females. Finally, neurologic, hematologic, and renal toxicity may occur rarely and disappear when the drug is discontinued.

SULFONES IN DERMATOLOGY

Sulfones (3) were first synthesized early in this century, but their place in medicine was not established until 1940 when they were shown to be active against the tubercle bacillus and ultimately the leprosy bacillus.

All disubstituted sulfones act in vitro thru the release of the parent compound diaminodiphenyl sulfone (DDS, dapsone). Therefore, most physicians prefer to treat dermatologic disease with dapsone. The mechanism of action of sulfones in infectious diseases such as leprosy probably relates to interference with folate metabolism and is reversible upon administration of *p*-aminobenzoic acid (PABA). In noninfectious inflammatory disease, the action of the drug is highly speculative and is irreversible even upon administration of PABA.

Indications

Leprosy. Dapsone, when used for the treatment of this disease, is bacteriostatic and is often not curative. Indeterminant as well as tuberculoid leprosy is treated with 25–50 mg/day of dapsone over a 2-year period while dimorphous leprosy is treated with similar doses for up to 10 years. Patients with lepromatous leprosy must be given 50–100 mg/day of dapsone for life. Current evidence suggests that dapsone is most effective when it is combined with a second drug such as rifampin or ethionamide.

Dermatitis Herpetiformis. This autoimmunologic disease is described completely in the chapter on bullous eruptions. Dapsone may be used to treat this condition in initial doses of 200–400 mg/day until control of the disease is obtained at which time the dose can be reduced to 50–100 mg/day.

Acne Conglobata. This highly inflammatory form of acne often results in severe scarring. When acne conglobata is refractory to other therapy, dapsone may be begun in initial doses of 50–100 mg daily increasing the dose every 5 days until significant side effects occur, the disease comes under control, or a maximum daily dose of 300–400 mg of the drug is given. Improvement may be dramatic in very severe forms of the disease on as little as 300 mg weekly over a 3-month treatment period.

Pyoderma Gangrenosum. In this process, recalcitrant ulcers occur primarily on the lower extremities often in conjunction with ulcerative colitis or regional enteritis. Pyoderma gangrenosum has been controlled successfully with combination systematic corticosteroids and orally administered dapsone.

Other Diseases Treated with Dapsone

Sulfones also have been suggested for the treatment of benign familial chronic pemphigus, recalcitrant eczemas, subcorneal pustular dermatosis, Mucha-Habermann disease, pustular psoriasis of Von Zumbusch, and mycetomas.

Side Effects

Hematologic side effects of dapsone include hemolytic anemia, methemoglobinemia, and agranulocytosis. Hemolytic anemia may occur in normal subjects at doses of 200–300 mg/day and its severity is dose-related. Those with glucose-6-phosphate dehydrogenase (G6PD) deficiency will develop hemolysis at a much lower dapsone dose than will normal subjects.

Other side effects of sulfones include a reversible peripheral neuropathy, urticaria, morbilliform eruptions, erythema multiforme, toxic epidermal necrolysis, exfoliative dermatitis, psychosis, and liver abnormalities including drug-induced hepatitis, cholestatic jaundice and liver function abnormalities. These drugs can induce entirely unique side effects in leprosy patients including so called "lepra reactions", erythema nodosum leprosum, and caseous necrosis of nerves.

Evaluation prior to treating a patient with sulfone should include a complete blood count (CBC), G6PD, liver function tests, urinalysis, and reticulocyte count.

RETINOIDS

Retinoids (4) are synthetic analogs derived from vitamin A or its naturally occurring derivative, all-*trans*-retinoic acid. They are presumably helpful in treating diseases for which vitamin A was previously prescribed while decreasing the incidence of side effects such as nyctalopia, xerophthalmia, keratomalacia, and liver toxicity. Retinoids are not yet approved by the Federal Drug Administration, but initial studies indicate that they may prove useful in the treatment of severe acne conglobata (5), psoriasis (6), Darier's disease (7), actinic keratoses, and erythrokeratoderma variabilis and other genodermatoses.

CIMETIDINE

Cimetidine (8) is a histamine (H_2) receptor antagonist ordinarily used to treat duodenal ulcers and Zollinger-Ellison syndrome. Recent case reports indicate that, in doses of 300 mg by mouth four times daily, cimetidine may be effective in treating bath pruritus, a common symptom of polycythemia vera and chronic urticaria.

ZINC

Acrodermatitis enteropathica is a rare hereditary disease characterized by acral dermatitis, alopecia, and diarrhea which responds to orally administered zinc sulfate. Likewise, acrodermatitis-like rashes may appear after intravenous hyperalimentation or malabsorption and these also respond to zinc administration (9). Michaëlsson (10) reported a patient with acrodermatitic enteropathica whose acne cleared on oral zinc therapy. He then treated 64 acne patients with oral zinc sulfate for 12 weeks with a significant decrease in the numbers of inflammatory as well as noninflammatory lesions per patient. More recently, however, Weimar (11) administered zinc sulfate to 52 acne patients with generally no improvement of their acne. Therefore, zinc sulfate is the treatment of choice for acrodermatitis enteropathica but its value for patients with acne is currently the subject of debate.

β-CAROTENE

β-Carotene is a carotenoid pigment present in fruits and vegetables which is useful in the treatment of photosensitivity reactions especially in patients with erythropoietic protoporphyria. It is not recommended as a sun screen for normal individuals since it causes yellow pigmentation of the skin. The usual adult dosage is 30–300 mg daily.

ANTIMALARIAL AGENTS

Antimalarial agents (12) including chloroquine, hydroxychloroquine, amodiaquin and quinacrine have been known to be beneficial in the treatment of discoid lupus erythematosus since the 1950s. They are indicated for cases of discoid lupus erythematosus which do not respond to topical corticosteroids. Hydroxychloroquine and chloroquine are most commonly used in doses of one to two tablets daily. Side effects include leukopenia and thrombocytopenia, pigmentary changes, and retinopathy. Chloroquin is effective therapy for porphyria cutanea tarda in very low dosages.

ANTIHISTAMINES

Antihistamines are commonly grouped into six classes (Table 23.3) and are indicated for

Table 23.3
Common Antihistamines

Class	Generic Name	Brand Name	Form	Dosage
Ethanolamines	Diphenhydramine hydrochloride	Benadryl	Capsules Elixir	25, 50 mg 12.5 mg/5 cc
Ethylenediamines	Tripelennamine hydrochloride	PBZ Pyribenzamine	Tablets Elixir	25, 50 mg 37.5 mg/cc
Alkylamines	Chlorpheniramine maleate	Chlor-Trimeton	Tablets	4 mg 2 mg/5 cc
Piperazines	Meclizine hydrochloride	Bonine	Tablets	25 mg
Phenothiazines	Promethazine hydrochloride	Phenergan	Tablets	12.5, 25, 50 mg
			Syrup Suppositories	25 mg/5 cc 12.5, 25, 50 mg
	Trimeprazine tartrate	Temaril	Tablets Syrup Spansules	2.5 mg 2.5 mg/5 cc 5 mg
Miscellaneous	Cyproheptadine hydrochloride	Periactin	Tablets Syrup	4 mg 2 mg/5 cc
	Hydroxyzine hydrochloride	Atarax	Tablets	10, 25, 50, 100 mg
			Syrup	10 mg/5 cc

the treatment of urticaria and histamine-induced pruritus. Many of these agents are sedatives as well as antihistamines and must be used cautiously in individuals who drive a car or who are required to remain alert during the day. The choice of an antihistamine depends upon the incidence of side effects (mainly the degree of sedation), the drug's cost, and its relative effectiveness in treating the patient's disease. Often, if an antihistamine from one group is not effective, drugs from other groups may be tried alone or in combination. Certain diseases respond more dramatically to specific antihistamines. For instance, hydroxyzine hydrochloride is particularly effective when administered to a patient with dermographism (13) or histamine-induced pruritus while cyproheptadine hydrochloride (Periactin) works best for cold urticaria (14). The correct dosage is variable depending upon the disease being treated as well as the patient's age and physical condition.

ANTIBIOTICS FOR ACNE

Erythromycin and tetracycline are the common antibiotics administered to patients with acne vulgaris and acne rosacea. The average acne patient can be controlled on doses as low as 250–1000 mg daily or every other day administered over a period of months. This important treatment modality is discussed more fully in the chapter on acne (see *Chapter 7*).

METHOTREXATE

Methotrexate (15) is occasionally employed by the dermatologist for the treatment of recalcitrant psoriasis vulgaris or for acute pustular psoriasis. At times, it has been used to treat patients with Reiter's syndrome, Mucha-Habermann disease, pemphigus, and mycosis fungoides. Many dosage schedules may be employed depending upon the disease being treated. For instance, methotrexate is administered to psoriatic patients using either a once weekly oral or intramuscular dose of 15–50 mg, or 2.5–7.5 mg of the drug orally every 12 hours for three doses once a week. In either case, administration of the drug is followed by a "rest" period in order to minimize possibly severe hepatotoxicity and bone marrow suppression. Use of the drug is discussed more fully in the chapter on psoriasis (see Chapter 8).

PSORALENS AND PSORIASIS

Psoralens are plant derivatives which, when administered with ultraviolet-A (UVA) light, are effective in treating psoriasis, mycosis fungoides, and Sezary syndrome. PUVA (psoralen plus UVA) has not yet been approved for general use by the Federal Drug Administration and is described more completely in the chapter on psoriasis (see Chapter 8).

References

1. Storrs, F.J.: Use and abuse of systemic corticosteroids therapy. J. Am. Acad. Dermatol., *1:* 95, 1979.
2. Crounse, R.G.: Human pharmacology of griseofulvin. J. Invest. Dermatol., *37:* 529, 1961.
3. Lorincz, A.L., and Pearson, R.W.: Sulfapyridine and sulfur drugs in dermatology. Arch. Dermatol., *85:* 2, 1962.
4. Bollon, W., and Hanck, H.: From vitamin A to retinoids. Modern trends in the field of oncology and dermatology. Acta Vitaminol. Enzymol., *131:* 113, 1977.
5. Pech, G.L., Olsen, T.G., Yoder, F.W., et al: Prolonged remissions of cystic and conglobate acne with 13-*cis*-retinoid area. N. Engl. J. Med., *300:* 320, 1979.
6. Orfanos, C.E., and Runn, U.: Systemic use of a new retinoid with and without local dithranol. Treatment in generalized psoriasis. Br. J. Dermatol., *95:* 101, 1976.
7. Orfanos, C.E., Kurka, M., and Strunk, U.: Oral treatment of keratosis folliculosis with a new aromatic retinoid. Arch. Dermatol., *114:* 1211, 1978.
8. Easton, P., and Galbraith, P.R.: Cimetidine treatment of pruritus in polycythemic vera. N. Engl. J. Med., *299:* 1134, 1978.
9. Bernstein, B., and Leyden, J.J.: Zinc deficiency and acrodermatitis after intravenous hyperalimentation. Arch. Dermatol., *114:* 1070, 1978.
10. Michaëlsson, G., Lennard, J., and Anders, V.: Effects of oral zinc and vitamin A in acne. Arch. Dermatol., *113:* 31, 1977.
11. Weimar, V.M., Puhl, S.C., and Smith, W.H.: Zinc sulfate in acne vulgaris. Arch. Dermatol., *114:* 1776, 1978.
12. Tuffanelli, D.L.: Management of the patient with lupus erythematosus. Dermatol. Foundation Bull., *8:* 5, 1974.
13. Matthews, C.N.A., Kirby, J., and James, J., et al.: A comparison of hydroxyzine pamoate with chlorpheninamine in the treatment of dermographism. Br. J. Dermatol., *88:* 279, 1973.
14. Wanderer, A.A., and Ellis, E.F.: Treatment of cold urticaria with cyproheptadine. J. Allergy Clin. Immunol., *55:* 180, 1971.
15. Roenigk, H., Maibach, H.I., and Weinstein, G.: Guidelines: methotrexate therapy for psoriasis vulgaris. Arch. Dermatol., *105:* 363, 1972.

CHAPTER 24

DRUG ERUPTIONS

RICHARD GIACOBETTI

The skin is the most frequent target of clinically recognizable adverse reactions to drugs. Therefore, in any clinical practice, knowledge of the different types of drug eruptions and the relative frequency of adverse reactions caused by particular drugs is of great significance. The magnitude of this problem becomes evident when it is realized that up to 20% of hospitalized patients have experienced various drug reactions, and approximately 3% of patients are admitted because of an adverse drug reaction. In the Boston Collaborative Drug Surveillance Program, allergic skin eruptions occurred in 2% of hospitalized patients. From this study it is calculated that there are 3 allergic skin eruptions per 1000 drug courses.

The following is a systematic account of the different morphological types of primary drug eruptions (Table 24.1) and cutaneous disorders induced or aggravated by drugs (Table 24.2). With the exception of acneform eruptions, the mechanisms of the primary drug eruptions involve a hypersensitivity phenomenon. That is, they can be precipitated by challenging an individual with a drug to which there has been previous sensitization. The mechanisms for the reactions induced or aggravated by drugs are not understood, nevertheless, an immune response is also postulated.

A principle which is paramount in any discussion of drug reactions is that a drug which has been tolerated for days, months, or years, even administered in low doses, may suddenly cause an adverse reaction.

In the broadest sense, a drug is any substance used in the treatment of disease. Realizing this, the evaluation of a patient with a suspected drug eruption requires a comprehensive history. Specific questions must be asked about vitamins, over-the-counter preparations, and substances kept in the medicine cabinet as well as certain food and beverages which an individual may not consider "medicine." Drugs routinely taken over a long period of time may understandably be overlooked, i.e., oral contraceptives.

For the sake of brevity, twelve of the most common classes of drugs causing adverse cutaneous reactions are listed in Table 24.3. Several specific drugs will be discussed; however, an extensive review is beyond the scope of this chapter.

A general comment on the therapy of drug eruptions: it is imperative that the responsible drug be discontinued. In reality, this may be difficult since an individual may be taking

Table 24.1
Primary Drug Eruptions

Exanthematous
Urticarial
Eczematous
Photosensitive
Purpuric
Vasculitic
Acneform
Pigmentary
Bullous
Lichenoid
Fixed drug

Table 24.2
Disorders Induced or Aggravated by Drugs

Erythema nodosum
Lupus erythematosus
Porphyria
Alopecia
Erythema multiforme
Toxic epidermal necrolysis

Table 24.3
The Most Common Classes of Drugs Causing Reactions

Antibiotics
Anticoagulants
Anticonvulsants
Antimalarials
Barbiturates
Cytostatics
Diuretics
Halogens
Heavy metals
Hormones
Major tranquilizers
Thyreostatics

many medications, some of which are life saving. In this case, after the elimination of the most dispensable drugs, appropriate substitutions should be made for priority medications. Discontinuation of all drugs may be impractical and unwise. Good judgement and knowledge of a drug's capacity to cause an adverse reaction are essential.

PRIMARY DRUG ERUPTIONS

Exanthematous Eruption

The exanthematous pattern is the most common of all drug eruptions. Clinically, there are two presentations: morbilliform and scarlatiniform.

The morbilliform rash (resembling measles) is evidenced by a symmetrically distributed, usually generalized, erythematous maculo-papular eruption as shown in Figure 24.1 (see color Plate IV). The macular component var-

ies from pink to red and only partially blanches on diascopy. The papular component consists of distinctly palpable lesions of less than 1 cm which later become confluent over large areas of the body. The scarlatiniform pattern, resembling the rash of scarlet fever, is a diffuse finely papular and fiery red erythematous eruption which blanches with pressure as shown in Figure 24.2 (see color Plate IV). Lesions have a predilection for the trunk and purpura may occur in dependent areas. Involvement of palms, soles, and mucous membranes is variable. Both forms can be pruritic. Fever is the most common, and usually the only, constitutional symptom. Generally, the exanthematous rash occurs within 8 days after drug administration. Healing occurs with a fine desquamation approximately 3 days to 3 weeks after the responsible drug is discontinued. It has been estimated that a drug has a 1–5% chance per dose of causing an exanthematous eruption. The penicillins are the most common offenders, with ampicillin having the highest incidence of rash occurring in 3–8% of recipients. In patients with infectious mononucleosis, the incidence of exanthematous reactions caused by ampicillin approaches 50–80%. A higher incidence is also seen in patients with cytomegalovirus infections, respiratory viral infections, and lymphatic leukemias. A higher incidence occurring in patients taking allopurinol is controversial.

In addition to most antibiotics, nearly every class of drug has been associated with this reaction pattern.

Exfoliative dermatitis is a major complication sometimes seen when the offending drug is continued.

Treatment.   Cessation of drug.

Topical
1. Soothing cool baths with or without oatmeal: (Aveeno or Aveeno Oilated)
2. Calamine lotion with or without 0.25% menthol, two or three times a day
3. Steroid creams, ointments, or emollients of medium potency: (Kenalog Ointment 0.1%, Cream 0.1%; Synalar Ointment 0.25%, Cream 0.2%; Cordran Ointment 0.05%; Cream 0.05%; Aristocort Ointment 0.1%) two or three times a day

Systemic

1. Atarax Tablets 10 mg, 25 mg, by mouth, twice a day, and at bedtime as needed for itching and mild sedation
2. Systemic steroids are not indicated when the presentation is uncomplicated.

Urticarial Eruption

Urticaria is the second most common type of primary drug eruption. It consists of well circumscribed, discrete wheals with erythematous, raised, serpiginous borders and blanched centers as shown in Figure 24.3 (see color Plate IV). Lesions are intensely pruritic. Uncomplicated urticaria usually occurs within 12–36 hours after drug administration. If it is part of an anaphylactic reaction, the onset will be immediate and there may be associated angioedema. If it is part of a serum sickness syndrome, the onset will not be until 7–10 days later. The penicillins lead the long list of offending drugs. Remarkable is aspirin, both in causing and exacerbating urticaria. Twenty to forty percent of patients with chronic urticaria are made worse by aspirin. This effect can persist for many weeks after ingestion.

Treatment.   Cessation of drug.

Topical

1. Cool compresses or cool baths with oatmeal (Aveeno)
2. Calamine lotion with or without 0.25% menthol.

Systemic

1. Atarax 25 mg by mouth, three times a day, or every hour, as needed
2. Epinephrine 1:1000 subcutaneously or intramuscularly every 1–2 hours (severe reaction)
3. Ephedrine 25 mg by mouth or sublingual isoproterenol (Isuprel), four times a day (severe reaction)
4. Corticosteroids, 40–60 mg prednisone every day for 2 weeks (severe reaction).

Eczematous Eruption

The acute eczematous eruption secondary to drugs is similar to contact dermatitis (see Chapter 6). It is characterized by intense, relatively well dermarcated erythema soon accompanied by edema, papules, vesiculation, oozing, and sometimes bullae (Fig. 24.4). There is intense burning and pruritus. It occurs in individuals sensitized by external exposure to a drug and challenged by the internal administration of the same drug or a chemically related one. The eruption starts approximately 1 or 2 days thereafter, and usually involves sites of previously existing contact dermatitis.

This pattern is considered an "occupational dermatitis" of medical personnel who dispense medication, i.e. antibiotics, tranquilizers, diuretics, and antihistamines. Notable in this latter category, is the over-the-counter preparation Caladryl which, in addition to calamine, contains Benadryl, a potent sensitizer when applied topically. Subsequent systemic administration of Benadryl may result in an eczematous eruption.

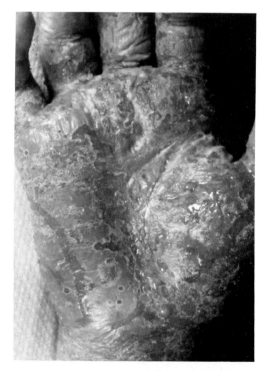

Fig. 24.4.   The intense eczematous reaction displays the hallmark of vesiculation oozing.

Treatment.   Cessation of drug.

Topical and Systemic Therapies are outlined in Chapters 5 and 6 on eczema and contact dermatitis.

Photosensitive Eruption

The morphology of this eruption is protean. It may be eczematous, papular, plaque-like, urticarial, vesiculo-bullous or merely resemble a common sunburn (Fig. 24.5). It characteristically appears in areas receiving the most sun exposure. This includes the malar area, tops of the ears, "V" of the neck, extensor surfaces of the arms and dorsa of the hands. The areas that are spared are the eyelids, the infranasal area, the groove of the chin, and the triangular area of the neck shielded by the mandible. The photosensitive reactions are divided into two categories: phototoxic and photoallergic. In practice, it may be very difficult to make this distinction.

The phototoxic reaction is nonimmunologic. It will occur in any individual given an adequate dose of drug and sunlight. The wavelength of sunlight needed to produce the reaction is dependent upon the absorption spectrum of the drug. Clinically, the toxic reaction is manifested as an exaggerated sunburn. Heading the long list of drugs causing this reaction are the diuretics, tetracyclines, and furocoumarins. Dimethylchlortetracycline has caused reactions in greater than 40% of recipients, while reactions to tetracycline are infrequent. Onycholysis, separation of the nail plate from the nail bed, has been associated with some phototoxic reactions.

The photoallergic reaction is a hypersensitivity phenomenon. It most commonly assumes an eczematous pattern, however, other forms are seen. There is sensitization and a latent period intervening between the sensitizing exposure and the development of the patient's capacity to react to a subsequent exposure. Once established, only minimal amounts of drug with sun exposure will trigger the reaction, i.e. not dose-dependent. The most commonly incriminated drugs causing photoallergy are topically applied sulfonamides, halogenated salicylanilides and chlorpromazine. See Chapter 6 for photopatch testing.

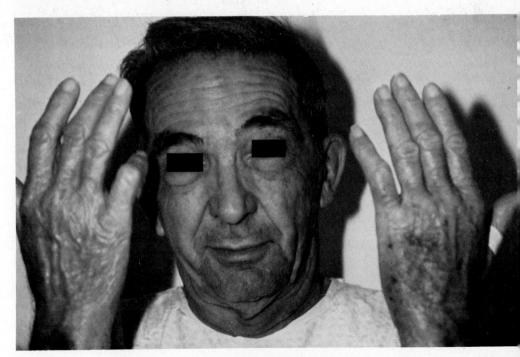

Fig. 24.5.   The photosensitivity reaction characteristically appears over sun-exposed areas i.e. face and dorsal aspects of upper extremities. Pattern resembles a severe sunburn.

Treatment. Cessation of drug.

Topical

1. Appropriate management of the eczematous eruption, i.e. soaks, steroids
2. Sunscreens containing 5% *p*-aminobenzoic acid (PABA) in 50–70% alcohol (Pabanol, PreSun Lotion and Gel)
3. Use of over-the-counter remedies containing caine derivatives (benzocaines) should be avoided to prevent the risk of sensitization.

Systemic

1. Aspirin 325 mg, 2 tablets by mouth every 4–6 hours as the occasion arises may relieve discomfort of sunburn
2. Prednisone 40 mg by mouth every day for 1 week (severe reaction).

Purpuric Eruption

Purpura is the extravasation of red blood cells into the skin (Fig. 24.6). It does not blanch on diascopy and it is not palpable. This distinguishes it from vasculitis. It occurs symmetrically and in areas of dependency. Of the two types of purpura, thrombocytopenic and nonthrombocytopenic, the reaction caused by drugs is of the allergic thrombocytopenic variety.

The drug acts as a hapten which combines with platelets rendering them autoantigenic. Reacting with antibody, the platelets agglutinate and undergo lysis. Drugs which are commonly involved in immunologically induced purpura are quinine, quinidine, chlorothiazide, Sedormid, meprobamate and PAS. Coumarin derivatives which may cause purpura because of excessive anticoagulation may also cause a rare and severe reaction consisting of petechiae, ecchymosis and hemorrhagic infarcts which lead to extensive necrosis. This occurs within the first week of anticoagulation therapy. The mechanism is unknown, however, a direct toxic effect of coumarin on the endothelial cells or a hypersensitivity reaction are postulated. There is a 27% incidence of this reaction with bishydroxycoumarin (Dicumarol) and a 3% incidence with sodium warfarin (Coumadin).

Vasculitis Eruption

Vascular alterations are present in most drug eruptions as part of the inflammatory process. Usually there is a perivascular infiltrate consisting of white blood cells. In contrast, vasculitis denotes vascular lesions characterized by fibrinoid necrosis and a segmented inflammatory reaction in vessel walls.

The clinical spectrum of vasculitic diseases is great. However, the pattern seen most frequently caused by drugs is a leukocytoclastic hypersensitivity angiitis.

This form of vasculitis is also seen in association with many systemic diseases, especially lupus erythematosus. Therefore, more than any other type of drug eruption discussed herein, a patient with vasculitis requires a thorough systemic evaluation.

Leukocytoclastic hypersensitivity angiitis affects small blood vessels less than 0.1 mm in diameter in the skin and viscera. Clinically, there are purpuric papules usually on areas of dependency, i.e. the distal lower extremities, thighs or buttocks, or posterior aspect of the body in a recumbent patient (Fig. 24.7). Ini-

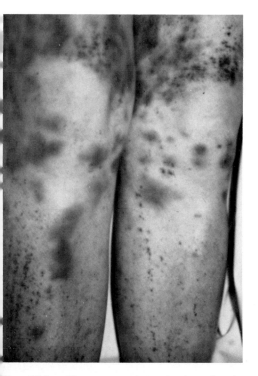

Fig. 24.6. The purpuric eruption is the nonpalpable, nonblanching extravasation of blood into the skin.

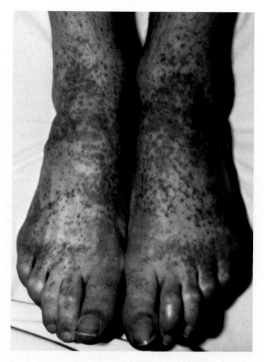

Fig. 24.7. Vasculitis, typically, is palpable purpura which occurs in dependent areas.

tially the lesions are flat, erythematous macules or urticarial lesions which progress to purpuric papules. The eruption may be polymorphic with superficial erosions, hemorrhagic bullae, or cutaneous infarcts. Papular lesions may be associated with burning or itching. Larger destructive lesions may be very painful. Dependent edema is common. Systemically, there may be malaise, athralgia, myalgia, and fever. Specific organ involvement is not uncommon, with renal failure being the most serious complication.

In addition to a clinical history and physical examination, skin biopsy is very helpful in diagnosing leukocytoclastic hypersensitivity angiitis. On routine staining, there is endothelial swelling, fibrin deposition, extravasation of red blood cells, and a polymorphonuclear cell infiltrate with the presence of nuclear fragments called nuclear dust. This results from the disintegration of neutrophils, i.e. leukocytoclasis. A skin biopsy for immunofluorescent staining is also helpful in establishing the diagnosis since immunoglobulins and complement are deposited about vessel walls.

Because these immune fractions are present for a short period of time, it is necessary to biopsy a new lesion not more than 18–24 hours old.

A few of the many drugs causing vasculitis are penicillins, sulfas, aspirin, phenylbutazone, quinidine, gold, and azo dyes.

After withdrawing the drug, certain baseline tests should be performed to rule out systemic involvement. These include a complete blood count with a differential white blood count, sedimentation rate, liver function tests, and urinalysis. If uncomplicated, itching and burning can be treated like the exanthematous eruptions. When the presentation is severe, systemic steroids could be administered only after a thorough medical evaluation has been made.

Acneform Eruption

Acneform eruptions vary in morphology and in distribution depending on the inciting drug.

With corticotrophin and corticosteroids, an acneform eruption occurs only after puberty. Acne is seen with both endogenous and exogenous glucocorticoids, but is less frequent with the latter. Occlusive application of fluorinated steroids also has produced an acneform eruption. In contrast to common acne vulgaris, there is neither sebaceous hyperplasia, nor limitation to sebaceous areas. Typically, the acne is distributed over the trunk, shoulders, and upper arms. Lesions are papulopustular and are usually in the same state of evolution. Comedones are characteristically absent and cysts and scarring are unusual (Fig. 24.8). Follicular hyperkeratinization is the proposed mechanism.

Testosterone, in contrast to the glucocorticoids, produces hypertrophy of sebaceous glands and, therefore, an eruption which is identical to common acne vulgaris.

It is known that the estrogen-dominant oral contraceptives are beneficial in the acne-prone patient. These include Enovid-E, Enovid-5, Ovulen, and Demulen. However, progesterone-dominant birth control pills which also can elicit androgenic effects are potentially acnegenic. These include Ovral, Ortho-Novum 1/50, 1/80 and 2 mg, Norinyl 1 + 50,

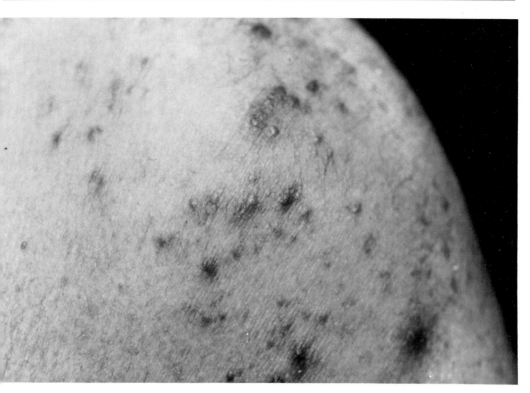

Fig. 24.8. Steroid acne is a papulopustular eruption which lacks comedones and cysts. Lesions on the shoulders are typical.

1 + 80 and 2 mg and Norlestrin 1 and 2.5 mg.

An eruption similar to common acne vulgaris can be seen after prolonged treatment with iodides and bromides which are contained in some sedatives, expectorants, and vitamins.

The antiepileptic drugs, phenobarbital, trimethadione, and diphenylhydantoin, are capable of exacerbating existing acne, the latter because of presumed androgenic effects. The antituberculous drug, isoniazid, may either exacerbate or cause acne de novo by stimulating sebaceous gland hypertrophy.

Treatment. The treatment of acneform eruptions secondary to drugs is similar to that of common acne vulgaris and is discussed in Chapter 7 on acne.

Pigmentary Eruptions

Pigment changes secondary to drugs may be a direct effect of the chemical substance or, more commonly, an induced disturbance in melanization. A classic example of the former is argyria, where silver is deposited in the lamina propria of sweat glands and other adenexal structures giving the skin a diffuse slate-blue color. Other examples of direct pigmentary alterations are seen with gold, bromides, bismuth, and mercury. Like argyria, the color change is irreversible. Mercury, paradoxically, may also cause hypopigmentation by inhibiting melanin synthesis.

The drugs which are noted for their effects on melanization are oral contraceptives, anticonvulsants, antimalarials, antimetabolic agents, and tranquilizers. Chloasma or melasma, which is seen in pregnancy, are also caused by oral contraceptives. This is a pattern of hyperpigmentation seen over the forehead and temporal areas, sometimes extending across the cheeks (Fig. 24.9). It darkens with sun exposure. In contrast to the pattern seen in pregnancy, the hyperpigmentation caused by oral contraceptives is rarely reversible.

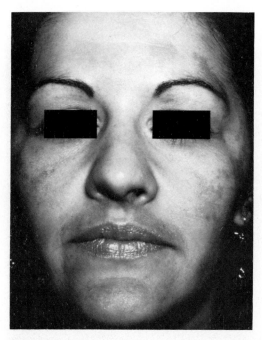

Fig. 24.9. Chloasma is increased pigmentation which occurs over the forehead, temporal, and malar areas of the face.

Ten percent of individuals on prolonged anticonvulsant therapy (diphenylhydantoin and related compounds) will develop a patchy brown pigmentation over light-exposed areas. In women, the pattern may resemble chloasma.

Pigmentary changes develop in about 25% of patients receiving antimalarials for more than 3 or 4 months. The color varies from gray to blue-black and is commonly seen over the pretibial area. It is imperative that all patients who develop hyperpigmentation have an eye examination since corneal pigmentation and retinal damage are associated findings.

The antimetabolic drugs busulfan, 5-fluorouracil, cyclophosphamide, and topical nitrogen mustard produce a diffuse hyperpigmentation especially in dark-complected individuals. The pattern resembles the increased pigment seen in Addison's disease, yet, endocrine studies are normal. Bleomycin may cause linear hyperpigmentation of the chest and back.

The tranquilizers, chlorpromazine and related phenothiazines cause a slate-gray to vi-

olaceous color limited to light-exposed areas. Pigment deposition also has been observed in the eye, the reticuloendothelial system, and in parenchymal organs. After the drug is discontinued the pigmentation may slowly disappear, but usually it is permanent.

Treatment. Cessation of drug.

Topical
1. Hydroquinone 3–5% cream two to three times a day for a week or month will bleach epidermal melanin
2. Sunscreens.

Systemic
1. Chelating agents are unsafe and ineffective in treating pigmentation secondary to metals.

Bullous Eruption

Bullae and vesiculobullous lesions are commonly a component of acute eczematous, photosensitive, and fixed drug eruptions as well as part of the drug-induced disease complexes of prophyria, erythema multiforme, and toxic epidermal necrolysis. Drug-induced coma, however, is one situation where blisters are seen as the sole manifestation. Originally described with barbiturate coma, bullous lesions also have been observed in comatose states due to methadone, hydrocodone, meprobamate, imipramine, glutethimide, and nitrazepam. Tense vesicles on erythematous indurated bases and large tense clear bullae sur-

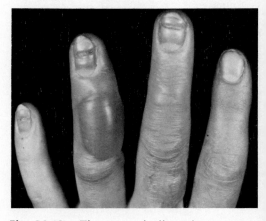

Fig. 24.10. The tense bullous lesion seen in drug-induced coma occurs in pressure areas and areas of trauma.

rounded by a narrow rim of erythema are localized to areas of pressure or trauma (Fig. 24.10). The mechanism is believed to be tissue anoxia which causes subepidermal and intraepidermal separation with sweat gland necrosis. Logistically, the comatose state, rather than a direct drug effect, causes the pathophysiological alteration. This is supported by the observation that skin lesions were found in 4% of 50 patients with barbiturate overdose and no patient developed bullae who had not been unconscious. Lesions heal with scarring in 10–14 days.

Lichenoid Eruption

Morphologically, the lichenoid drug eruption resembles lichen planus with lesions that are flat-topped angulated papules (Figure 24.11). Unlike lichen planus, however, an eczematous component may be present. Also, involvement of the flexor surface of the wrists and glans penis is absent and oral involve-

ment is rare. A few of the more common drugs causing this eruption are heavy metals, antimalarials, phenothiazines, and diuretics.

Treatment. Cessation of drug.

Topical
1. Steroids of medium to strong potency (Lidex 0.05% Cream or Ointment, Halog Ointment, Topicort Emollient Cream 0.25%) two to three times a day.

Systemic
1. Atarax 25 mg by mouth, two to three times a day.

Fixed Drug Eruptions

The fixed drug eruption is a rare, yet classic, dermatologic entity. It may be generalized, but it more commonly presents as one or more localized, sharply demarcated, circular areas of macular erythema 10–20 cm in diameter. Less commonly, the lesions may be papular,

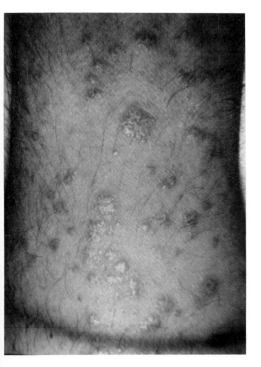

Fig. 24.11. The lichenoid drug reaction resembles lichen planus with flattopped angulated papules.

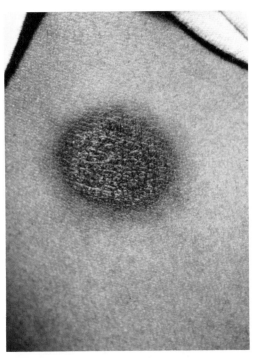

Fig. 24.12. The residual hyperpigmentation secondary to fixed drug eruption will increase in intensity with repeated challenges of drug.

vesiculo-bullous or urticarial. Although usually asymptomatic, a mild burning sensation may be experienced. When the responsible drug is withdrawn, the lesion(s) fades leaving hyperpigmentation (Fig. 24.12). If the drug is reintroduced, the reaction will occur in the same location. Therefore, the reaction is "fixed." With recurrences, the residual pigmentation becomes darker. It is interesting that skin from an affected area temporarily retains its capacity to react if transplanted to an unaffected area. Conversely, normal skin which is grafted to an affected site will react. Antibodies have not been identified. However, a serum factor has been isolated which causes lymphocyte blast transformation. This factor increases its activity in the presence of the responsible drug.

The most common drugs implicated in causing fixed drug eruptions are phenolphthalein (contained in laxatives), barbiturates, pyrazolon derivatives, phenacetin, tetracyclines, sulfonamides, and chlordiazepoxide. Cross-sensitivity has been demonstrated with the tetracycline and pyrazolon derivatives.

Treatment. After withdrawal of the drug, the hyperpigmentation may be treated with bleaching agents (see Pigmentary Eruptions).

DISORDERS PRECIPITATED OR AGGRAVATED BY DRUGS

Erythema Nodosum

More common in women, erythema nodosum presents with bright, round, warm, tender nodules in the subcutaneous fat. Lesions are usually multiple and symmetrically located on the anterior tibial surfaces. Ankle edema may be prominent. Fever, malaise, and arthralgias also may be present. After 10 days, lesions become bluish and assume a bruise-like appearance. Complete healing may occur in 3 weeks, however, many patients are affected with recurrent lesions for several months.

Erythema nodosum is commonly associated with sarcoidosis, inflammatory bowel disease, and streptococcal, deep fungal, and mycobacterial infections. Drug-induced erythema nodosum is apparently less common and the association is difficult to prove. Nevertheless, the major drugs incriminated are oral contraceptives, codeine, sulfonamides, penicillin, salicylates, bromides, and iodides.

Systemic Lupus Erythematous

Lupus and lupus-like syndromes have been reported after the administration of drugs (see Chapter 15, Lupus Erythematosus). It has been estimated that 3%–12% of the cases have been activated or caused by drugs. Usually, the syndrome has followed the use of the drug in high doses for at least 2 months.

Clinically, drug-induced lupus is similar to idiopathic lupus with a few important exceptions. Cutaneous manifestations occurred in 18.2% of the drug-induced patients compared with 71.5% in idiopathic cases. Lack of adenopathy and renal involvement is a significant observation in drug-related disease. The two major drugs which "trigger" this complex are procainamide and hydralazine. Fifty percent of patients taking procainamide will develop antinuclear antibodies and half of these will develop overt disease. The antibodies are single-stranded rather than double-stranded DNA. It is postulated that both drugs are capable of complexing with DNA or nucleoprotein, rendering it antigenic. Other drugs which are less frequently associated with this syndrome are hydantoin, pencillamine, methyldopa, sulfonamides, and oral contraceptives. Interestingly, chlorpromazine and isoniazid induced antinuclear antibodies without precipitating clinical disease.

Discontinuing the drug will result in a clinical remission for over half of the affected patients. The approach to therapy for persistent reactors is discussed in Chapter 15 on lupus.

Porphyria

Many drugs are known to precipitate different forms of hepatic porphyria. Acute intermittent porphyrin with no cutaneous manifestations has been associated with the ingestion of barbiturates, anticonvulsants, griseofulvin, and oral contraceptives.

Porphyria cutanea tarda presents with vesiculobullous, and ulcerative lesions usually in light-exposed areas. The disease is "triggered" by alcohol, estrogens, hexachlorobenzene, and chlorinated phenols. Other cutaneous signs of porphyria cutanea tarda include moderate to severe photosensitivity, facial hypertrichosis, increased skin fragility to mechanical trauma, hyperpigmentation, sclerodermoid plaques, and scarring alopecia. The biochemical defects are increased urinary excretion of uroporphyrin, 7-carboxylporphyrins, and isocoproporphyrin which is also increased in the feces. Enzymatically, there is a uroporphyrinogen decarboxylase deficiency in the liver and red blood cells. It is suggested that drugs causing porphyria cutanea tarda may inhibit this enzyme system. However, the true mechanism is unknown and complicated by the observation that ingestion of griseofulvin and oral contraceptives may cause increased excretion of porphyrins in normal individuals.

Alopecia

Alopecia induced by drugs is usually localized to the scalp in a diffuse or masculine pattern. It is usually reversible. Like alopecia in general, hair loss caused by drugs can be divided into anagen and telogen effluviums, or hair loss. Anagen is the growing phase and interruption during this stage results in very abnormal hairs. The hair bulb is small and deformed. The diameter of the shaft varies and tapers to a ragged point at the proximal end where breakage occurs. Drugs classically causing this type of alopecia are the antimetabolic cancer chemotherapeutic agents. These inhibit the mitotic activity of growing hair and include alkylating agents, antimetabolites, antibiotic cytostatics, and alkaloid cytostatics.

Telogen is the resting phase. With telogen hair loss, the hair bulbs are normally clubbed and lack pigment. The hair shaft is uniform. Alopecia occurs in a diffuse pattern 3–4 months after the insult, i.e. drug, physical, or emotional stress. The drugs which have been associated with telogen hair loss are oral contraceptives, coumarin, heparin, and thioureas. After a telogen effluvium, regrowth should be appreciated in about 2 months.

Erythema Multiforme

A patient with erythema multiforme could present with urticarial-like lesions, erythematous macules, papules, vesicles, or bullae. The pathognomonic sign is the target or iris lesion which consists of a blister surrounded by a pale zone which is enveloped by an erythematous halo. Stevens-Johnson syndrome designates a form of erythema multiforme with severe mucous membrane involvement. See Chapter 17 on bullous diseases.

Drugs are only one of the many suspected causes of erythema multiforme. Responsible drugs are antibiotics (penicillin, sulfonamides, tetracycline), phenytoin and pyrazolon derivatives, metals, barbiturates, hydralizine, and phenolphthalein.

Toxic Epidermal Necrolysis

It is estimated that only 25% of all cases of toxic epidermal necrolysis are due to drugs. Sulfonamides, penicillin, barbiturates, diphenylhydantoin, and allopurinol are a few of the many drugs which are responsible.

Approximately 1–2 weeks after ingesting the drug, a patient will experience a prodromal period of malaise, fever, and exquisite tenderness of the skin. This is followed by diffuse erythema. Within the next 24 hours the full thickness of epidermis is sloughed from the dermis. There may or may not be flaccid bullae formation. Histologic differentiation from staphylococcal scalded skin syndrome and approaches to therapy are discussed under bullous diseases (Chapter 17).

SUMMARY

Drug eruptions constitute a significant amount of morbidity in both inpatient and outpatient populations. Therefore, it is imperative that all physicians be aware of the many patterns of primary drug eruptions and syndromes precipitated by drugs. A thorough history of "medications" used by a patient is of utmost importance. Good judgement and knowledge of a drug's capacity to cause an adverse reaction are essential.

References

1. Arndt, K.A., and Jick, H.: Rates of cutaneous reactions to drugs. A report from the Boston Collaborative Drug Surveillance Program. JAMA, *235:* 918, 1976.
2. Baer, R.L., and Harris, H.: Types of cutaneous reactions to drugs. Importance in recognition of adverse reactions. JAMA, *202:* 150, 1967.
3. Bruinsma, W.: A guide to drug eruptions. Excerpta Med. Int. Congr. Ser., Amsterdam, 1973.
4. Hurwitz, N.A.: Admissions to hospitals due to drugs. Br. Med. J. *1:* 539, 1969.
5. Hurwitz, N.A., and Wade, O.L.: Intensive hospital monitoring of adverse reactions to drugs. Br. Med. J. *1:* 531, 1969.
6. Jackson, R.: Systemic drug rashes: pitfalls in diagnosis and treatment. Cutis, *17:* 386, 1976.
7. Parker, C.W.: Drug allergy. N. Engl. J. Med., *292:* 511, 732, and 957, 1975.
8. Seidl, L.G., Thornton, G.F., Smith J.W., and Cluff, L.E.: Studies on the epidemiology of adverse drug reactions. III. Reactions in patients on a general medical service. Bull. Johns Hopkins Hosp., *119:* 299, 1966.
9. Wintroub, B.V., Shiffman, N.J., and Arndt, K.A.: Adverse cutaneous reactions to drugs. *In* T.B. Fitzpatrick, A.L. Eisen, and K. Wolff, et al., (Eds), *Dermatology in General Medicine*, Ed 2. McGraw-Hill, New York, 1979.

CHAPTER **25**

PLASTIC PRINCIPLES IN DERMATOLOGIC SURGERY

PETER McKINNEY

SCAR PLACEMENT

The direction of the dermal incision is the major determinant of the final scar. The type of suture, characteristics of the skin, and the handling of the tissues are not without influence on the result but these play a minor role in comparison to the placement of the incision. In the 1860s, Karl Langer's experiments focused attention upon "skin tension" lines which gave us the first clue to lines of elective incisions (1). Langer's lines are not always useful for elective incisions, however, because they focused only on skin and excluded the influence of the underlying muscular forces.

Three principles determine the direction of reliable incisions for producing an optimal result:

1. Placing incision at right angles to direction of muscle pull
2. Allowing the scar to bend
3. Use of fixed anatomical points.

Muscle Pull

An optimal scar is achieved by placing the incision at right angles to the direction of the major muscle pull. This prevents a hypertrophic scar which results from tension along

the long axis of the scar. These directions are readily identifiable in the adult but require knowledge of the underlying muscle anatomy in the younger patient, as the skin creases caused by the muscle pull are not yet defined. Voluntary muscular motion in the area will outline these creases. For example, the excision of a lesion of the cheek would parallel the nasolabial folds to correspond to the pull of the elevators of the mouth (smile action) while excision of a lesion of the lip would be in a radial fashion (pursing of the lips) (Fig. 25.1).

The excision is usually lenticular in shape measuring approximately 3–4 times as long as the diameter of the lesion to be excised (Fig. 25.2). This allows tapering of the edges to prevent redundant tissue at the ends ("dog ears"). Circular excisions can be closed by V-Y closure but this technique is an advantage only in larger wounds as it leaves too many scars for the smaller lesions (Fig. 25.3).

Allowing the Scar to Bend

As collagen cross-links, a scar contracts in all directions but the net result is a shortening from end to end. Therefore, closing a wound in a step, W, or Z fashion, or by excising in an irregular fashion ("haptoplasty") (Fig. 25.4, 25.5), provides a spring to a scar by

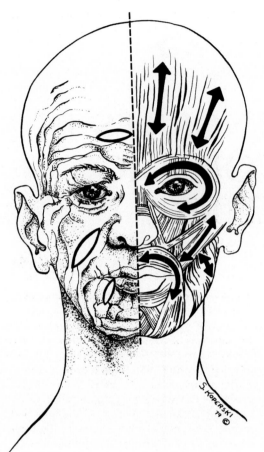

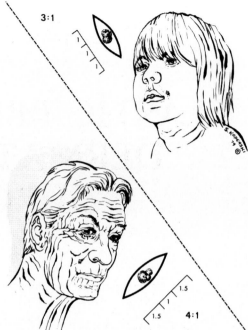

Fig. 25.2. The excision for inelastic or older skin may require a ratio of excision of 4 times the diameter of the lesion whereas, in excisions in the younger patient with elastic skin, a 3:1 ratio may be sufficient.

Fig. 25.1. This illustrates the changes in the direction of incisions necessary to correspond to the underlying muscle pull. The excisions on the *left* are at right angles to the muscle pull illustrated on the *right*.

allowing the scar to "bend." This circumvents the inability of the scar to stretch and prevents hypertrophic scarring.

This technique of bending the scar is used whenever the scar has to run counter to skin tension lines. Some of the irregular lines of the incision are placed in skin creases and this creates the optical illusion of making the scar appear shorter.

For the purposes of this text, however, since we are emphasizing excisions of lesions with simple closure, only the "haptoplasty" would be useful as Ws, and Zs would apply mainly to scar revisions. The exception would be

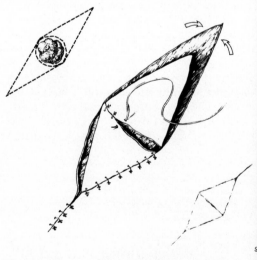

Fig. 25.3. The V-Y advancement technique sacrifices less skin by saving the triangle at the corners. However, it creates more scars and is useful only for larger lesions.

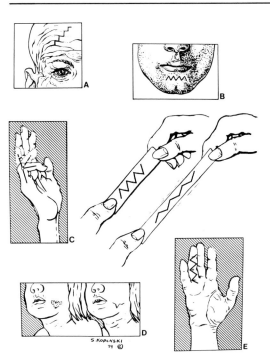

Figure. 25.4. Various techniques of "bending a scar." Closure of a wound in a broken line fashion also allows the scar to bend ("stretch") (*center, C* and *E*) preventing a scar contracture or hypertropic scar. A step or broken line closure (*A, B, D*) also gives the optical illusion of a shorter scar.

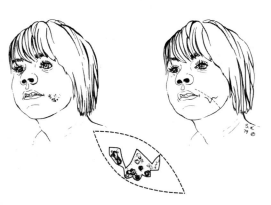

Fig. 25.5. A "haptoplasty" preserves the most tissue in an excision as it skims the lesion (*left*). When the pieces (*center*) are fit together one has a broken line (*right*). Compare the length with the *dashed line* which would illustrate a lenticular excision.

where the proposed excision "turns a corner," i.e. around the earlobe, or an edge, or around the edge of the mandible as where the band-like contractions of the scar result in a depressed scar (Fig. 25.6).

Placing a scar in a line point-to-point in a

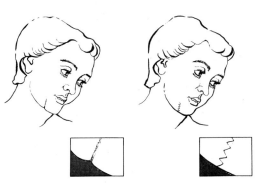

Fig. 25.6. The shortening of a scar is very apparent where the scar goes around a curve causing a bowstring effect and a depression of the scar (*left*). A broken-line closure prevents this by allowing the scar to bend or "stretch" (*right*).

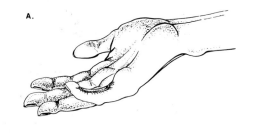

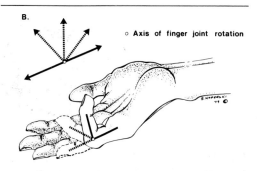

Fig. 25.7. Another technique of allowing the scar to bend prevents a bandlike contracture (*A*) by placing the limbs of the scar in the joint axis (*B*). (See also Fig. 25.4 *C*)

joint axis also allows it to bend. If this scar were placed across the flexor creases, a hypertrophic scar would develop as extension of the finger stimulates the cycle of formation of additional collagen which contracts shortening the scar still further (Fig. 25.7).

Use of Fixed Anatomical Points

Certain anatomical points in the body by experience allow incisions in fixed directions; for example, incisions around the nipple, in the long axis of the midline body such as the sternum (longitudinal), around the ear, in mucous membranes and in the loose skin of the genitalia. All of these areas heal well because they are disguised by pigment changes (areolar—breast junction) or anatomic structures (curves of the ear). In addition, the thin skin in these areas allows a fine scar (Fig. 25.8).

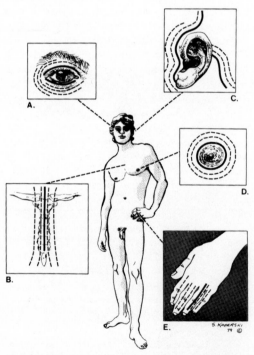

Fig. 25.8. Even though these anatomical points do not correspond to the direction of muscle pull they are reliable for scar placement. *Dashed lines* represent Langer's lines which would be incorrect. *Solid lines* represent preferred lines of incisions.

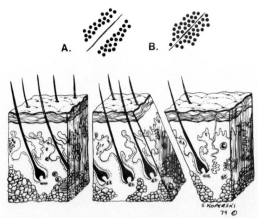

Fig. 25.9. Beveling of the incisions preserves the hair roots and prevents the "widening" of the scar which is, in fact, an area of alopecia from damage to the hair roots surrounding the scar. *A* is the result in going straight down. Note the surrounding "wide scar" which is really alopecia. *B* gives a "narrow" scar by preserving the hair.

Incisions are always made perpendicular to skin except in hair-bearing areas when the skin is purposely beveled to preserve the hair roots (Fig. 25.9). Beveling in non hair-bearing areas results in a depressed scar.

WOUND MANAGEMENT

Hemostasis and environment are the most important aspects in managing a wound. Hemostasis must be meticulous because a hematoma can prolong wound healing from weeks to months. Cautery is useful for all vessels up to 2 mm in size but must be used with pinpoint accuracy to reduce damage to surrounding tissue. Wound environment is controlled by careful technique such as isotonic solutions, moist environment, and delicate instruments. Antiseptics, the crushing force of a large clamp, or even a hot operating room light can be damaging to a wound. Fine instruments, including hooks when possible, should be used instead of crushing forceps, and also small hemostats that grasp only the vessel instead of the surrounding tissue. If irrigation is needed to keep the wound moist, warmed isotonic plain saline or Ringer's lactate is recommended. Above all, no harm should be done. The use of strong solutions in a wound or large instrument-damaged tissue left behind in a wound may be a culture media for subsequent infection.

WOUND CLOSURE

The overriding principle in wound closure is to close a wound without tension on the wound edges. How often we have heard the phrase, "the wound got infected," when, in fact, it became devascularized by a tight closure, creating a culture media, which then allowed infection. This is an important distinction. One can determine if there is enough skin prior to the resection by pinching the skin together, giving an idea of how much one will be able to draw it together. If the wound is moderately tight, undercutting the skin by detaching its dermal fascial attachments allows some advancement of the skin. If the wound will not close without tension, however, then a flap or graft should be outlined ahead of time. If caught short, a thin graft of skin can close a wound temporarily and subsequent contracture of the wound may allow serial excisions of the graft.

Fine sutures can be used because there is no tension on a properly closed wound. Interrupted sutures give the best alignment of skin and they can be removed in 3–4 days preventing notching. This technique is useful on the face; however, on the leg or trunk, where healing is slower, subcuticular sutures are preferred as they will not leave suture marks (Fig. 25.10).

Excision of Benign Lesions

The lines of elective incisions are used to outline excisions of small lesions. Larger lesions can be excised in the "haptoplasty" fashion (Fig. 25.5), which both breaks up the scar line and keeps it as short as possible. In removing benign lesions, excisions of one cell width of normal tissue are theoretically sufficient to eradicate the growth. Practically, however, this is not realistic and 0.5-1 to 1.0-mm borders are used for lesions such as nevi, fibromas, angiomas and xanthelosma. Sebaceous cysts in areas other than the scalp are

excised with the epidermal attachment puncta. In the scalp, the cyst is excised by incision to expose the growth which then dissects easily from the loose areolar tissue and shells out like a pea.

Patients with ill-defined lesions such as multiple sebaceous cysts should be warned that they will develop new ones in the future, frequently in the area of previous resection. These are often new cysts and not recurrences. The same occurs in patients with recurrent deep keratosis that require resection. Most of these can be treated topically. Lipomas are excised by incision, dissection, and enucleation as they have no dermal attachment. Care should be taken to remove all the cells to avoid recurrence. The fat of the lipoma is in larger segments and usually is distinguishable from the surrounding lipoma by a slight difference in color.

Excision of Malignant Lesions

The three common skin tumors, melanoma, squamous cell carcinoma and basal cell carcinoma are handled differently. Melanoma requires wide local excision and reconstruction and probably will require local node resection. Squamous cell carcinoma requires less radical resection but may involve the lymph nodes as well as requiring reconstruction, except for the very small ones where small resection is sufficient. Basal cell carcinoma is one of the most common malignant skin tumors. It practically never goes to the local nodes and can almost always be handled by local excision. Chemosurgery, x-ray, and topical 5-fluorouracil also have a place in management of these tumors but the subject under discussion is surgical management. Although some texts list many types of basal cell carcinoma, from a practical standpoint there are two that concern us:

1. Isolated pea-like mobile basal cell carcinoma with sharp distinct borders, which are exophytic in nature. These can be removed with less than a 1-mm border which is sufficient. This author uses ×2.5 loop magnification to define the border.
2. Ill-defined, vague, scaly, endophytic lesions which need a 5-mm border as these basal cells have a higher recurrence rate.

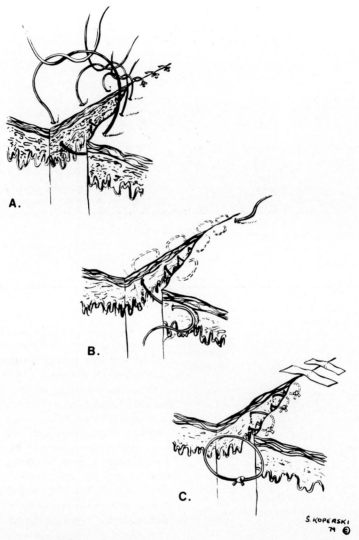

Fig. 25.10. Interrupted sutures give the best skin alignment but must be removed in 2–4 days to prevent suture marks *A*. Subcuticular sutures can be left indefinitely and no suture marks will be apparent (*B* and *C*).

SUMMARY

Three principles offer a guide to the direction of elective incisions on the body—these are made at right angles to skin, except in hair-bearing areas. Gentle handling of the tissues and closure without tension complete the requirements for an optimal scar on the body.

References

1. Langer, K.: On the anatomy and physiology of the skin. Conclusions. Br. J. Plast. Surg., *31:* 277, 1978.
2. McKinney, P. and Griffith, B.H.: Appraisal of treatment of basal cell carcinoma of skin. Plast. Reconstr. Surg., *51:* 565, 1973.

CHAPTER 26

HOW TO SET UP FOR OFFICE EXCISIONAL SKIN SURGERY

BRYAN C. SCHULTZ

To obtain good cosmetic results, one must pay meticulous attention to the general principles of skin surgery as discussed in the previous chapter. Proper instrumentation and selection of appropriate lesions amenable to office surgery are equally important. This chapter will discuss the basic set-up and instrumentation for outpatient office surgery. Several common lesions may or may not be treated in the office.

Postoperative Evaluation and Instructions

A good history and physical examination are essential to preoperative evaluation of any surgical patient. For office surgery, an extensive evaluation questionnaire is often helpful. Blood pressure is especially important on all patients since hypertensive patients will frequently bleed profusely, especially when doing surgery of the scalp. Any irregularities of pulse should be noted. A record of all allergies and present medications should be noted. The patient should be specifically asked about any history of epilepsy. The physician should be aware of the fact that larger doses of local anesthetic may induce convulsions. The patient also should be questioned about the use of a cardiac pacemaker since electrocoagulation should not be used in such patients. The physician should examine the entire skin surface to rule out bacterial or viral skin disease at distant locations. The patient should be instructed to maintain all necessary medications, *including* the day of surgery. It is especially important that the patients continue antihypertensive medications in contrast to what is done for patients undergoing general anesthesia.

Allow the patient to have a light breakfast with juice in the morning of the procedure. This seems to avoid syncope, and vomiting has rarely been a problem with small outpatient procedures. The patient should avoid caffeinated beverages the day of the procedure since they may precipitate hypertension. The patient should be warned specifically about ingestion of any aspirin or aspirin-containing products. He should be aware that only one aspirin tablet within 7–10 days before the procedure may induce prolonged bleeding. Tylenol or codeine may be used as substitutes, depending on the severity of pain. This may be a significant problem when dealing with patients with severe arthritis.

HOW TO SET UP FOR OFFICE SURGERY

The Room

Most offices can easily have one room set up for excisional skin surgery. It would be preferable to have this room used exclusively for surgery of the skin. If this is not possible, meticulous attention to cleaning of all surfaces within the room is mandatory. Patients known to be carrying pathogenic bacteria or viruses should definitely be kept out of the room at all times. This is especially true in a busy dermatologic practice. Patients with generalized skin disease, such as atopic eczema and psoriasis, are known to frequently harbor *Staphylococcus aureus.* Any patients with draining or crusting lesions should definitely be kept out of this room. Drainage of furuncles or acne cysts should obviously not be done in this room.

One should be sure there is adequate space, ventilation, and cooling in the surgery room. This is important for both patient and physician, since active perspiration during the procedure may lead to extreme discomfort and contamination of the wound. If the physician is operating with an assistant, there will be at least three people within a small area. If a cool light source is not used, this will also add to increased temperature in the operative area. High quality surgical lighting may be mounted on the ceiling or wall of the surgical room (Fig 26.1). One may also obtain cool surgical lighting from various floor stand models (e.g. Burton lamp).

Several factors should be considered when choosing an operating table. A high quality power table is preferable. Separate controls for table height and head elevation should be included. It is also helpful if the table can be placed in a Trendelenberg position. Some tables may also rotate 180° on their base (e.g. Ritter table) (Fig. 26.1). This feature is rarely necessary in most offices. If the physician wishes to operate from a sitting position, the tables should adjust to the appropriate height and also with a head piece smaller than the rest of the table for easy accessibility. Several dental and podiatry chairs are quite comfortable, but should be carefully scrutinized. They may be well suited for surgery of one area and totally inadequate for another area. If operating on the trunk, this area of the body would be in flexion during surgery if the chair had a permanent curvature here. Some tables have a permanently attached footrest, perpendicular to the table, making surgery of the foot almost impossible.

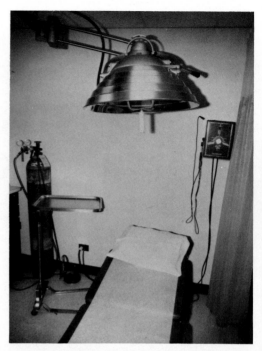

Fig. 26.1   A typical out-patient surgical set-up. Overhead lighting, Ritter power table, Bovie electrocoagulator and Mayo stand are seen. Tank with compressed gas for Stryker dermabrader is seen in the background.

Shelving and other surfaces should be of stainless steel if possible, facilitating cleaning and disinfection. A Mayo stand of adjustable height should be placed in close proximity to the operating area. A fully equipped emergency kit should be in the operating room whenever surgery is being performed (Table 26.1). Individual components of an emergency kit may be purchased at a reduced cost compared to the cost of a premade kit.

Emergency treatment should be directed toward maintaining vital functions with rapid transport of the patient to the nearest hospital. One employee should have the job of immediately notifying the nearest paramedic-ambulance team in the area. The physician should personally acquaint himself with such facilities.

Sterilization and Skin Preparation

It is suggested that surgical packs be prepared and autoclaved with steam under pres-

Table 26.1
Essentials for Emergency Kit

Oxygen supply system
"Ambu" resuscitating bag with adult and pediatric masks and tubing for connection to oxygen
  system.
Intravenous equipment
  Tourniquet
  No. 18 needles and Angiocath or Intracaths
  Tape and arm board
  Tubing and 500 ml bags of normal saline and D5W
  Scalpel, hemostats, and suture for "cut-down" if needed (these may already be on excision kit).
    Sterile gloves and Betadine prep also should be available.
Head board to place under patient for cardiac massage
Medications
  NaHCO$_3$, Prepackaged 50 ml syringes, at least two
  Epinephrine 1:1000 (1-ml ampule) for allergic reactions 1:10,000 (10-ml ampule with intracardiac
    needle)
  50% Dextrose (50-ml Ristojet ampules), for hypoglycemic reactions
  Lidocaine 2% (5-ml syringe, 100 mg)
  Aminophylline (10 ml., 250 mg ampules)
  Narcan (0.4 mg/ml) only if narcotics used before or during surgery
  Valium (10-mg ampule for I.V. use)
  Benadryl (50-mg ampule)

sure. It is best to obtain an autoclave with a separate door used for dry heat sterilization (e.g. Pelton-Crane). There is less damage to sharp instruments if they are wrapped in aluminum foil and sterilized by dry heat. These instruments may be placed on the open excision pack by means of a transfer forceps.

Prior to sterilization, all instruments should be scrubbed with an ordinary detergent to remove visible debri. Further cleaning of cracks and crevices may be done with several of the available ultrasonic cleaners.

Mechanical scrubbing of the skin surface before surgery has been shown to adequately remove surface bacteria. The iodophors are most commonly used for this purpose. Seventy percent isopropyl alcohol may also be used. A more effective solution may be obtained by adding 1% iodine to the isopropyl alcohol. In one prospective study, 807 plastic surgical cases were prepped with a physiologic solution (similar to saline) (1). The overall infection rate was 0.62%. The authors suggested that a gentle cleansing was adequate, provided that meticulous attention was given to handling of tissues during surgery. It is also most important to be sure that the patient is not harboring a skin or mucosal infection at a distant sight (e.g. herpes simplex or furunculosis).

The Surgical Pack

The surgical pack may be wrapped in suitable cloth material (e.g. surgical towels) or in autoclave paper. If autoclave paper is used, the Mayo stand must be covered with a sterile impermeable sheet (e.g. Barrier Field). This is to prevent contamination if the paper becomes moistened (e.g. with Xylocaine) during the procedure. Autoclave tape should be used to close the pack. This will turn color when sterilization is complete. The following should be contained in the surgical pack (Fig. 26.2):

1. An adequate number of 4- by 4-inch gauze sponges
2. A pointed wooden toothpick for drawing the line of excision
3. A glass syringe, 5 cc (optional)
4. Towel drapes (disposable fenestrated drapes are optional)
5. A No. 3 Bard-Parker handle with centimeter markings on one side
6. A 4½-inch needle holder (Webster type-smooth jaws)
7. Two or three short, curved, mosquito hemostats
8. A small medicine cup (glass or metal, optional)
9. Small tissue forceps with medium teeth
10. One forceps without teeth (Adson)
11. One or two skin hooks (optional)
12. One dissecting scissors (optional).

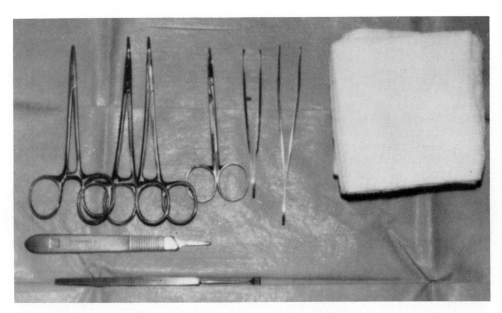

Fig. 26.2. Surgical pack. Other items may be added to this basic set-up.

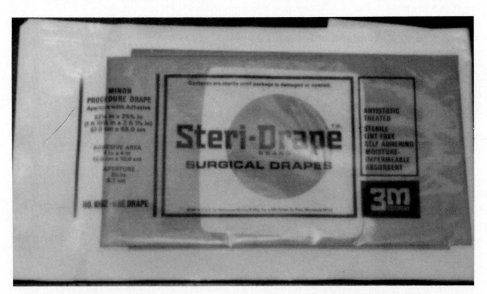

Fig. 26.3. Steri-Drape with fenestration and adhesive backing.

Disposable plastic syringes (5 cc) may be added to the excision set at the time of surgery. These should be obtained without needles attached and a 18- and 30-gauge needle added to the kit at the time of the surgery.

Xylocaine can be drawn up with an 18- gauge needle and infiltration accomplished with the 30-gauge needle. Whenever possible, the 30-gauge needle should be used for infiltration, since the pain involved is significantly less than that with larger needles. Disposable towel drapes are available with various size fenestrated holes or the fenestrated drape with adhesive on one side (3M Steri-Drape). (Fig 26.3). The Steri-Drape has the advantage of not allowing blood to run under the drape onto the patient. All fluid during the procedure will run from the operative down the drape. It is important to draw your lines of excision before placing the drape, since anatomic markings are lost at that time. Either gentian violet solution or methylene blue may be added to the medicine cup for this purpose.

For most skin surgery, a 4½-inch needle holder is adequate. Since 5-0 and 6-0 suture material will be most commonly used, a smooth-jaw needle holder (e.g. Webster type) should be used, so suture material will not slip.

Instruments and Other Additions to Surgical Pack

The following may be added to a routine excisional pack:

1. No. 15 Bard-Parker blade.
2. One short, curved, sharp iris scissors (dry sterilized in aluminum foil to maintain sharpness).
3. A disposable hot cautery unit (e.g. Concept unit), may be used directly. Coagulation of blood vessels can be also accomplished by clamping vessels with mosquito hemostats and use of an electrocoagulation unit in the surgery room. Such a unit should have a ground plate (e.g. Bovie or Electricator).
4. Suture material.

5. Steri-Strips should be added to the excision pack. White or skin-colored Steri-Strips are available in various sizes.

Absorbable sutures for subcutaneous suturing may be added. Synthetic absorbables such as Dexon (Davis & Geck) or Vicryl (Ethicon) may be used. Even though these suture materials may come braided, they should be double-knotted on the first tie. Chromic cat gut may also be used. Nonabsorbable synthetics should be used for skin suturing (either subcuticular or interrupted). There is little reason to use silk suture in skin surgery. The most commonly used suture materials would be 5-0 and 6-0 Prolene (or nylon). Prolene is possibly slightly less reactive than nylon and seems to be somewhat more stretchable. This suture has great memory and must be tied with at least 4 or 5 knots. For surface and subcuticular sutures, a ⅜ or ½ circle, P-3 plastic needle is suitable. A half-circle needle may be used for subcutaneous suturing. Reverse cutting, sharp, plastic needles should be used for all skin work. These needles are approximately 3 times as expensive as ordinary cuticular needles; however, they are much less traumatic to tissue.

References

1. Johnson, H.A., and Edwards, L.D.: A more physiologic skin prep. Ill. Med. J., p. 352, 1980.
2. Epstein, E., and Epstein, Jr., E.: *Skin Surgery.* Ed. 4. Charles C Thomas, Springfield, Ill., 1977.
3. Zoltan, J., Wilgis E.F., and Hansen, F. et al.: *Cicatrix Optima—Techniques Wound Healing.* University Park Press, Baltimore, Md., 1977.

CHAPTER 27

EXCISION OF COMMON BENIGN SKIN LESIONS

BRYAN C. SCHULTZ

NEVOCELLULAR NEVI

Any nevus with recent change in color, size, or sensation should be excised. Recently traumatized, bleeding, or ulcerated lesions should also be excised and sent for histologic examination.

When one is relatively confident that the lesion is benign and only to be removed for a cosmetic reason, two techniques may be used. The lesion (Fig. 27.1) may be shaved flush to the surface. When using this technique, a sharp curette can be used to even out the borders of the lesion or an irregular scar may result. If the lesion is heavily pigmented, significant pigment may be left after the shaving process. The patient should always know that part of the nevus has been left within the skin, if there was any intradermal component to the nevus. One must realize that such a biopsy can evaluate only the removed portion of the nevus. If there is a surrounding border with macular pigment, (indicating a junctional epidermal component) the shaving technique would leave a depressed area if one attempts removal of this portion. Since histologic examination of this junctional component may be necessary, excision is preferable here (Fig. 27.2). Hemostasis may be adequately achieved with a 35% solution of aluminum chloride (Figs. 27.3, 27.4). Cautery is not necessary for hemostasis and may cause added scarring in susceptible individuals.

Cosmetic removal of benign nevi also may be obtained through excision surgery. If a lesion is 4 mm or less in diameter, a circular punch may be used. This should be used only in areas where tissue is loose and easily approximated. If the skin is stretched slightly perpendicular to the line of intended suturing, an oval will result after removing the lesion with a circular punch (Figs. 27.5–27.7). This oval may be closed with one or two sutures with no evident dog-earring effect. The skin should be stretched prior to infiltration with anesthetic to determine if the diameter of the nevus will exceed 4 mm with stretching.

Circular punch excision over 4 mm in size usually cannot be closed adequately without a dog-ear effect at both ends of the suture line. One also should be careful not to infiltrate a large amount of Xylocaine into the superficial dermis or the nevus may be expanded in diameter, no longer being amenable to removal with a 4-mm punch.

Routine elliptical excision is ideal for removal of both benign and suspicious nevi (Figs. 27.8, 27.9). If there is any suspicion of malignancy, careful marking of the skin with exact borders should be carried out. The chart should clearly indicate the location and size of a lesion and the exact dimensions of the excision. This is of utmost importance if extensive excision is to be done in the future. Although there is no solid evidence of cancer spread from punch biopsy of malignant mel-

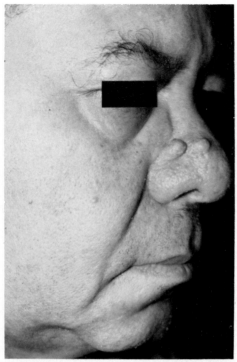

Fig. 27.1. Two small nevocellular nevi on the nose.

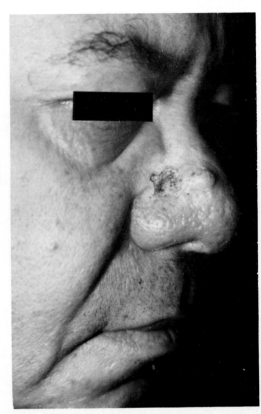

Fig. 27.3. Successful hemostasis after shave excision by application of 35% aluminum chloride.

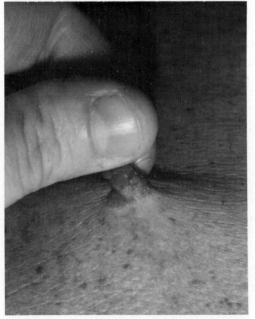

Fig. 27.2. Nevus with junctional component.

anoma, most surgeons would prefer total excisional biopsy if melanoma is expected.

Congenital, giant, hairy nevi are well known to have an increased incidence of malignant degeneration. Total excision of these lesions, when feasible, is recommended. A current controversy exists, however, as to whether congenital nevi of smaller size have increased malignant potential. It has been suggested by some that only congenital lesions greater than 1.5 cm be excised. Since controversy still exists, it would seem reasonable also to excise lesions less than 1.5 cm in diameter. These lesions are usually the easiest to remove with excellent cosmetic results.

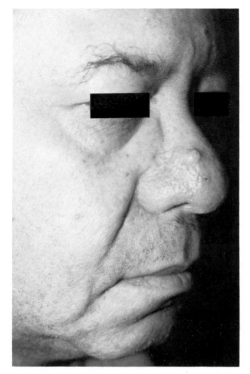

Fig. 27.4. Two weeks after shave.

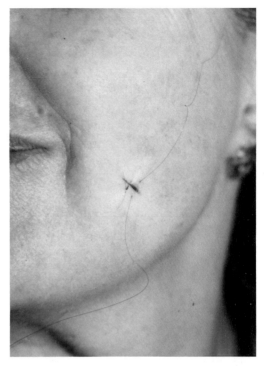

Fig. 27.6. One suture in place.

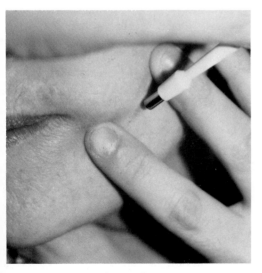

Fig. 27.5. Stretching skin prior to punch excision.

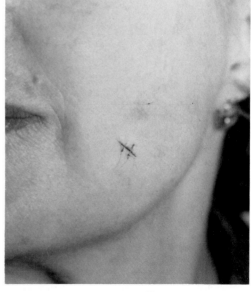

Fig. 27.7. Two nylon sutures to close oval.

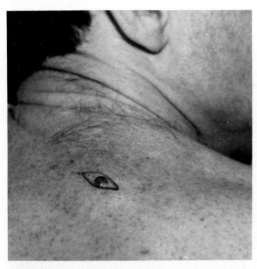

Fig. 27.8. Black nevus with elliptical excision drawn with gentian violet.

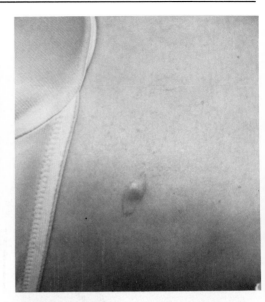

Fig. 27.10. Dermatofibroma on the trunk.

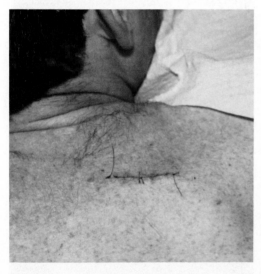

Fig. 27.9. Closure with subcuticular stitch showing interruption through skin in the center. This suture may be left in place for 2 weeks.

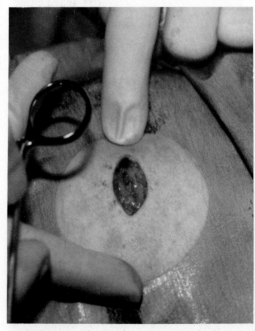

Fig. 27.11. Elliptical excision including superficial subcutaneous tissue.

EPIDERMAL NEVI

Small epidermal nevi are most satisfactorily removed by excisional surgery. Although shaving and dermabrasion has been done for these lesions, they are not usually flush with the surface.

DERMATOFIBROMAS

Dermatofibromas are common intradermal tumors frequently seen on the extremities (Figs. 27.10, 27.11). Depending on their size, these lesions may be removed with the punch excision technique or a simple elliptical excision. Biopsy should always be done.

CAPILLARY HEMANGIOMAS

Small capillary hemangiomas (e.g. cherry angioma) may be removed by excision. (Fig. 27.12). This is usually for cosmetic purposes only. These lesions are frequently small enough to be excised with a small punch.

PYOGENIC GRANULOMA

Pyogenic granuloma is a rapidly enlarging hemangioma that can usually be excised with

a simple ellipse. Electrodessication and curettage is an alternative treatment for this lesion, as shown in Figure 27.13 (see color Plate V). Biopsy should always be done.

EPIDERMAL CYST

Another very common lesion seen in the office is the *epidermal cyst*, (Fig. 27.14). Before removal of these lesions, a punctate aperture should be searched for on the surface of the lesion. This is usually a grayish or blackish color. Frequently, slightly squeezing the surrounding cyst may accentuate this aperture, (Fig. 27.15). This will frequently assure preoperative diagnosis. This prevents attempted excision of other cystic lesions with possible deeper extension, such as dermoid cysts. If epidermal cysts are small in size, a small opening may be placed over the central part of the cyst. A curved iris scissors may be used

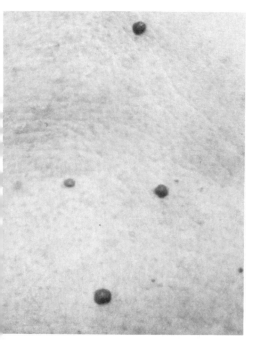

Fig. 27.12 Capillary angioma.

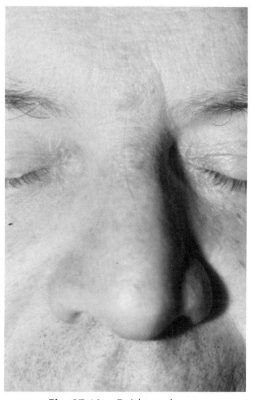

Fig. 27.14. Epidermal cyst.

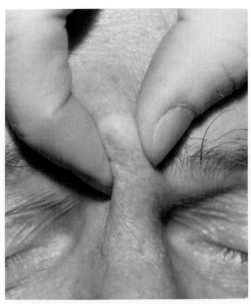

Fig. 27.15. Squeezing cyst to accentuate aperture.

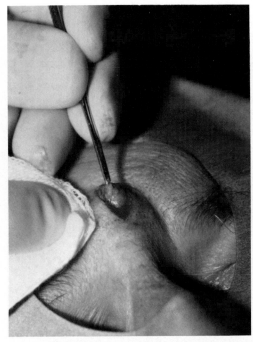

Fig. 27.17. Excision of cyst.

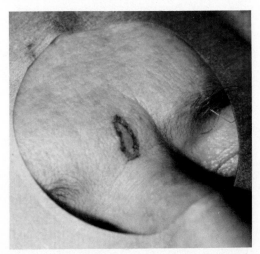

Fig. 27.16. Vertical incision lines follow existing skin furrows.

to dissect and deliver the cyst through this aperture, (Figs. 27.16, 27.17). An alternative method is by making a small aperture with a No. 11 blade, and squeezing out the contents of the cyst. The cyst wall is then delivered with a tissue forceps and iris scissors. Cysts occupying significant space should be approached with an elliptical excision over the central portion of the cyst. If this is not done, there will be a significant dead space left after removal.

Pilar tumors of the scalp may be removed in a similar fashion, (Fig. 27.18). Special attention should be paid to closing off dead space in these tumors, since a hematoma may accumulate within such space in the scalp. One should be aware of significant calcification of these tumors.

LESIONS THAT SHOULD NOT BE EXCISED IN THE OFFICE

Many epidermal lesions (e.g. seborrheic keratosis, actinic keratosis, senile lentigo, wart, etc.) are simply removed with superficial curettage, electrodessication, or cryosurgery. In most circumstances, superior results will be obtained with such methods (with the exception of epidermal nevi).

A seborrheic keratosis is easily curetted off (Figs. 27.19, 27.20). Aluminum chloride or light cautery may be used for hemostasis. These lesions should *never* be excised. Lentigines may be treated adequately with cryo-

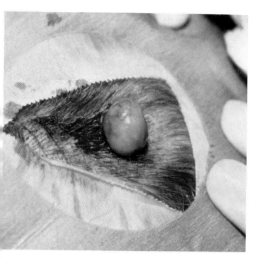

Fig. 27.18. Delivery of pilar cyst from elliptical excision.

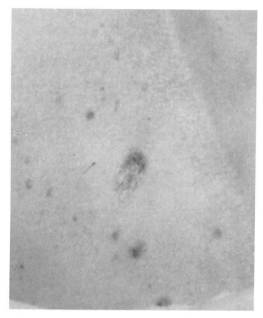

Fig. 27.20. Immediately after removal with hemostasis achieved with 35% aluminum chloride.

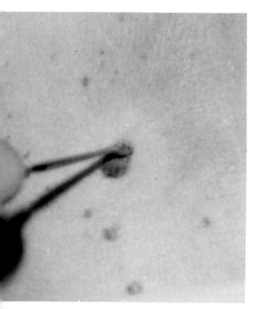

Fig. 27.19. Sharp curette in place to remove seborrheic keratosis.

therapy and should not be excised unless lentigo maligna is suspected.

One probably should refrain from attempting removal of any lesion that could possibly penetrate beyond the subcutaneous tissue level. Such poorly defined lesions as lipomas probably should not be attempted in the office. The same holds true for large or deep hemangiomas.

Lymphangioma circumscriptum frequently has deeper extensions and is notorious for recurrence after excision. Such lesions should be handled by a competent plastic surgeon.

One should be suspicious of any lesions lying over, or close to, the spinal cord. Such lesions may frequently have communications to the spinal canal. Although such lesions may appear to be rather benign and easily approached, they should not be done in the office. Common sense would seem to dictate that very long procedures should not be performed in the office. Such procedures are better performed in the operating room.

CHAPTER **28**

EXCISION OF COMMON MALIGNANT TUMORS OF THE SKIN

BRYAN C. SCHULTZ

BASAL CELL CARCINOMA

Excision or curettage and electrodessication are perhaps the most popular forms of treatment for this most common of skin malignancies. Radiation and cryosurgery may also be used. Microscopically controlled surgery (Mohs' surgery) is frequently the treatment of choice for recurrent tumors of this type. The advantage of excisional surgery for this and other malignancies is the removal of the entire excisional specimen. A microscopic check can be done to determine the adequacy of excision. Such a specimen is not available with radiation, electrodessication, and cryosurgery.

Before excising a basal cell carcinoma, several factors should be assessed. Different clinical types are known to frequently follow different invasion patterns and growth rates. For the purpose of determining treatment modality and extent, one should differentiate noduloulcerative, fibrosing, or morphea-like, and superficial basal cell carcinoma.

Noduloulcerative basal cell carcinoma is by far the most common type. It most frequently is found on sun-exposed skin, especially the face. If a primary lesion has well defined margins and is not greater than 1 cm in diameter primary excision is a reasonable approach (Figs. 28.1–28.3). There is some con-

troversy over what constitutes an adequate margin when excising such tumors. In one study evaluating 634 basal cell carcinoma, two plastic surgeons compared cure rates using different margins of normal tissue (1). One surgeon took a 2- to 3-mm border routinely while the other used margins "of grossly normal tissue on all sides at least as wide as the diameter of the tumor." Similar cure rates at 3 years or later were obtained (approximately 98.6%). In another study, excised lesions with at least one high power field of normal tissue between specimen edge and tumor showed a 1.2% 10-year recurrence rate (2). Lesions with tumor at the surgical margin showed a 33% recurrence rate. If there are recurrences, they usually occur in the first few years after excision. One study showed 60% of recurrences within 2 years after excision and 76% of recurrences within 3 years.

Superficial basal cell carcinoma usually presents as a slightly elevated scaling reddish plaque, frequently on the trunk. It may be very slowly growing with a characteristic thready, pearly, border at some edges. One such patient of ours had a 4-cm plaque that had been growing for more than 20 years without deep extension or metastasis. These patients should be questioned about arsenic ingestion as long as 20 or more years previ-

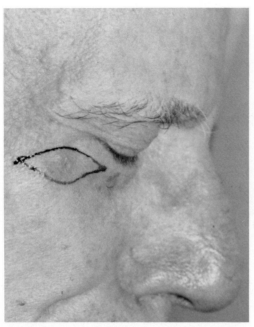

Fig. 28.1. Conservative 3-mm border for a primary basal cell carcinoma.

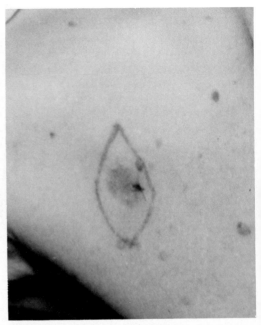

Fig. 28.3. Three-millimeter border for superficial basal cell carcinoma.

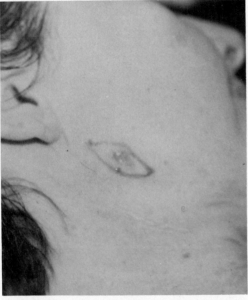

Fig. 28.2. Conservative 3-mm border drawn for a primary nodular basal cell.

ously, (e.g. Fowler's solution, Asiatic pills, contaminated well water). The physician should also look carefully for other arsenical lesions such as arsenical keratosis, Bowen's disease,

and squamous cell carcinoma. The lesion can easily be excised with a 3-mm border from the clinical edge. Microscopic examination shows numerous tumor islands coming off the epidermis without evidence of deep dermal or subcutaneous extension. This lesion also can be treated with curettage and electrodessication or cryotherapy. This is the only basal cell carcinoma that could reasonably be approached with topical 5-flourouracil. With so many other definitive time-tested methods, it is difficult to accept this form of treatment.

Sclerosing or morphea-like basal cell carcinoma is relatively uncommon. It frequently presents as a poorly defined yellowish plaque on the face. Telangiectases may sometimes be seen if the skin is stretched. Histologically, a particularly thick connective tissue stroma with thin threads of basal cells in the dermis may be seen. Since definition of borders may be difficult both clinically and microscopically, some dermatologists consider this a primary indication for Mohs' microscopically controlled surgery. If excised, a larger border should be used and careful microscopic examination of tissue edges done. Curettage and electrodessication seem to be inadequate here since tumor tissue is not as easily distinguished with the curette.

Location of basal cell carcinoma may influence technique, border of tumor-free tissue, and likelihood of recurrence. The nasolabial fold seems particularly prone to recurrence. Electrodessication seems to leave a higher incidence of hypertrophic scars in this area and the adjacent upper lip. Excision of the ala nasi is frequently done with placement of a skin graft or rotation flap. Recurrences also seem to be higher near the eye and ear (3), possibly because of the difficulty in taking significant tumor-free margins.

Recurrent basal cell carcinoma probably should be treated with Mohs' microscopically controlled surgery (see Chapter 31). Although metastasis is distinctly rare, local extension of tumors with significant destruction of adjacent skin, cartilage, or bone is not uncommon. Death may even be seen with destruction of skull and extension to the brain.

Most studies show similar cure rates for primary basal cell carcinoma using excision or curettage and electrodessication (4, 5). Curettage and electrodessication is easier and quicker, but the healing time is definitely longer than for excision and primary closure. The curette may find soft tumor masses in the dermis not detected with the razor-sharp scalpel but, if the tumor or a previous punch biopsy has penetrated the subcutaneous tissue, the curette cannot distinguish this from tumor. In some situations, the frequently shorter, but wider, scar from curettage is preferable to the longer thin scar of excision. Properly placed excision lines will often be cosmetically superior. A scar from curettage or Mohs' surgery on the ala nasi may look better than a graft after surgical excision. Tumor recurrence may be more difficult to assess after healing by granulation tissue since the result is frequently sclerotic and studded with telangiectasia. Excision and Mohs' surgery provide a complete histologic specimen, whereas curettage, radiation, and cryosurgery do not.

If excision is chosen to treat basal cell carcinoma, the clinical appearance is often diagnostic enough to proceed with total excision before biopsy. Any suspicion as to alternative diagnoses (especially benign conditions such as sebaceous hyperplasia with surrounding telangiectatic skin) should prompt an initial 3-mm punch biopsy.

Excision of basal cell carcinoma or any malignant skin tumor should at least extend to the complete depth of subcutaneous tissue.

SQUAMOUS CELL CARCINOMA OF THE SKIN

Only squamous cell carcinoma in areas of actinic damage should be excised in the office. These lesions have a low incidence of deep invasion and rarely metastasize. This is in contrast to the more malignant nature of squamous cell carcinoma arising de novo from burn scars, chronic draining sinuses or ulcers, and mucous membranes. Squamous cell carcinoma arising from Bowen's disease also has greater tendency to metastasize and should be excised with larger margins. A careful search should be made histologically for adjacent actinic keratosis in squamous cell carcinoma of the skin. This enables one to more definitively categorize the squamous cell carcinoma. Margins similar to those for basal cell carcinoma may be used in most instances of squamous cell carcinoma arising in actinic keratosis.

Careful physical examination for other possible squamous cell carcinomas should be done in all these patients. They almost invariably will have other actinic keratoses which should be treated. Curettage and electrodessication, cryosurgery or topical 5-fluorouracil are all acceptable methods of treatment for actinic keratosis. Any lesion not resolving should be biopsied to rule out squamous cell carcinoma. These patients should be checked at least twice a year for new lesions.

SOLITARY KERATOACANTHOMA

A careful histologic diagnosis of this tumor should be made by an experienced skin pathologist. It may be difficult to differentiate this lesion from squamous cell carcinoma. Complete excision should be performed as soon as the diagnosis is made clinically for the following reasons: 1) a complete surgical specimen ensures a more accurate histologic diagnosis, with characteristic buttressing seen at tumor margins; 2) the lesion may continue to rapidly enlarge causing more tissue destruction eventuating in a larger scar; 3) the cos-

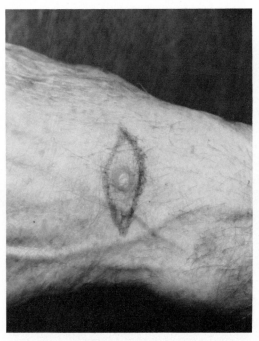

Fig. 28.4. Solitary keratoacanthoma on wrist with conservative border drawn.

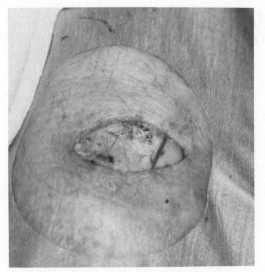

Fig. 28.5. Complete excision.

metic result from surgical excision is usually distinctly superior to the scar left after natural involution; and 4) squamous cell carcinoma is frequently a possibility even with careful histologic examination. Tumor margins

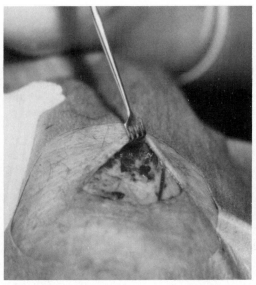

Fig. 28.6. Undermining to loosen tissue.

should ensure removal of the entire lesion with excision extending to the complete depth of subcutaneous tissue (Figs. 28.4–28.6).

DERMATOFIBROSARCOMA PROTUBERANS

This is a slowly growing tumor of the dermis, usually occurring on the trunk. It is notorious for extension (see Chapter 17) beyond clinically visible or palpable borders. It should never be excised in the office. In one study, metastasis occurred in 5 of 86 cases (6). Excision should be with a wide margin and include deep fascia. Mohs' microscopically controlled surgery has been used successfully for this tumor (7, 8).

MALIGNANT MELANOMA

It is not within the scope of this chapter to discuss the surgical treatment of malignant melanoma (see Chapter 19). Although there is no direct evidence that tumor may be spread by incisional biopsy through the tumor (9, 10), most surgeons would prefer a complete excisional biopsy where feasible. An accurate appraisal of type, level, and thickness of tumor

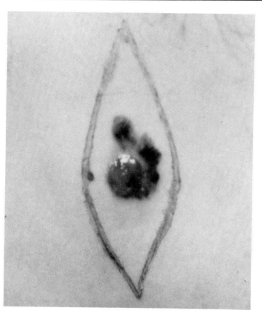

Fig. 28.9. Lines drawn for excisional biopsy.

is necessary to determine the treatment approach to melanoma. This is best done with serial sections throughout the entire tumor. Initial excisional biopsy should have a 3- to 10-mm border and extend to subcutaneous fat (11), as shown in Figures 28.7 and 28.9 (see color Plate V), and Figure 28.9. Exact measurements of all borders should be accurately recorded in the chart so that proper

margins may be used for subsequent surgery if the biopsy is positive. Photographs should be taken, especially if the surgeon has not seen the case first.

References

1. Griffith, B.H., and McKinney, P.: An appraisal of the treatment of basal cell carcinoma of the skin. Plast. Reconstr. Surg. *51:* 565, 1973.
2. Pascal, R.R.: Prognosis of "incompletely excised" versus "completely excised" basal cell carcinoma. Plast. Reconstr. Surg. *41:* 328, 1968.
3. Shanoff, L.B., Spira, M., and Hardy, S.B.: Basal cell carcinoma: a statistical approach to rational management. Plast. Reconstr. Surg. *39:* 619, 1967.
4. Kopf, A.W., Bart, R.S., and Schrager, D., et al.: Curettage-electrodessication of basal cell carcinoma. Arch. Dermatol., *113:* 439, 1977.
5. Bart, R.S., Schrager, D., and Kopf, A.W., et al.: Scalpel excision of basal cell carcinoma. Arch. Dermatol., *114:* 739, 1978.
6. McPeak, C.J., Cruz, T., and Nicastri, A.D.: Dermatofibrosarcoma protuberans: an analysis of 86 cases—five with metastasis. Ann. Surg., *116: (Suppl. 12):* 803, 1967.
7. Mohs, F.E.: *Chemosurgery.* Charles C Thomas, Springfield, Ill., 1978.
8. Mikhail, G.R., and Lynn, B.H.: Dermatofibrosarcoma protuberans. J. Dermatol. Surg. Oncol., *4:* 81, 1978.
9. Jones, N.M., Jones-Williams, W., and Roberts, M.M., et al.: Malignant melanoma of the skin: prognostic value of clinical features and the role of treatment in 111 cases. Br. J. Cancer, *22:* 437, 1968.
10. Epstein, E., Bragg, K., and Linden G.: Biopsy and prognosis of malignant melanoma. JAMA, *208:* 1369, 1969.
11. Kopf, A.W., and Bart, R.S.: Malignant melanoma. J. Dermatol. Surg. Oncol., *3:* 90, 1977.

CHAPTER **29**

HAIR TRANSPLANTS

HENRY H. ROENIGK, JR.

MALE PATTERN ALOPECIA

Hair is a completely useless vestige of our body; however, in modern society with our concerns for external appearance, people have become enormously sensitive about how they appear to others. Why do we worry about our hair? Hair loss of the male pattern type is partially due to the normal aging process. We fear aging! The constant desire to retain a youthful appearance may be important in retaining or obtaining a job in competition with younger people, sexual attractiveness, or just a sense of good feeling and personal attractiveness.

The average scalp contains approximately 100,000 hairs and 25,000 hairs must be lost before an unmistakable thinning is noticed. The growth of hair is a dynamic process in which many new hairs are regrowing at the time of shedding of old hairs. The average daily loss is 100 hairs per day.

Male pattern alopecia is due to androgen hormones, genetic predisposition, and aging. None of these factors can satisfactorily be modified by any known medical treatment. Therefore, if the proper conditions are present, most males and some females will eventually show certain degrees of baldness. The male pattern baldness takes certain patterns (Figs. 29.1, 29.2).

METHODS OF COVERING BALDNESS

There are many techniques used to cover the balding area to give the illusion of a youthful head of hair:

Hair Styling—changing the method of combing or allowing hair from side to grow long and then covering the crown or frontal areas.

Hair Toupee—Hair pieces made from natural hair or artificial fibers can be made to match one's normal hair. These must be attached by tape or glue.

Hair Weaves—Hair pieces are attached to lateral normal hair by a small loop of hair from sides. As hair grows, the loops need to be reformed. There is also a tendency to pull hair out and damage hair roots.

Hair Implants—Pieces of silicone suture or loop of normal scalp are created to anchor the hair piece to the scalp.

Fiber Implants—Individual fibers with anchoring knot are injected into the scalp. Because there is no hair root, these fibers eventually fall out or create infection due to foreign body reaction in the scalp.

HAIR TRANSPLANTATION

Orentreich (1) described the technique of hair transplantation over 20 years ago. He demonstrated that hair follicles, when transplanted from a hair-producing to a bald region of the scalp, continued to function and grow normally as if they were still in their original location. He devised a technique for transplantation of hair by means of multiple, small, full thickness autografts. After local anesthetic (Fig. 29.3) the recipient site is prepared with 3.5- to 4.0-mm round punches

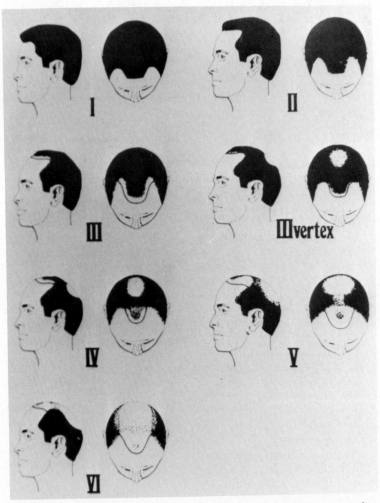

Fig. 29.1.   Classification of male pattern alopecia (Norwood).

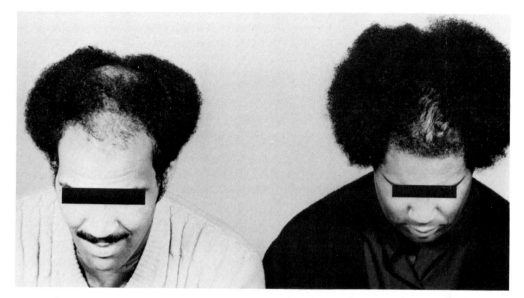

Fig. 29.2. Genetically determined male pattern alopecia in two brothers.

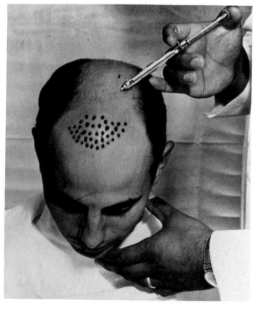

Fig. 29.3. Preparation for hair transplantation with local anesthetic. The previous transplants had been performed 2 weeks earlier.

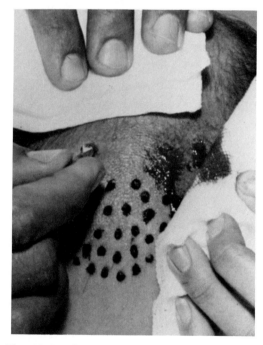

Fig. 29.4. Recipient area is prepared with round punch.

(Fig. 29.4). The donor area is the occipital or lateral aspect of the scalp using 4.0- to 4.5-mm round punches (Fig. 29.5). After removal of the plugs, they are placed in sterile normal saline and all hair, foreign matter, and part of the fat are removed (Fig. 29.6). The plugs are then placed in the frontal bald area in a preplanned method to create a natural appearing area of hair growth (Fig. 29.7).

Dressings are applied which can be re-

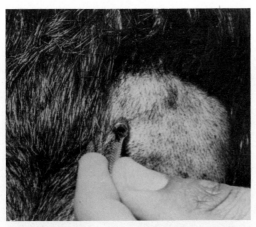

Fig. 29.5. After partial trimming of hair, the donor area in occipital scalp is taken with a slightly larger (0.5 mm) round punch.

moved in 24 hours. Small crusts form on each plug which fall off in 10 days to 2 weeks. The hair in the transplanted plugs falls out soon after the procedure, but the hair roots are still present so new hair will reach the scalp surface in 2–3 months following hair transplantation.

The clinical results depend on the skill of the surgeon, proper selection of patients, good follow-up, completion of fill-in transplants and lack of any complications (Figs. 29.8–29.11). Patients should be given an honest evaluation of what can be expected from the procedure. Although the transplant cannot give a perfect return to a youthful head of hair, it can make a marked improvement in the patient's appearance.

The procedure also may be adapted for scarring alopecia and loss of eyebrows (Figs. 29.12–29.15).

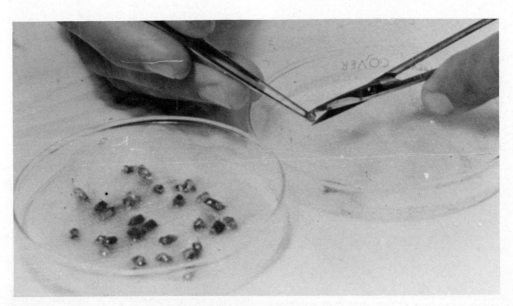

Fig. 29.6. Donor transplant plugs are placed in Petrie dish with sterile saline and cleaned of blood and subcutaneous fat.

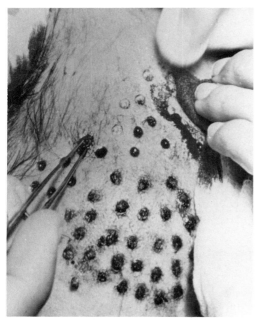

Fig. 29.7. Donor plugs are then placed into the frontal bald area.

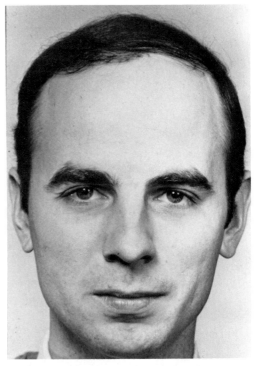

Fig. 29.9. Appearance of scalp after 400 hair transplants.

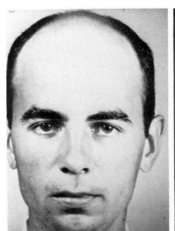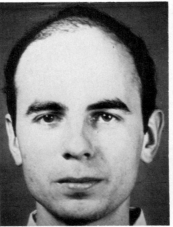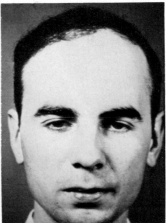

Fig. 29.8. Complete baldness of top of scalp (*left*) and after 400 hair transplants there is progressive change in appearance (*center* and *right*).

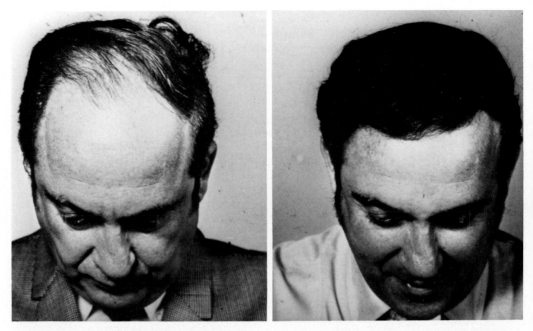

Fig. 29.10. Before (*left*) and after (*right*) hair transplantation and the changing of hair style.

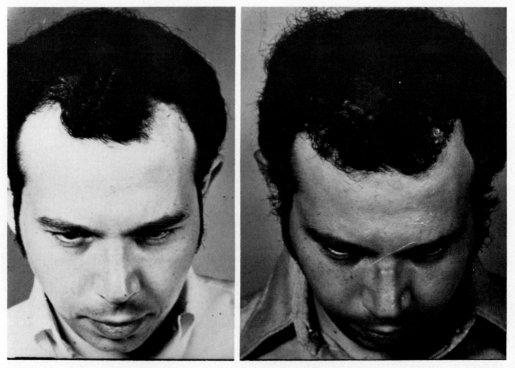

Fig. 29.11. Bilateral temporal alopecia (*left*) corrected with as little as 60 hair transplants (*right*).

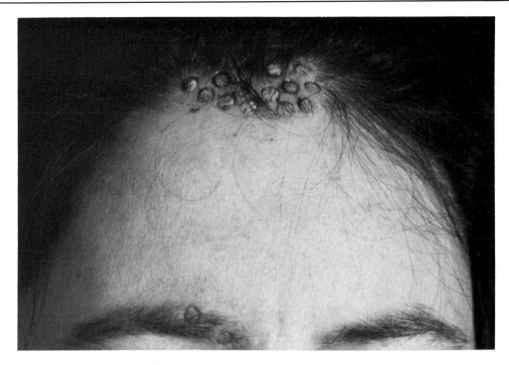

Fig. 29.12. Traumatic frontal hair loss from scalp and right eyebrow repaired with hair transplant plugs.

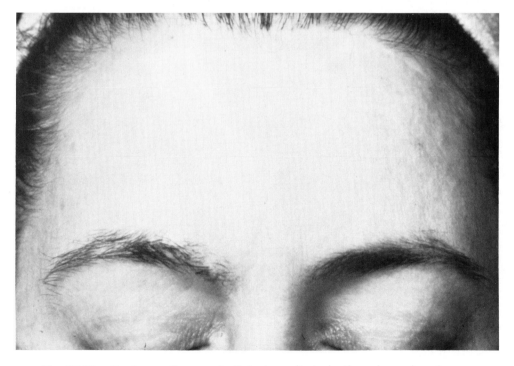

Fig. 29.13. Postoperative good clinical results in both scalp and eyebrow.

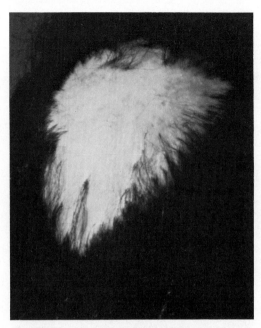

Fig. 29.14.   Scarring alopecia due to a burn.

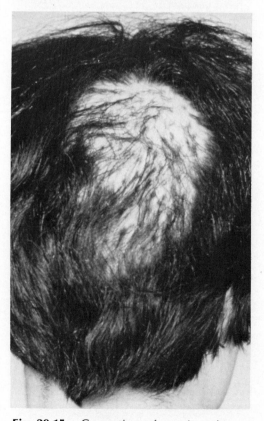

Fig. 29.15.   Correction of scarring alopecia with hair transplants.

References

1. Orentreich, N.: Autografts in alopecia and other selected dermatological conditions, Ann. N.Y. Acad. Sci., *83:* 463, 1959.
2. Unger, W.: *Hair Transplantation*, Marcel Dekker, New York, 1979.

CHAPTER 30

DERMABRASION

HENRY H. ROENIGK, JR.

Dermabrasion is a technique of planing off the epidermis and a portion of the dermis using a motor or pneumatic-driven metal brush or diamond fraise. This procedure can be done as an office procedure, but requires skill and judgement on the part of the operator. Mild preoperative sedation is necessary, but anesthesia is obtained with either ethyl chloride spray or 1% Xylocaine injectable local anesthetic. No general anesthetic is necessary and although operating room facilities are desirable they are not required for dermabrasion.

Postoperative care includes the application of topical antibiotic and a Telfa dressing or Debrisan beads followed by a full-face gauze dressing. This dressing is removed in 24 hours and a firm crust is allowed to form which begins to peel off in 7–10 days. Erythema persists for about 30–60 days and sunlight exposure is restricted during this period.

Complications can include: hyperpigmentation or hypopigmentation of the dermabraded areas, keloid or hypertrophic scar, milia, reactivation of original disease (acne, discoid lupus erythematosus, persistent erythema, purpura, and herpes simplex infection.

Indications for dermabrasion include: acne scars (Figs. 30.1, 30.2), tattoos (Figs. 30.3, 30.4), multiple trichoepitheliomas (Brooke's tumors) (Figs. 30.5–30.7), linear epidermal nevus (Figs. 30.8, 30.9), rhinophyma (Figs. 30.10, 30.11).

Other indications for dermabrasion may include: syringoma, adenoma, sebaceum, recurrent basal cell carcinoma, nevus angiomatosus, hypertrophic scars, traumatic tattoos, actinic damaged skin, and Darier's disease.

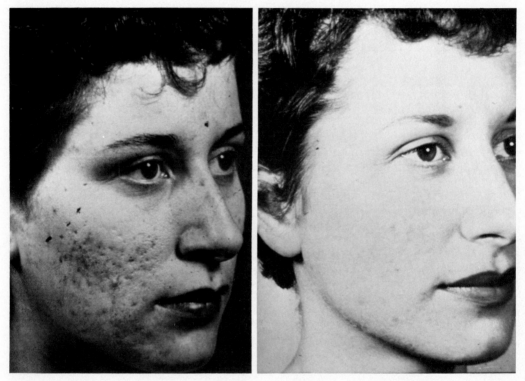

Fig. 30.1.   Preoperative (*left*) and postoperative (*right*) results of dermabrasion for acne scars.

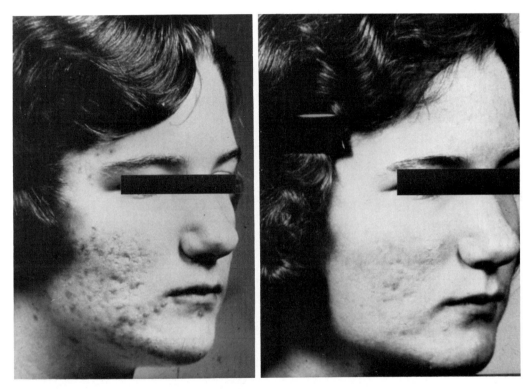

Fig. 30.2. Acne scars (*left*) have improved in the postoperative photo (*right*) but perfect results may not always be achieved. A second dermabrasion may be necessary.

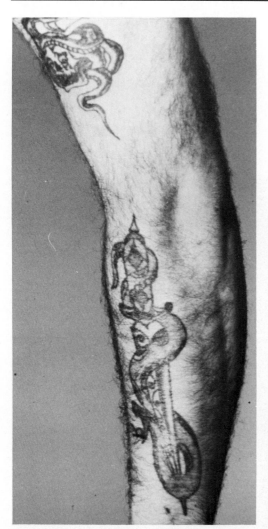

Fig. 30.3.   Preoperative tattoo on arm.

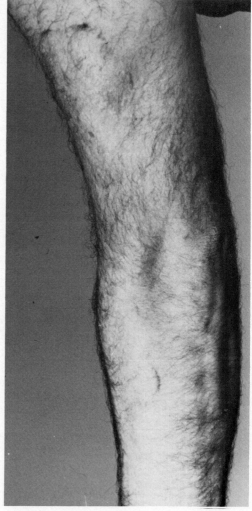

Fig. 30.4.   Postoperative tattoo after several superficial dermabrasions to remove pigment in dermis without creating much scar tissue (same patient as in Fig. 30.3).

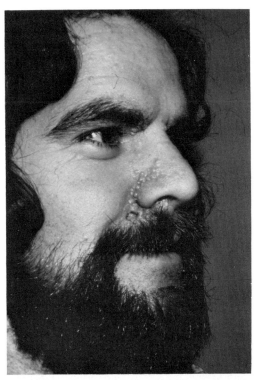

Fig. 30.5. Multiple trichoepitheliomas of paranasal area, nose, and forehead.

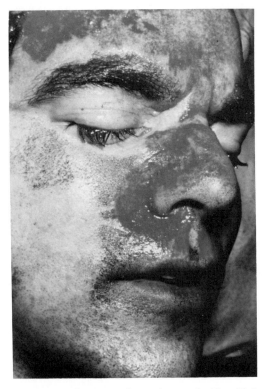

Fig. 30.6. Same patient shown in Fig. 30.5 immediately after facial dermabrasion.

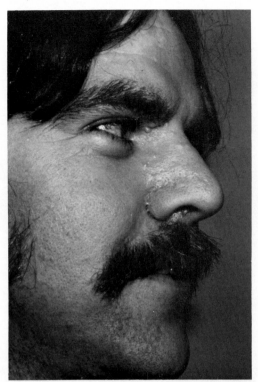

Fig. 30.7. Six weeks after dermabrasion the tumors are gone and may remain gone for many years (same patient as in Figs. 30.5 and 30.6).

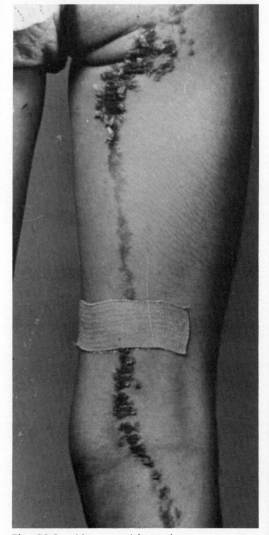

Fig. 30.8. Linear epidermal nevus present since birth.

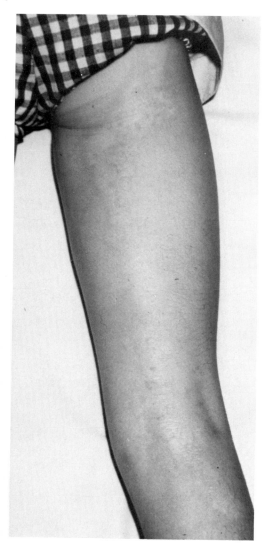

Fig. 30.9. One year postdermabrasion there is a good cosmetic result with no scar and no recurrence of the nevus (same patient as in Fig. 30.8).

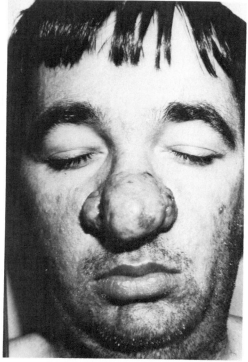

Fig. 30.10. Bullous enlargement of nose from rhinophyma.

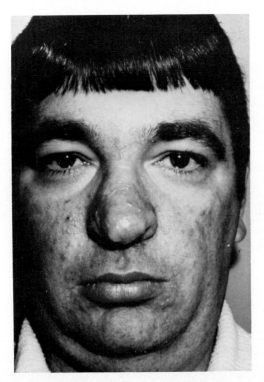

Fig. 30.11. Postoperative, after combining both cutting electrocautery of the bullous tissue and dermabrasion (same patient as in Fig. 30.10).

References

1. Burks, J.W.: *Dermabrasion and Chemical Peeling in the Treatment of Certain Cosmetic Defects and Diseases of the Skin.* Charles C Thomas, Springfield, Ill., 1979.
2. Epstein, E.: *Skin Surgery*, Charles C Thomas, Springfield, Ill., Fourth Edition, 1978.
3. Roenigk, Jr., H.H.: Dermabrasion for miscellaneous cutaneous lesions (exclusive of scarring from acne): J. Dermatol. Surg. Oncol., *3:* 3 322, 1977.

CHAPTER 31

MOHS' SURGERY FOR SKIN CANCER: MICROSCOPICALLY CONTROLLED EXCISION

JUNE K. ROBINSON

Basal cell carcinoma is the most common skin cancer in the white population. It is estimated that 300,000 new skin cancers, exclusive of malignant melanoma, are diagnosed in the United States each year. Skin cancer is most frequent on the head and neck and is often multiple. Ultraviolet light, exposure to arsenic ingestion, exposure to x-ray, and genetic factors (i.e. the nevoid basal cell carcinoma syndrome and xeroderma pigmentosum) are important in its etiology. While it is generally a cancer of the middle to later years, it is becoming increasingly more common in people in their twenties. Certainly, a clinically suspicious lesion should not be overlooked on the basis of the patient's age.

A number of modalities are effective in the treatment of skin cancers: excisional surgery, radiation therapy, cryosurgery, and electrodesiccation and curettage; however, a significant number of lesions resist the standard therapeutic methods and result in clinical recurrences. The Mohs' technique (1) is particularly effective in radiated recurrent basal cell carcinomas, in large and deeply invasive tumors with subcutaneous extensions difficult to eradicate by surgical means, in morpheiform basal cell carcinomas, in multicentric

and "field-of-fire" basal cell carcinomas, and in recurrent squamous cell carcinoma.

The fundamental principle of Mohs' surgery is serial excisions, with careful microscopic examination of the entire undersurface of the tissue specimen and precise mapping of malignant cells within the specimen. While sacrificing the least amount of normal tissue, the technique results in ablation of the malignancy. There is an extremely low operative risk because general anesthesia is not required nor are there problems from the need for excessively radical excision.

IDENTIFICATION OF A SKIN CANCER

On clinical morphological grounds, there are three types of basal cell carcinomas:

Nodular basal cell carcinomas. These are firm and raised from the surrounding skin. The pearly papule often has an ulcerated or crusted center with surrounding superficial telangiectasia. Smaller tumors may be mistaken for a nevus, molluscum contagiosum, or sebaceous hyperplasia (Fig. 31.1).

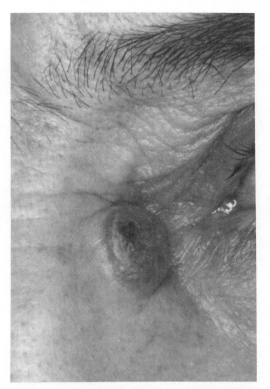

Fig. 31.1. A nodular basal cell carcinoma with central crusting is located adjacent to the inner canthus.

Superficial basal cell carcinomas, or "field-of-fire" lesions. These are flat, eczematous, crusted lesions with an active border and central clearing. They may have a well demarcated pearly, thread-like border. Many have pigmentation. This can be mistaken for fungal infection, eczema, or psoriasis. If it is located on the scalp, it may be thought to be seborrheic dermatitis, ordinary dandruff (Fig. 31.2).

Fibrous basal cell carcinomas. Morpheiform basal cell carcinomas, clinically resembling morphea (localized scleroderma), is often mistaken for scars or benign fibrous growths. The area is often depressed and has a waxy superficial appearance with telangiectasia. The borders are not clinically discernable as shown in Figure 31.3 (see color Plate V).

Large basal cell carcinomas occur, but quite uncommonly. More dramatic are those basal cell carcinomas that are so invasive

locally as to destroy structures. Lesions on the face may invade through the orbit, sinuses, or large vessels of the neck. These rare tumors need to be recognized and treated early.

Unlike basal cell carcinoma, squamous cell carcinoma has an easily diagnosable premalignant stage of actinic, or solar keratosis which is readily treated. The most common clinical manifestation of squamous cell carcinoma is a shallow ulcer of extensively actinically damaged skin. Squamous cell carcinoma metastasizes more readily than basal cell carcinoma, but some locations show metastasis less frequently than others. While squamous cell carcinoma arising from actinic keratosis rarely, if ever, metastasizes, squamous cell carcinoma on mucosal surfaces is more aggressive. Because of this, it is necessary that an adequate lymph node examination be performed on every patient with squamous cell carcinoma. This is repeated on each follow-up visit. A lymph node dissection is done when palpable nodes are present.

HISTORICAL PERSPECTIVE

In the 1930s, Dr. Frederic E. Mohs, as a medical student and research assistant, developed a method to fix tissue in situ without

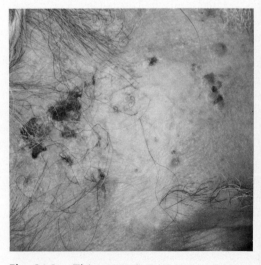

Fig. 31.2. This superficial basal cell carcinoma has not been treated previously. The active border and central clearing may lead to a faulty diagnosis of a fungal infection.

altering the architecture of the tissue. Application of a paste containing 40% zinc chloride in stibnite gave adequate fixation of tissues. Thus, the fixed-tissue technique of Mohs' chemosurgery permitted scalpel excision of tissue in a bloodless field. This method is still required for advanced and complicated skin cancers.

More recently, it has been demonstrated that the same excellent results can be obtained without the use of the chemical fixative. The fresh-tissue technique, in which the layers are excised without the use of the chemical fixation in situ, still requires complete microscopic examination by a modified frozen-section technique. These steps are repeated as often as is necessary to remove the residual tumor in serial stages. The fresh-tissue technique is preferred for lesions of moderate extent. This variation in the original form of Mohs' surgery spares the patient the considerable discomfort associated with the use of the chemical fixative. It also allows more rapid excision of residual tumor layers, thus saving time and travel for the patient. Not only is time saved because of the shorter time between excisions, but also because there is often no need for the patient to return in 7–14 days to debride the wound as the eschar is sloughed.

The sparing of tissues that is possible with the fresh-tissue technique is often very important. A cancer that has not quite eroded through the nasal ala may be removed without perforation, but the extra tissue killed by the fixative might produce a hole when the tissue sloughs. Cartilage or bone exposed during excision of the cancer by the fresh-tissue technique will be covered with granulations without removal of an extra strip of cartilage or layer of bone as is necessary with the fixed-tissue technique.

The fresh-tissue technique was used by Dr. Theodore Tromovitch (2) in the late 1960s in the periorbital area as zinc chloride paste applied to this area could irritate and damage the globe with the fixative.

As the chemical fixative paste is not used in most cases now, the name chemosurgery is not as accurate a description for the technique as it once was. Also, many patients find the term chemosurgery a confusing one. They expect it to mean systemic chemotherapy as is used in treating leukemia. The term suggests to the patient a prolonged course of chemical treatments causing hair loss, weight loss, nausea, and vomiting. It takes quite a bit of effort to dispel these ideas once they are formulated by the patient. It would seem to be easier to change the name of the technique at this time. For these reasons, many have adopted the more accurate term microscopically controlled excision or, in honor of Dr. Mohs, Mohs' surgery.

TECHNIQUE OF MOHS' SURGERY

All patients treated by either fixed- or fresh-tissue techniques of Mohs' surgery must have a biopsy of the tumor processed by routine paraffin-embedded histologic methods and stained with hemotoxylin and eosin stains. This biopsy will allow the most accurate diagnosis of the tumor type. The Mohs' technique is then applied to a biopsy-proven malignancy of the skin and traces that malignancy through the skin until a tumor-free plane is reached.

The following steps are performed:

1. The area is anesthetized by a regional or local block.
2. As much of the clinically detectable malignancy as possible is scraped away with a small curette.
3. A tissue section of the remaining base is excised in a saucer-like manner. This piece of tissue has a thickness of 2–3 mm.
4. Hemostasis is obtained with the use of electrodesiccation and fulgeration as well as a variety of chemical compounds: aluminum chloride 35% in isopropyl alcohol 50%, or Monsel's solution, (ferric subsulfate solution).
5. The excised tissue is cut into 1-square centimeter pieces bearing identifying numbers. Indelible dye markings are applied to opposing cut edges of the sections. Accurate mapping of the tissue segmentation and dyeing allow the jigsaw puzzle to be reassembled under the microscope.
6. Frozen sections are cut from each section. The histochemical staining process does not distort the dye markings.
7. Upon microscopic examination of the undersurface of the tissue, the Mohs' surgeon pinpoints the exact position on the map of the tissue of any remaining malignancy.

This microscopic control allows the Mohs' surgeon to formulate a three-dimensional view of the tumor extension, which often extends considerable distances beyond the clinically apparent margins of the neoplasm. A surgeon or a radiotherapist must excise or irradiate blindly and more extensively destroy normal tissue than the Mohs' surgeon who minimizes the removal of normal tissue.

INDICATIONS

The prime indication for Mohs' surgery is the extensive tumor which has recurred after previous treatments. Other indications include:

1. Primary lesions in "dangerous areas", such as the eyelids, canthi, pinnae, nasolabial folds, and alae nasi. In these locations, as much normal tissue as possible must be preserved. In some locations, basal cell carcinoma will invade more deeply than is clinically apparent on the surface. In the nasolabial fold, it dissects along embryonic fusion planes and follows nerve sheaths toward the brain. On the alae and the pinnae, the skin lies close to cartilage which permits tumor migration along the perichondrium. In these "dangerous areas," there is a high recurrence rate for skin cancers treated by the conventional methods (Figs. 31.4–31.7).
2. Tumors with ill-defined clinical borders, as morpheiform basal cell carcinoma (see Figure 31.3 in color Plate V).
3. Tumors with unusually large diameters (Figs. 31.8, 31.9).
4. Tumors arising primarily in areas of extensive radiodermatitis, i.e. patients who have received x-ray for epilation of the face. The dense collagen robs the hand of the operator of the ability to feel the soft malignant tissue with the curette.
5. Areas in which maximal preservation of normal function is sought. For instance, with squamous cell carcinoma of the penis or erythroplasia of Queyrat of the penis, Mohs' surgery may avoid the more radical procedure, a penectomy (Figs. 31.10, 31.11). So, too, with Bowen's disease or squamous cell carcinoma of the digits, Mohs' surgery may prevent amputation of a vital digit such as the thumb.

When recurrent basal cell carcinomas are treated by excisional surgery, radiation, or curettage and electrodesiccation, the like-lihood of another recurrence is in the range of 50% (3). This is probably best explained by the formation of scar tissue in recurrences, which entraps and buries malignant cells. This scar tissue, acting as a barrier, prevents upward migration of malignant cells, forcing them to migrate horizontally before surfacing far beyond the original site of the neoplasm. When a recurrent lesion finally is seen clinically at the periphery of the scar, it must be remembered that its origin is probably somewhere beneath the scar. Removal of the grossly detectable recurrence alone without examining the scar, will result in another recurrence.

CURE RATES

Three centers have submitted their records to statistical analysis. The 5-year cure rates of Dr. Frederic Mohs at the University of Wisconsin have been borne out by Dr. Theodore Tromovitch at the University of California, San Francisco and by Dr. Perry Robins (4) at the New York University Skin and Cancer Unit. Dr. Mohs' statistics are highly valid because he has had an unusually high percentage of his patients return for follow-up examination. In his series, only 1.3% of those

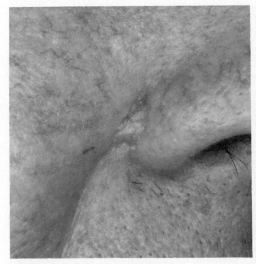

Fig. 31.4. Before treatment with Mohs' surgery, this primary basal cell carcinoma of the nasolabial fold has a clinical size of 1.8 cm.

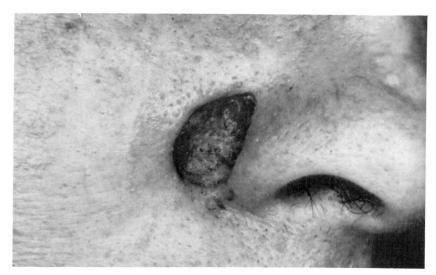

Fig. 31.5. After completion of Mohs' surgery, the defect (same patient as in Fig. 31.4) measures 2.0 cm. in the greatest diameter.

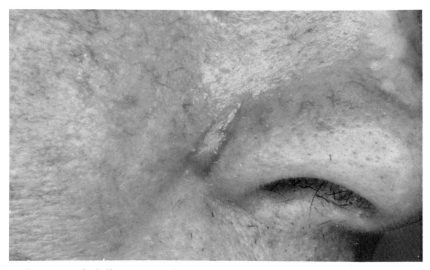

Fig. 31.6. One month following Mohs' surgery, the wound (same patient as in Figs. 31.4 and 31.5) has closed totally by secondary intention.

with basal cell carcinomas and 1.4% of those with squamous cell carcinomas have been lost to continuing observation. In over 9000 cases of basal cell carcinoma, the 5-year cure rate is 99%. Of this series, 18.3% were cases of recurrent basal cell carcinoma after previous unsuccessful therapy. In a series of over 3000 cases of squamous cell carcinoma of the skin, of which 15.8% were recurrent after previous treatment, the 5-year cure rate was 94%.

Of all modalities of therapy, Mohs' surgery offers the highest cure rate in the treatment of malignancy of the skin.

In summary, the advantages of Mohs' sur-

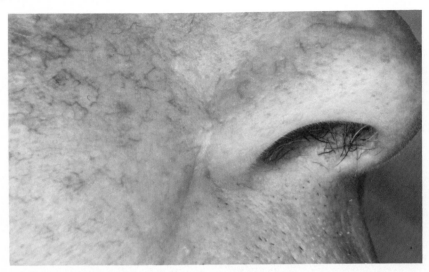

Fig. 31.7. After 6 months, the surgical scar is barely discernable (same patient as Figs. 31.4–31.6). This result should be compared with the result of radiotherapy in the same location. (see Fig. 32.5 of Chapter 32, Treatment Modalities).

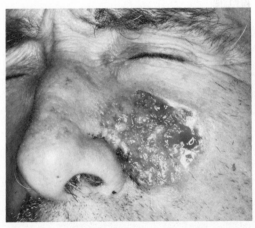

Fig. 31.8. This previously untreated basal cell carcinoma had a well defined border with a diameter of 3.5 cm.

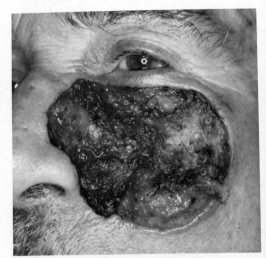

Fig. 31.9. In five stages of excision of tissue, 75 sections of tissue were examined microscopically before a tumor-free plane was achieved. The final defect is 7 × 4.5 cm. The tumor followed the sheath of the infraorbital nerve into the infraorbital foramen. The nasal bone is exposed at the base of the wound (same patient as Fig. 31.8).

gery in the treatment of cancer of the skin are:

1. High degree of reliability
2. Conservative removal of normal tissue
3. Low operative risk
4. Extension of operability to those patients who are unable to withstand general anesthesia and extensive surgical procedures because of general medical problems
5. Healing by granulation tissue formation in most instances
6. Extension of operability to patients with extensive tumors who have no hope of a cure with other methods
7. Patients remain ambulatory, thus decreasing the risk of a pulmonary embolus.

References

1. Mohs, F.E.: *Chemosurgery: Microscopically Controlled Surgery for Skin Cancer.* Charles C Thomas, Springfield, Ill., 1978.
2. Tromovitch, T., and Stegman, S.: Microscopic-controlled excision of cutaneous tumors: chemosurgery, fresh tissue technique. Cancer, *41:* 653, 1978.
3. Menn, H., Robins, P., Kopf, A.W., and Bart, R.S.: The recurrent basal cell epithelioma. Arch. Dermatol., *103:* 628, 1971.
4. Mohs, F.E.: Chemosurgery for Microscopically Controlled Excision of Skin Cancer. *J. of Surg. Oncol. 3(3):* 257, 1971.

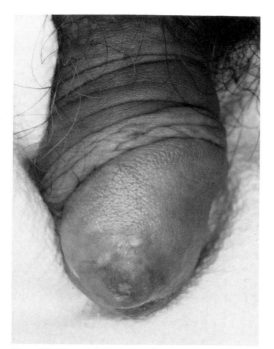

Fig. 31.10. A 40-year-old man has a biopsy-proven squamous cell carcinoma of the glans penis.

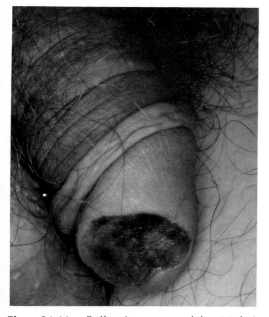

Fig. 31.11. Following removal by Mohs' surgery, the wound healed by granulation tissue formation without loss of function (same patient as Fig. 31.10).

CHAPTER 32

TREATMENT MODALITIES: CURETTAGE AND ELECTROSURGERY, CRYOSURGERY, AND RADIOTHERAPY

JUNE K. ROBINSON

There are currently three modalities of physical therapy in use in treating dermatologic problems. Electrosurgery and curettage, cryosurgery, and radiation therapy have been used to treat a variety of benign and malignant dermatologic problems. Today radiotherapy is reserved for malignant problems in dermatology. Electrosurgery and curettage, and cryosurgery, are performed extensively in the office for a large gamut of cosmetically displeasing problems, as well as in treating cutaneous malignancies.

CURETTAGE AND ELECTROSURGERY

The spectrum of usefulness of electrosurgery ranges from cosmetic problems to the skillful destruction of cutaneous malignancies. This gamut includes the treatment of premalignant growths such as leukoplakia, actinic keratoses, and cutaneous horns.

Instruments

A curette (Fig. 32.1) is an instrument with a sharpened circular surface for scraping tissue. It is used to remove soft or necrotic tissue. The operator soon learns what size and which type he prefers for a given procedure. For small superficial lesions, he may select a curette with a small cup about 3 mm in diameter, for a larger more indurated lesion a curette with a larger cup is more appropriate, about 5 mm in diameter. Curettes are available in a range of sizes, from 1 mm to 6 mm seems to be used most often by dermatologists.

In performing the procedure of curettage, the surgical setup should include:

1. Instruments for local anesthesia
2. Dermal curettes of varying sizes
3. A hemostat (a small mosquito will do)
4. A scissor (either a curved iris or a straight iris)
5. A forcep (an Adson tissue forcep is very nice)
6. Sponges

327

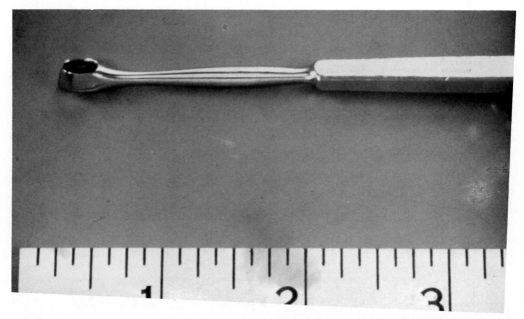

Fig. 32.1. A curette is an instrument with a sharpened circular surface for scraping soft or necrotic tissue.

7. A small bottle with 10% formalin to submit a specimen for histologic examination.

The electrosurgical unit contains a transformer and a rheostat for controlling the current (Figs. 32.2–32.4). The intensity of the current can be regulated by adjusting the rheostat on the face of the instrument. The spark gap generators used in earlier years have given way to solid state equipment, but all produce current with wave characteristics which can be adjusted either for cutting or tissue coagulation. These electrosurgical units produce an alternating current in a range between 0.5 and 3 megahertz (Hertz is the term for cycles per second). Continuous high frequency waves produce cutting while increased damping, or separation of the waves, yields increased hemostatic effects and tissue coagulation without cutting. Both cutting and coagulation are a result of the heat generated by the concentrated transfer of electrical energy to tissue. With cutting current, a minute electric arc forms and tissue is vaporized over a fraction of a millimeter. With coagulating current, tissue either boils or chars, depending on whether contact is made over a wide area, as with a disc electrode, or at a point, as with a needle. The workhorse unit in use in many

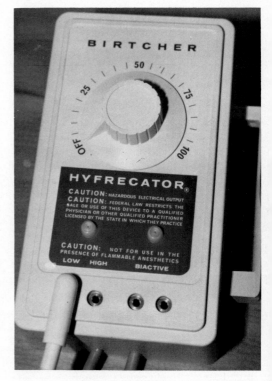

Fig. 32.2. Birtcher Hyfrecator type of electrosurgical unit. Foot pedal to control cautery.

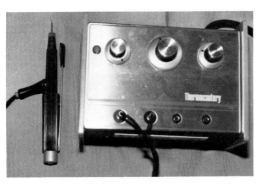

Fig. 32.3. Hot tip electrocautery unit with hand piece for control.

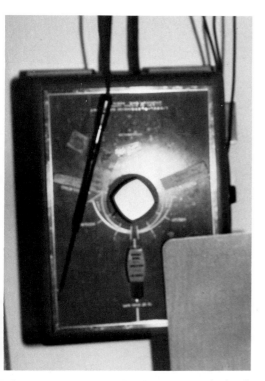

Fig. 32.4. Bantum Bovie unit with both cutting and coagulation capabilities. Foot pedal, and grounding for patient.

offices of dermatologists is the Bantum Bovie model (Fig. 32.4).

Procedure

The area is cleansed with 70% alcohol and dried thoroughly. The application of the desiccating spark to an area moistened with alcohol will ignite the inflammable alcohol. Strict asepsis is not necessary, as the wound heals by secondary intention and the heat produced by the electrosurgery kills any bacteria on the surface. Sterile instruments are employed, but the operator prepares his hands by simply washing with soap and water. The operator must be careful not to hold a blood-soaked sponge in an ungloved hand in a wound while using electrosurgery with the other hand. If he does this, he will receive the full impact of electrosurgery without the benefit of anesthesia.

Curettage is performed after the anesthetic is injected. The skin around the lesion is fixed in a position of stretch between the operator's index finger and thumb. The abnormal tissue is removed with a scraping motion of the curette. In treating malignancies, the curette moves over the surface of the lesion from the periphery to the center, criss-crossing the lesion repeatedly in several directions. The neoplastic tissue has the feel of the center of a ripe banana. The scraping action is continued until the curette comes into contact with the firm feel of normal tissue which feels like the gritty pulp of a not yet ripe pear. Often heavy bleeding, encountered early in the removal of a basal cell carcinoma, will be followed by less vigorous oozing as the diseased tissue is removed. In treating malignant and premalignant conditions, electrodesiccation follows curettage to insure destruction of an additional margin of tissue. The depth of electrodesiccation will vary with the extent and depth of the lesion. When the lesion is removed for cosmetic purposes, such as a nevus, a minimum of desiccation should be performed as a depressed scar may be as disfiguring as the nevus itself. In treating a basal cell carcinoma, cure is the essential purpose and the cosmetic result is of secondary importance. In a malignant lesion, an electrodesiccating spark of medium intensity is applied to the entire operative field in a "point to point" fashion. In desiccating small lesions such as spider angiomas or verucca planae, a small depressed scar may result. In these instances, it might be better to treat by lightly curetting or doing a shave removal and then achieving hemostasis with a chemical styptic agent, such as Monsel's solution (ferric subsulfate solution) or aluminum chloride 35% in isopropyl alcohol 50%, applied with constant moderate pressure for 5–10 minutes.

As the skin of elderly patients is often friable, thin, and tears easily, special care must be taken. In this circumstance, the curette may yield false information about the extent of the lesion. For such fragile skin, excisional surgery or radiation therapy may provide a better form of therapy.

All procedures are performed under local anesthesia in the physician's office. Dressings are often not necessary or no more than a simple BAND-AID may be required. Cosmetic results are excellent to acceptable.

Clinical Application

CONDITIONS TREATED BY ELECTRODESICCATION ALONE

Electrodesiccation without curettage may be employed for treatment of lesions which do not require pathologic examination. With these small lesions, the cosmetic result necessitates destruction of as little tissue as possible. The clinical diagnosis is readily apparent beyond a shadow of a doubt. Spider angioma, filiform warts, flat warts, small condyloma accuminata, small nevi, seborrheic keratosis, actinic keratosis, and xanthelasma can be treated with a light "sparking" of electrodesiccation. The charred tissue can be rubbed off with a gauze sponge or simply remains on the patient to be shed at a later time.

CONDITIONS USING ELECTRODESICCATION AND CURETTAGE

This technique is employed when a specimen is necessary for pathologic examination. The curette removes all of the diseased tissue first. The operator learns the feel of soft pulpy malignant tissue and is able to discriminate it from the feel of normal skin. Usually the process of curettage is continued until there is no soft tissue remaining. When treating a malignancy, electrodesiccation is then used. Curettage is carried out again with a small curet (1 or 2 mm) to get into any pockets of tumor remaining. Electrodesiccation is repeated. This is followed by one additional curettage and electrodesiccation. This makes a total of three separate cycles of curettage and electrodesiccation. With experience, the well trained physician is able to produce high cure rates in selected cases of basal cell carcinoma.

Leukoplakia of the lips and oral mucosa may be electrodesiccated and curetted but a biopsy must be performed to ensure that malignant transformation has not occurred. Leukoplakia should always be biopsied prior to treatment as many white lesions on the mucosa may actually represent other conditions.

For seborrheic keratosis, in which the differential diagnosis includes pigmented lesions such as malignant melanoma, a biopsy is necessary. An adequate specimen for pathologic examination can be obtained by a shave biopsy followed by electrodesiccation of the base. The curette can be used to smooth off any elevation remaining after the shave biopsy has been completed. Keratoacanthoma (Figs. 32.5, 32.6) can be diagnosed and treated by this same method of a "deep" shave biopsy followed by electrodesiccation and curettage.

Postoperative Care

Most patients prefer to keep the wound covered and there is some evidence that wound healing proceeds at a faster rate in an occluded wound. The wound is cleansed twice a day with 3% hydrogen peroxide and dried. A thin layer of an antibiotic ointment, such as Bacitracin Topical Ointment or Polysporin Ointment is applied to the wound surface and covered with a BAND-AID. It is wise to inform the patient that there will be exudation and later crusting. Healing time is longer than in excisional surgery and may require 2–4 weeks, depending upon the size and extent of the lesion.

Postoperative Scar

Scars following electrodesiccation and curettage tend to improve progressively with time, reaching their best appearance in 1–5 years. This is in contrast to scars produced by radiation therapy, which worsen as time passes.

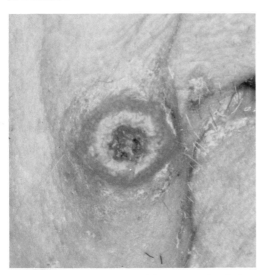

Fig. 32.5. An 80-year-old woman had this lesion appear over a period of 6 weeks. This rapidly growing tumor has the classic morphologic appearance of a keratoacanthoma.

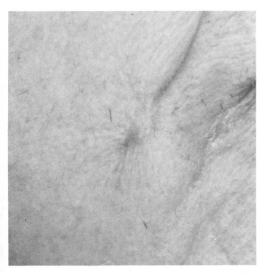

Fig. 32.6. Three months after treatment by "deep" shave biopsy for diagnosis, followed by electrodesiccation and curettage of the base of the wound, the surgical site has the appearance of a flat erythematous scar (same patient as Fig. 32.5).

At least 6 months should elapse before the clinician decides he has a satisfactory result. Hypertrophic scars, elevated and reddish, will take on an appearance approaching normal skin in 6 weeks. The scar may be sensitive. It may resemble the original tumor and the clinician may be uncertain as to whether a recurrence of the neoplasm has developed. The person who did the procedure is the best one to judge whether he has eradicated the lesion. Often, the final decision can be made only after several months of observation, and another punch biopsy may be necessary.

The end result in 2–5 years represents the molding of the skin to conform to normal contours. There is a marked tendency for even large residual scars to become linear in character. The scar usually appears whiter than the surrounding skin.

Complications

When treatment occurs in the vicinity of a small-sized arteriole, a late separation slough may result in minimal to vigorous bleeding. If the patient applies firm pinpoint pressure uninterrupted for 20 minutes, it will usually stop the bleeding.

Occasionally, hypertrophic scars and keloids arise. Some locations seem to give rise to keloids more frequently than others, the presternal and deltoid areas commonly give rise to keloids. Contracture scars or elevated extra skin folds are often seen following electrodesiccation and curettage of basal cell carcinoma on the nose adjacent to the inner aspect of the eyelids (Fig. 32.7).

RADIOTHERAPY

The role of radiotherapy in dermatology has been rapidly changing. Thirty years ago x-ray therapy was an indispensable part of dermatologic therapy. More than half of all skin diseases were listed as indications for radiotherapy in older textbooks. Now, dermatologists can utilize therapeutic methods that are more effective and safer than ionizing radiation for most of their patients. In view of proved or suspected potential side effects of ionizing radiation, some physicians advocate abandoning all forms of radiotherapy for benign conditions. New important fields of radiotherapy include the treatment of cutaneous lymphoma and mycosis fungoides. Re-

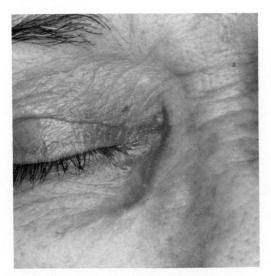

Fig. 32.7. An elevated extra skin fold is seen following electrodesiccation and curettage of a basal cell carcinoma of the nose adjacent to the lower lid and the inner canthus.

cent advances in electron-beam therapy of mycosis fungoides have shown that long-term remissions can be induced by ionizing radiation. Even though recent developments in surgical, cryosurgical, chemosurgical, and immunotherapeutic methods have narrowed down the indications for x-ray therapy of skin cancers, radiotherapy remains one of the methods of treatment for basal cell carcinoma and squamous cell carcinoma of the skin, in selected patients.

Although extremely superficial lesions may be treated by beams of very low penetration, a minimum energy of 100–120 kV filtered by 1–3 mm of aluminum should be employed. Field size rather than clinical lesion size determines fractionation and total dose of treatment. For field sizes ranging from 1.5–5 cm, 4500 rads in 10 fractions over 12 days are administered. In general, 5000 rads in 15 fractions over 19 days will be sufficient for most lesions. Since there is no good evidence for a difference in radiosensitivity between basal cell carcinoma and squamous cell carcinoma, the theoretical considerations and techniques are applicable for both malignancies. A minimum margin of at least 0.5 cm should be used on all occasions and will suffice for lesions that are easily and confidently

delimited. For malignancies less than 4 cm in diameter, whose borders are less easily defined, a margin of at least 1 cm should be used. For larger lesions, more generous borders should be employed.

Relative contraindications to the use of radiotherapy for skin cancers are:

1. Patients under the age of 55. Radiotherapy scars worsen in cosmetic appearance as time passes. A person under the age of 55 has an anticipated life span which will allow the development of an unacceptable cosmetic result from radiotherapy as shown in Figure 32.8 (see color Plate V).
2. Lesions that arise on areas of skin with extensive sun damage or radiodermatitis are best managed by surgical methods. The scar of excisional surgery opposes sun-damaged skin, resulting in a linear scar that tends to become less conspicuous with the passage of time.
3. Radiochondritis may occur on the pinnae and the nose if proper fractionation techniques are not used.
4. In order for radiotherapy to be effective in curing the cancer, the margins must be confidently delimited. This is not possible to do in many instances: morpheiform basal cell carcinoma, either squamous or basal cell carcinoma recurrent in a scar.

Indications for the use of radiotherapy include:

1. older patients who may not be able to tolerate surgical procedures and those who fear injections and surgical procedures.
2. In primary tumors with clearly demarcated borders on the eyelid, radiotherapy offers excellent cosmetic results with little loss of function. This also applies to the lips (Figs. 32.9, 32.10).

CRYOSURGERY

In use since the late 1800s, cryotherapy includes ethyl ether, ethyl chloride, carbon dioxide stick, liquid air, liquid oxygen, and liquid nitrogen. Cryotherapy is the destruction of tissue by the application of intense cold, causing tissue death by rapid freezing. Because of its ability to freeze quickly and deeply with greater control than carbon dioxide, liquid nitrogen is the best and most widely used refrigerant.

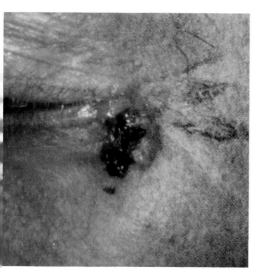

Fig. 32.9. This 80-year-old man has a previously untreated basal cell carcinoma of the outer canthus.

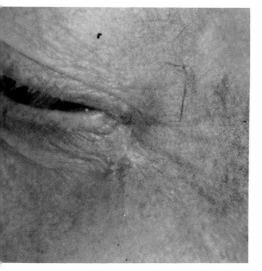

Fig. 32.10. Eight weeks following radiotherapy he (the patient seen in Fig. 32.6) has a mild ectropion and a good cosmetic result.

This is a very versatile method of therapy. The method of delivery can be as unsophisticated as a cotton swab immersed into a thermos bottle (Fig. 32.11) containing liquid nitrogen or it can be very sophisticated, consisting of probes, discs, sprays (Fig. 32.12), and thermal couples. Naturally, the more ad-

vanced technology delivers a deeper and more reliable freeze of the tissue. The simpler methods of delivery are usually applicable to benign lesions such as warts or to premalignant conditions such as actinic keratosis.

Compared to soft tissue, bone and cartilage are more cryoresistant. Melanocytes are easily damaged, and this may explain the occurrence of postoperative hypopigmentation after deep freezing. Nerves are especially susceptible to cold and neuropathy, which may develop following cryosurgery, is slow to recover. Pain is generally tolerated, but some patients complain when multiple lesions are treated.

Technique

Cotton-tipped applicators soaked in liquid nitrogen produce rapid freezing of the skin but only to a depth of 1–2 mm. The depth of freezing is limited by two factors: cotton has a low specific heat, and there is rapid vaporization of liquid nitrogen. The blood flow in the dermis and the frozen tissue act as barriers to prevent deeper freezing. Pressure with the

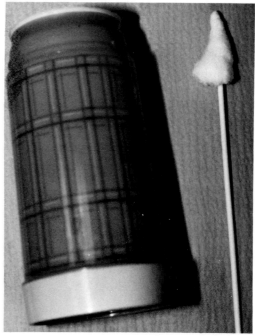

Fig. 32.11. Liquid nitrogen application with cotton tip applicator in thermos bottle.

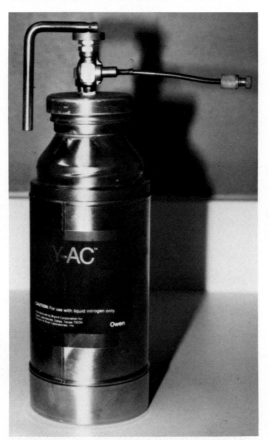

Fig. 32.12. Cryospray unit for application of liquid nitrogen to the skin.

swab is indicated for more rapid, superficial freezing. Although treatment time varies with the type, size, and depth of the lesion, only a few seconds are required. This technique is excellent for the treatment of warts, actininc keratosis, and seborrehic keratosis.

In malignant lesions, tissue should be frozen rapidly and allowed to thaw slowly. This quick-freeze slow-thaw cycle should be repeated twice, or more, to produce tissue response necessary to result in cryonecrosis for malignant tumors. The necrosis of tissue becomes apparent in 24 hours. There may be a considerable amount of swelling in the initial period. Slough of the tissue will occur in 7–14 days. It is generally agreed that $-20°$ C is sufficient to cause destruction of cancer cells. Thus $-30°$ C will almost certainly provide an

adequate margin of safety. This intensity of freezing can be achieved by the use of probes or sprays of liquid nitrogen. The more exact details of the procedure can be found in a larger work than this chapter.

Effects of Freezing of Tissue

The application of the cold produces a stinging, burning pain. This is practically unbearable in the subungual, periungual, and plantar locations. Pain increases with thawing and may require postoperative analgesics. In treating lesions on the scalp, headache persisting for several hours may result. Swelling may be a problem in any location, but especially on the eyelids, ears, and lips.

Complications

The most common complication of deeply freezing a lesion is hypopigmentation. While dilated blood vessels and milia may appear in scars, hypertrophic scarring is seldom seen. Periorbital edema may develop from 1 to 4 days after cryosurgery of the lids, forehead, and paranasal areas.

Advantages

It is a quick, effective method of treatment and causes relatively little inconvenience. It does not require local anesthesia and rarely causes hemorrhage or infection.

It is invaluable in treating a range of benign problems such as acne cysts and acne scarring, actininc keratosis, warts, and hemangiomas. Cryosurgery also is useful in selected cases of skin cancers, but a cotton tipped applicator dipped into liquid nitrogen has no place in the treatment of carcinoma.

References

1. Epstein, E.: *Skin Surgery*. Lea & Febiger, Philadelphia, 1962.
2. Zacarian, S.A.: *Cryosurgical Advances in Dermatology and Tumors of the Head and Neck*. Charles C Thomas, Springfield, Ill., 1977.
3. Goldschmidt, H.: *Physical Modalities in Dermatologic Therapy*. Springer-Verlag, New York, 1978.

CHAPTER 33

HAIR DISEASE

WILMA F. BERGFELD

CLASSIFICATION OF HAIR DISORDER

Nonscarring
  Alterations in hair growth cycles
    Telogen shed
    Anagen shed
  Abnormalities of hair shaft—fragile hairs
    Congenital hair abnormalities
    Tinea capitis
    Acquired
      Trichotillomania
      Physical and chemical damage
Scarring
  Associated with skin disease
    Lupus erythematosus
    Lichen planopilaris
    Follicular mucinosis
    Scleroderma
    Sequela of suppurative skin inflammation
  Physical and chemical damage
    Infections—viral, bacterial, fungal
    Neoplasm
      Primary
      Metastatic
      Cysts
      Granulomatous disease

Hair disorders are a perplexing and frustrating dilemma to both the clinician and the involved patient. If the hair disorder is not immediately recognized by the clinician, it frequently means that the clinician must engage in a detailed evaluation of the patient's medical history, examination of scalp and body hair, physical examination, and multiple laboratory tests as indicated by history and physical examinations.

The most valuable step in the evaluation is to first determine whether the patient has a true hair disorder. The complaints indicative of such a hair problem might be "my hair is coming out by the roots, my hair does not seem to grow, the texture of my hair has changed, my hair breaks off, or my scalp hair is thinning." Any one of these complaints is a meaningful one and points to a hair disorder. The common hair disorders are broadly classified as alterations in hair growth cycles, hair shaft abnormalities, scarring alopecias, and cutaneous neoplasms.

To fully understand hair disorders or systemic diseases which induce hair loss, it is always essential to be aware of the normal scalp conditions of maturation and growth of hair. Scalp hair grows in an asynchronous pattern with 90% of the hair in an anagen growth phase (growing phase), and 15–20% in a telogen phase (resting phase). Any alteration of the growing phase and the telogen phase presents itself as increased shedding of scalp hair. In addition, variations of hair growth are normally observed with age, sex, and seasons (Table 33.1) (1–4).

Office techniques that aid one in diagnosing hair disorders include visual examination of the scalp, skin, body hair, and nails. Specific techniques employed to diagnose include hair pull, hair pluck, and scalp biopsy. A hair pull consists of stroking the patient's scalp hair with one's fingers and removing loose hair. The amount of hair shed as well as abnormalities of hair shafts and hair bulbs as demonstrated under light microscopy are frequently diagnostic (Table 33.2).

The hair pluck is a quick, painful extraction of 20–50 growing or anchored scalp hairs with

Table 33.1
Normal Scalp Hair Growth Patterns

Average total volume of scalp hair—100,000 hairs
Fastest growth between 15 and 30 years
Slow growth in the elderly
Average rate of growth 0.35 mm/day
Faster growth in summer than winter
Active growth period 2–5 years prior to replacement
Average daily loss 25–100 hair/day
Female hair grows faster than male
Fiber diameters and shapes vary in different races and nationality groups

Table 33.2
Hair Disorders—Examination

Local examination
    Pattern of hair loss
    Length and diameter of hair fiber
    Scalp skin condition
    Hair pull
    Hair pluck
    Light microscopy examination of hair
    Fungal culture
    Scalp biopsy
Laboratory examination—screen
    Complete blood count (CBC), differential, SMA-12
    Serology
    Serum iron
    Thyroid screen
    Special studies as indicated by history and physical

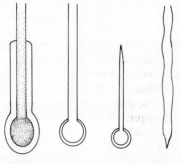

	Anagen	Telogen	Vellus Telogen	Dystrophie Anagen
Normal	90%	15–20%	—	—

Fig. 33.1. Hair pluck hair types. Diagramatic description of anagen, telogen, vellus, and dystrophic hair.

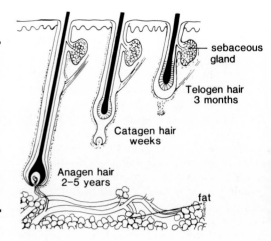

Fig. 33.2. Scalp hair growth cycles. Skin, cyclic hair growth phases.

a rubber tipped hemostat. Examination of these plucked hairs by light microscopy will allow one to determine the anagen-telogen ratio of cyclic hair growth in the involved patient. Examination of the plucked hair shafts for keratinizing hair or structural abnormalities is also valuable. Both the hair pull and the hair pluck are helpful in diagnosing alterations of scalp hair growth cycles as well as congenital or acquired structural abnormalities of the hair shafts (Fig. 33.1).

The scalp biopsy is often employed for diagnosis of scalp hair disorders which are not diagnosed by hair pulls or plucks. Evidence of scalp skin changes; for example, erythema, scarring, or palpable masses are a definite indication for a diagnostic scalp biopsy (Fig. 33.2)

ALTERATIONS OF HAIR GROWTH CYCLES

The complaint that "my hair is coming out by the roots" represents an alteration in the cyclic growth pattern of scalp hair (5–29) and may present as either a telogen or anagen shed. The long terminal anagen hair grows from 2–5 years. The anagen germinal center matrix is constantly undergoing active protein synthesis, metabolism, and keratinization. This matrix is exquisitely sensitive to many internal and external stimuli or insults (Fig.

33.3). A minimal insult will initiate the formation of an early telogen or resting hair while a maximum insult will reduce or totally interrupt the active metabolism of the anagen matrix. This latter insult produces an anagen arrest or cessation of growth with subsequent abrupt shedding of the deformed anagen hair. Shedding of these deformed anagen hairs has been called an anagen dystrophic shed.

The telogen sheds are the most common sheds observed in any clinical condition and result in a minimal to moderate insult of the growing anagen matrix with early transformation of this anagen hair to a telogen resting hair. On hair pluck, this is expressed as a 25–35% telogen hair count which is above the normal accepted level of 15–20%. Thus, a diagnosis of telogen shed can be established. These sheds are observed 4–6 weeks after the insult to the growing anagen matrix (Table 33.3). Telogen sheds are the most common cause of hair falling out by the roots.

Multiple causes of telogen sheds include drugs, chronic illness, high fevers (Fig. 33.4), childbirth, major surgery, anesthesia, crash

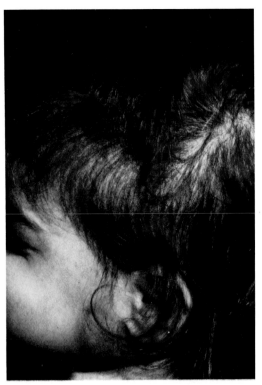

Fig. 33.4. Telogen shed of 25% of scalp hair; secondary to high fever; 2-year-old child.

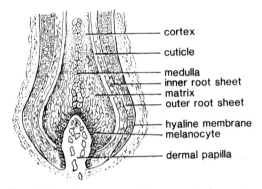

Fig. 33.3. Anagen matrix germinal center growth, the area of active protein metabolism (keratinization).

cortex
cuticle
medulla
inner root sheet
matrix
outer root sheet
hyaline membrane
melanocyte
dermal papilla

Table 33.3
Hair Loss

Clinical Picture	Anagen Shed	Telogen Shed
Onset-insult	1–3 weeks	2–4 months (latent)
Hair pluck	Normal	Increased telogen
Hair shed	Marked	Moderate
Dystrophic hair	+	−
Seborrheic dermatitis	−	+

diets, inadequate protein intake, severe psychological stress, hereditary genetic, hypo- or hyperthyroidism (Tables 33.4, 33.5). The telogen shed is usually a self-limiting process, especially if the precipitating cause is eliminated or treated. This is true in drug-induced telogen sheds as well as telogen sheds induced by crash diets and thyroid disease. However, androgenetic alopecia or common baldness may be irreversible and present as episodic telogen sheds over a period of years.

Androgenic Alopecia

Androgenic alopecia is the most common form of baldness which is observed in genetically predisposed individuals whose hair follicles are highly sensitive to androgen hormones as compared to normal individuals. Essentially, in the genetic predestined individual, male or female, there is a gradual reduction of scalp hair density as well as a transfor-

Table 33.4
Telogen Shed

Acute (8–16 weeks)
  Childbirth
  Hormones
  High fever
  Physiological in neonates
  Androgenetic—hereditary
  Surgical shock
  Anesthesia
  Drugs
  Alopecia areata

Chronic (greater than 16 weeks)
  Nutritional, crash diets (inadequate protein)
  Metabolic disorders
  Endocrinopathies (hypo- hyperthyroidism)
  Collagen vascular disease
  Chronic illness
  Psychological and neurological disorders
  Androgenic alopecia
  Overwhelming infections

Table 33.5
Common Drugs Causing Telogen Shed

Heparin
Coumadin
Triparanol
Thiouria
Carbamazepine
Indomethacin
Lithium carbonate
Furadantin
Haldol
Azulfidine
Propranolol
Probenecid
Allopurinol
Vitamin A

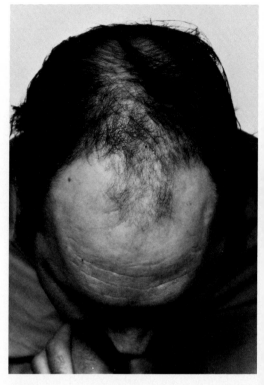

Fig. 33.5. Androgenetic alopecia (common baldness); adult male.

mation of terminal anagen hair to small, fine vellus anagen hair in a patterned distribution. This condition is an autosomal dominant and is observed in both males and females (Figs. 33.5, 33.6). The disorder may present in early teens or in late adult life. Clinically, the earlier the androgenic alopecia arises the greater the loss of scalp hair and the worse the condition. Males and females tend to display different patterns of hair loss. The male pattern may present as a variety of patterned hair loss, for example, patchy frontal, parietal, or occipital loss leaving only a horseshoe of hair around the parameter; whereas, the female pattern is more diffuse with some thinning of the sideburn area and some pronounced thinning of the parietal areas. Obviously, males may present with a female pattern and vice versa. The female androgenetic alopecia appears in females with strong family histories of baldness and a personal history of normal menses in the absence of virilization. In the female, androgenetic alopecia may present in youth as well as in the postmenopausal female.

The treatment available for androgenic alopecia is less than desirable. In the male, the treatment consists of creative hair styles, hair pieces, and hair transplantation. In the female, the same treatment modalities are available but in addition, antiandrogens are commonly employed. These include estrogen dominant products such as Enovid-E and Ovulen or topical estrogens in solution. Contraindications to antiandrogen therapy include a strong family history of carcinoma,

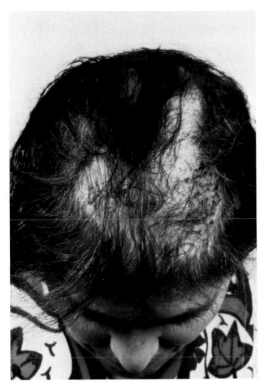

Fig. 33.6. Androgenetic alopecia; female pattern; adult female.

especially breast carcinoma, thrombophlebitis, and severe vascular headaches.

Physiologic Alopecia

Neonatal infants may demonstrate an acute telogen effluvium which is abrupt or insidious in nature. The onset occurs in the first few weeks of life with gradual replacement of hair over the ensuing months. This is a self-limiting disorder and is similar to the postpartum shed seen in the mother.

Syphilitic Alopecia

Syphilitic alopecia is observed as a secondary sign of syphilis. This condition presents as a patchy moth-eaten alopecia which involves the scalp, eyebrows, eyelashes, and beard. On the occasion when the first presenting sign is an acute telogen shed, the diagnosis is made by positive screening tests for syphilis such as VDRL or RPR which reflects elevated titers greater than 1:4. The treatment of choice is penicillin.

Anagen Shed

Anagen sheds are the result of an extreme alteration or cessation of growth of the growing anagen matrix. This results in a dystrophic or deformed hair shaft which is weak and easily shed from the scalp. These sheds are observed 1–2 weeks after the insult to the growing hair. The shed hair shows alterations in the fiber diameter with tapered areas as well as small nodular swellings (Fig. 33.7). The insults that cause cessation of growth are predominantly chemotherapeutic drugs, such as the antimetabolites, alkylating agents, and cytotoxic agents (Fig. 33.8) (Table 33.6). Alopecia areata also may present as an anagen dystrophic shed.

Alopecia areata is a classic representation

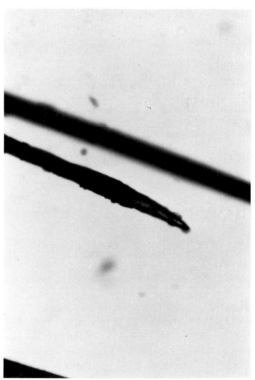

Fig. 33.7. Dystrophic anagen hair; proximal end; anagen shed.

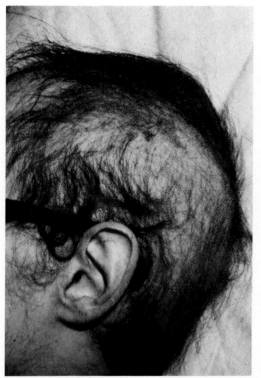

Fig. 33.8. Severe anagen dystrophic shed; telogen hair unaffected.

Table 33.6
Causes of Anagen Shed Secondary to Anagen Arrest

Drugs
  Antimetabolites
    Methotrexate
    6-Mercaptopurine
    6-Fluorouracil
  Alkylating agents
    Nitrogen mustard
    Chlorambucil
    Cyclophosphamide
    Triethylenethiophosphoramide
  Cytotoxic agents
    Actinomycin D
    Colchicine
    Vinblastine
Disease
  Alopecia areata
Miscellaneous
  High dose corticosteroids
  Vitamin A toxicity
  Triparanol
  Salicylate toxicity
  Thiouracil
  Anticoagulants (heparin)

of the anagen shed and is thought to be one of the autoimmune diseases. The acute onset of alopecia areata-totalis-universalis is that of an anagen dystrophic shed. If the disease, however, is chronic and insidious with a patchy discoid presentation, there is a combined telogen and anagen dystrophic shed observed on hair pull and hair pluck. The clinical presentation of alopecia areata varies and is patterned and may present as a patchy discoid type (Fig 33.9), marginal type, diffuse type, totalis type, and universal type (Fig. 33.10). Most often the condition is abrupt in its onset and the discoid presentation may proceed to totalis or universal loss of body hair within weeks or months. When the clinical presentation is patchy discoid; it is difficult to differentiate it from trichotillomania and/or tinea capitis. Diagnostic techniques include a scalp biopsy and fungal culture. The scalp biopsy demonstrates characteristic lymphocytic cuffing around the germinal center of the anagen hair. The fungal cultures are negative.

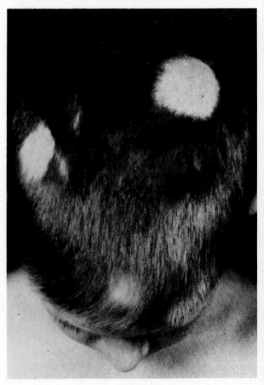

Fig. 33.9. Alopecia areata, discoid type; 4-year-old child.

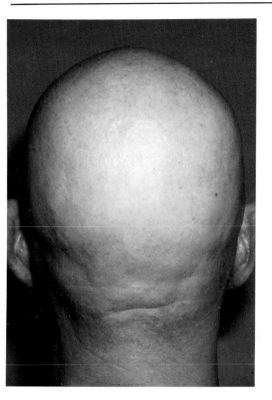

Fig. 33.10. Alopecia areata-universalis; adult.

The treatment of choice varies from topical irritant therapy to topical corticosteroids and oral corticosteroids. It is advisable in children to use topical medications rather than oral corticosteroids.

PHYSICAL AND CHEMICAL DAMAGE

Physical and chemical damage (30–41) to hair secondary to sunlight and to hair care techniques and chemicals frequently damage the hair shaft and produce a fragile hair which is broken easily with normal handling. These hair disorders may be corrected by discontinuing the inducing agent or practice for at least 12 months with gradual cutting off of the damaged hair. Shampoos and hair conditioners are helpful hair care agents but until the hair regrows and replaces itself, the damage remains.

Traction Alopecia

Hair loss secondary to traction, pulling, or prolonged tension on the scalp hair will also produce alterations in hair growth cycles as well as abnormalities of hair shafts. If the traction on the hair is repetitive and over a long period of time, it may become irreversible and present as a scarring alopecia. Hair techniques that commonly induce such disorders include braiding (Fig. 33.11), ponytails, elastic hair bands, hair rollers, and extreme teasing of hair.

Hot Comb Alopecia

Hot comb alopecia is a condition observed in the black race and appears to be secondary to cosmetic procedures of straightening the curly, thick, scalp hair. These procedures are initiated in the young adolescent and carried on at 2-week to 6-month intervals throughout adult life. In this condition there is both chem-

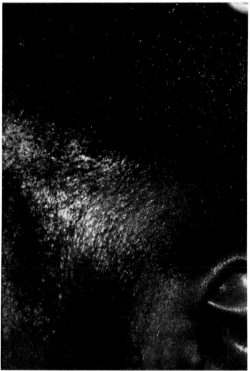

Fig. 33.11. Traction alopecia secondary to plaiting (braiding); temples of scalp.

ical and physical damage done to the hair shaft as well as alteration of growth cycles and skin inflammation.

Hair loss in this condition is first observed on the marginal peripheral areas of the scalp in the traction alopecia as well as on the vertex of the scalp. In the chronic states, hair loss may involve the entire central parietal scalp. Clinically, the patient presents as a traction alopecia with or without scarring. The older patients who have engaged in the damaging hair care techniques have a poor prognosis and generally present as a scarring alopecia. Diagnosis is made by history, clinical presentation, and light microscopy of hair shafts which demonstrate damaged hair shafts with horizontal fractures. A scalp biopsy demonstrates decreased anagen hair follicles as well as increased dermal scarring. In the early stages of this disorder, treatment includes discontinuation of the hair care procedures. In the late stages when scarring alopecia is evident, hair pieces, wigs, or hair transplantation are cosmetically helpful.

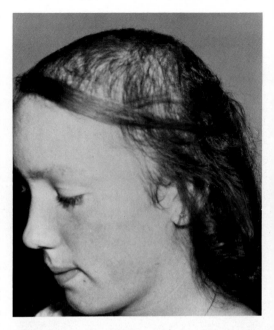

Fig. 33.12.   Trichotillomania, bizarre patterned hair loss; teenage female.

Trichotillomania

Trichotillomania is a traction alopecia which is produced by a patient who pulls, plucks, or cuts the hair in a bizarre clinical pattern (Fig 33.12). This condition is generally associated with psychological disorders and is seen frequently in children and in the elderly. Clinically, the patient is observed to have incomplete hair loss with a short stubble of hair on the scalp. If the eyelashes and eyebrows are involved, it is possible to have total loss of hair in these areas since the resting stages are long after hair plucking. Diagnosis is confirmed by light microscopy of the clipped hair which demonstrates fracture of the terminal depigmented ends. A scalp biopsy is also helpful in identifing the increased numbers of resting hair as well as follicular cysts and perifollicular scarring. Therapy is psychological counseling or psychiatric treatment.

Tinea Capitis

Tinea capitis is a condition usually observed in the prepubital children. However, it

is seen as a patchy hair loss with broken hairs which are observed as black dots on the scalp. Inflammation may or may not be present. In the adult male and female, it is observed as a diffuse loss of hair with some fine scaling of the scalp. Examination of plucked hairs for endothrix and ectothrix fungus by KOH preparation is diagnostic. The causative agents include *Trichophyton mentagrophytes*, *Trichophyton tonsurans*, *Microsporum canis* and *Microsporum audouinii*. Diagnostic procedures include KOH preparation of scales and hair, Wood's light examination, and fungal cultures. Therapy consists of topical antifungal agents as well as oral griseofulvin.

CONGENITAL HAIR ABNORMALITIES

Congenital hair abnormalities (42–53) are observed and recognized in children as genetic markers as well as markers of cutaneous and systemic disease. Frequently, children present with funny, light-colored straw-like hair which is lusterless, unmanagable, and may or may not be of normal density. The areas of involvement may be patchy or diffuse in nature. Other hairy areas of the body also may be involved such as eyebrows, eyelashes, pubic hair, and body hair. Frequently congenital hair abnormalities are associated with neurological and/or metabolic abnormalities. Associated cutaneous disorders include nail dystrophies, atopic dermatitis, and a variety of ichthyotic conditions.

The hair abnormalities are the result of defective keratinization of the hair shaft as well as the internal and external root sheath. On occasions, metabolic disturbances may induce an abnormal hair shaft. These hairs are fragile and "funny looking" clinically. Under light microscopy, the hair shafts frequently have nodal swellings and/or twisted hair or thin hair fibers.

Monilethrix is a rare congenital hair shaft abnormality which is inherited as an autosomal dominant trait. It presents on hair examination as a beaded hair (Fig. 33.13). There are usually multiple beads on a hair shaft. The beads represent normal hair while the constricted areas are representative of defects and keratinization. This condition may improve at puberty, pregnancy, or when taking oral contraceptives.

Trichorrhexis Invaginata

Trichorrhexis invaginata is also a rare congenital hair shaft abnormality which is autosomal recessive. The hair shaft abnormality is a cup and ball intussusception observed under light microscopy as a bamboo hair shaft abnormality. This condition is more frequently observed in females than males and may affect all the body hair. The hair defect is secondary to abnormal keratinization of the internal root sheath. This allows for the distal end of the hair to invaginate into the proximal portion of the ball and cup abnormality. This condition is generally self-limited and may improve at puberty.

Trichorrhexis nodosa is the most common hair shaft abnormality. This can be secondary to both the congenital or acquired defect of keratinization. The acquired defects are secondary to a variety of physical and chemical processes that induce a structural defect of intracellular cement of the cuticle and defective keratinization of the external root sheath (Fig. 33.14). On rare occasions, trichorrhexis nodosum may be associated with an inborne area of metabolism, aminoaciduria. Congen-

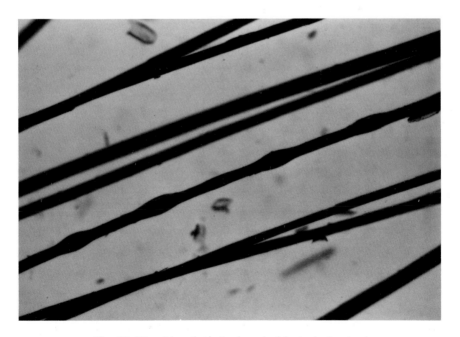

Fig. 33.13.   Monilethrix, beaded hair; hair pluck.

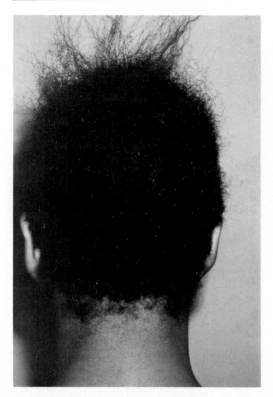

Fig. 33.14. Acquired trichorrhexis nodosa; patchy areas of fractured hair shafts (short hair); adult female.

combing, reverse permanents, and coloring procedures. Characteristically, the hair breaks off suddenly and becomes strikingly short in the affected areas which may be patchy or diffuse in nature. The treatment of choice is discontinuation of all hair care procedures except for normal shampooing and the use of hair conditioners. This condition may exist for 2–6 years.

Pili torti (twisted hair) is a rare autosomal dominant disorder of keratinization of affected hairs. On examination of involved hairs, one knows that the hair is flat and twisted with a rotational twist of 180–360°. Pili torti has been associated with monilethrix, keratosis pilaris, mental retardation, and deafness.

Pili annulati (ringed hair) is a rare familial-spread defect of the scalp hair shaft which does not produce fragility of the hair shaft. The abnormality is air-filled cavities interspersed within the hair keratin. These air spaces or cavities appear light by reflected light or dark by transmitted light. This hair shaft is structurally strong and the appearance of bright rings tend to highlight the scalp hair. Pseudopili annulati is an unusual variant of normal hair in which bright rings appear to be secondary to periodic twisting or curling of the hair shafts.

ital trichorrhexis nodosa is a familial disorder of hair and may have other associated abnormalities. The hair shaft nodal lesion is a genetic marker in patients with mental retardation and inborne areas of metabolism such as argininosuccinicaciduria. This immuno-acid easily can be identified in the urine, blood, and cerebrospinal fluid of the affected patient. The acquired form of trichorrhexis nodosa is the most common cause of hair loss secondary to physical and chemical damage to scalp hair. There are clinically two varieties which present 1) as a proximal nodal lesion and, 2) as a distal nodal lesion. Proximal lesions represent a distinct disorder of the black population, while the distal nodal lesions are observed mainly in the white race. The usual complaint is that the hair is short, of good density, but fails to grow. History reveals indulgence in a variety of hair care techniques such as hair straightening, hot

Hair Loss Secondary to Scarring

Any cutaneous or systemic disorder which induces destruction of the hair follicles and replacement of the normal dermal connective tissue by neoplastic proliferation or fibrosis will produce irreversible hair loss or a scarring alopecia (54–60). Conditions commonly observed to fall into the category of a scarring alopecia are discoid lupus erythematosus (DLE) (Fig. 33.15) lichen planopilaris, scleroderma, and suppurative inflammation secondary to viral, bacterial, and fungal infection, and cutaneous trauma secondary to physical agents such as chemicals, radiation, and thermal burns. Neoplastic proliferations are also frequently observed in the scalp skin and may represent primary malignant neoplasia, metastatic malignant neoplasia, benign adnexal cyst, or granulomatous disease.

Lupus erythematosus of the discoid type,

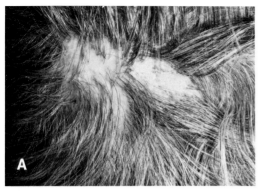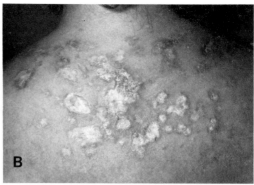

Fig. 33.15. *A*, Scarring alopecia, discoid lupus erythematosus (DLE), scalp: *B*, Cutaneous DLE on trunk in patient with scalp lesions of DLE.

with or without systemic disease, characteristically presents as a psoriasiform hairless plaque on sun-exposed surfaces as well as within the scalp skin. The diagnosis can be made by clinical presentation, skin biopsy, and direct immunofluorescence technique. Serological testing for connective tissue disease may be negative. Therapy frequently is topical high potency corticosteroids.

Lichen planopilaris is a rare inflammatory disorder of the follicular apparatus which produces a scarring hair loss condition. It is most commonly observed in adult females. Clinically and histologically, it differs from DLE, both by clinical presentation, skin biopsy, and direct immunofluorescent techniques of diagnosis. DLE demonstrates a band of fluorescence at the dermal-epidermal junction of IgG and C3 while lichen planopilaris demonstrates a globular deposition of IgG, IgA, and fibrinogen in the papillary dermis as well as adjacent to the follicular epithelium.

The treatment of DLE and lichen planopilaris is similar, but use of topical high potency steroids is indicated; however, on occasion, systemic corticosteroids as well as antimalarial therapy is helpful.

Scleroderma

Scleroderma, or morphea of the scalp, is a rare cutaneous disorder. The sclerodermatous process is destructive to the follicular apparatus and results in increased dermal connective tissue or scar. This condition is rarely associated with systemic progressive sclerosis or generalized scleroderma. Active lesions of localized scleroderma have been treated successfully with high potency topical steroids as well as oral antimalarials. The disease itself is self-limiting. Old quiescent lesions may be treated cosmetically by hair transplantation.

Neoplasia

Neoplastic proliferation either of benign or malignant types frequently produce a hair loss condition which is localized and focal in nature. The proliferating neoplasm frequently destroys or pushes aside the growing hair follicles thus producing the hair loss condition. A skin biopsy of the localized area of hair loss is diagnostic of the disorder. The most frequent benign neoplasia of scalp include pilar cysts, nevi, and organoid nevi. The malignant neoplastic lesions or scars are frequently metastatic from breast, lungs, and gastrointestinal tract and, on occasion, represent a cutaneous lymphoma.

SUMMARY

Hair diseases are indeed a perplexing and complicated problem for both the physician and the involved patient. The appropriate approach to the patient with hair disease will eliminate much of the frustration in dealing with these patients. Basically, the clinician deals with alterations in hair growth cycles,

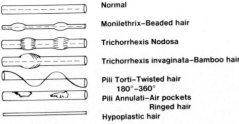

Normal

Monilethrix–Beaded hair

Trichorrhexis Nodosa

Trichorrhexis invaginata–Bamboo hair

Pili Torti–Twisted hair
180°–360°

Pili Annulati–Air pockets
Ringed hair

Hypoplastic hair

Fig. 33.16.   Hair shaft abnormalities

abnormalities of hair shafts (Fig. 33.16), inflammatory disorders of scalp skin, physical and chemical damage to the scalp, and neoplastic proliferations as well as systemic disease. Careful history taking, examination of scalp, skin, and hair, physical examination, and indicated laboratory tests will allow the physician to at least sort out this perplexing problem. It is hopeful that in categorizing the hair disease the physician can counsel the patient as well as develop an effective therapy for treatment of the hair disorder.

References

1. Adachi, K.: The metabolism and control mechanism of human hair follicles. *Curr. Probl. Dermatol. 5:* 37, 1973.
2. Adachi, K., Takaysau, S., Takashima, I., Kano, M., and Kondo, S.: Human hair follicles: metabolism and control mechanisms. J. Soc. Cosmet. Chem., *21:* 901, 1970.
3. Barman, J.M., Astore, I., and Pecoraro, V.: The normal trichogram of the adult. J. Invest. Dermatol. *44:* 233, 1965.
4. Brown, A.A.: The First Human Hair Symposium. New York Medical Commission, New York, 1974.
5. Blackburn, G.L.: Hair loss with rapid weight loss. Arch. Dermatol., *113:* 234, 1977.
6. Bradfield, R.B., Bailey, M.D., and Margen, S.: Morphological changes in human scalp hair roots during deprivation of problems. Science, *157:* 438, 1967.
7. Crounse, R.G., and Van Scott, E.J.: Changes in scalp hair roots as a measure of toxicity from cancer chemotherapeutic drugs. J. Invest. Dermatol., *35:* 83, 1960.
8. Ebling, F.J., Hale, P.A., and Johnson, E.: Hormonal influence on hair growth. In *Proceedings of Second International Congress of Endocrinology*, p. 441. Excerpta Medica Foundation, Amsterdam, 1965.
9. Frienkel, R.K., and Frienkel, N.: Hair growth and alopecia in hypothyroidism. Arch. Dermatol., *106:* 349, 1972.
10. Goette, D.K., and Odom, R.B.: Alopecia in crash dieters. JAMA, *235:* 2623, 1976.
11. Griffiths, W.A.D.: Diffuse hair loss and oral contraceptives. Br. J. Dermatol., *88:* 31, 1973.
12. Jackson, D., Church, R.E., and Ebling, F.J.: Hair dynamics in female baldness. Br. J. Dermatol., *87:* 351, 1972.
13. Jenkins, J.S., and Ash, S.: Metabolism of testosterone by human skin disorders of hair growth. J. Endocrinol. Metab., *59:* 345, 1973.
14. Johnson, A.A., Latham, M.C., and Roe, D.A.: Use of changes in hair assessment of protein calorie malnutrition. J. Invest. Dermatol., *68:* 311, 1975.
15. Kaidbey, K.H.: Hair growth inhibition as a method of screening drugs for local antimitotic activity. J. Invest. Dermatol., *68:* 80, 1977.
16. Kaufman, J.P.: Telogue effluvium secondary to starvation diet. Arch. Dermatol., *112:* 731, 1976.
17. Klein, A.W., Rudolph, R.I., and Leyden, J.: Telogen effluvium as a sign of Hodgkin's disease. Arch. Dermatol., *108:* 702, 1973.
18. Kligman, A.M.: Pathologic dynamics of human hair loss. I. Telogen effluvium. Arch. Dermatol., *83:* 175, 1961.
19. Ludwig, E.: Classification of the types of androgenetic alopecia (common baldness) occurring in the female sex. Br. J. Dermatol., *97:* 247, 1977.
20. Martin, C.M., Southwick, E.G., and Maibach, H.I.: Propanalol induced alopecia. Am. Heart J., *86:* 236, 1973.
21. Muller, S.A., and Winklemann, R.K.: Alopecia areata, an evaluation of 736 patients. Arch. Dermatol., *88:* 290, 1963.
22. Papa, C.M., and Kligman, A.M.: Stimulation of hair growth by topical application of androgen. JAMA, *191:* 521, 1965.
23. Papadopoulos, S., and Harden, R.: Hair loss in patients treated with carbimagol. Br. Med. J., *2:* 1502, 1966.
24. Pecoraro, V., Astore, I., and Barman, J.M.: Cycle of the scalp hair of the newborn child. J. Invest. Dermatol., *43:* 145.
25. Price, V.H.: Testosterone metabolism in the skin: review of its function in androgenic alopecia, acne vulgaris, and idiopathic hirsutism including recent studies with antiandrogens. Arch. Dermatol., *111:* 1492, 1975.
26. Rawnsley, H.M., and Shelly, W.B.: Salicylate ingestion and idiopathic hair loss. Lancet, *1:* 567, 1968.
27. Sulzberger, M., Witten, V., and Kopf, A.: Diffuse alopecia in women. Arch. Dermatol., *81:* 108, 1960.
28. VanScott, E.J., Reinertson, R.P., Steinmuller, R.: The growing hair roots of the human scalp and morphologic changes therein following amethopterin therapy. J. Invest. Dermatol., *29:* 197, 1957.
29. Wilburne, M.: Hair loss and pigmentation due to thiouracel derivatives. JAMA, *147:* 379, 1971.
30. Goldsmith, L.A., and Baden, H.A.: The mechanical properties of hair. J. Invest. Dermatol., *50:* 200, 1971.
31. Harman, R.R.: Traction alopecia due to hair extension. Br. J. Dermatol., *87:* 79, 1972.
32. Holder, W.: The broken ponytail. Arch. Dermatol., *103:* 101, 1971.
33. Kligman, A.M.: Facts and fancies on the cure of hair and nails. South. Med. J., *55:* 1001, 1961.
34. Lipnik, M.: Traumatic alopecia from brush rollers. Arch. Dermatol., *84:* 183, 1961.
35. LoPresti, P., Papa, C., and Kligman, A.: Hot comb alopecia. Arch. Dermatol., *98:* 234, 1968.
36. Muller, S.A., and Winkleman, R.K.: Trichotillomania: a clinical pathologic study. Arch. Dermatol., *102:* 129, 1965.

37. Orfanos, C.E., and Mahrle, G.: Human hair and how it changes under cosmetic procedures in vivo. Parfumeric Kostmetick, *52:* 203, 235, 1971.

38. Papa, C.M., Mills, O.H., and Hanshaw, W.: Seasonal trichorrhexia nodosa. Arch. Dermatol., *106:* 888, 1972.

39. Savill, A.: The nylon brush. Br. J. Dermatol., *70:* 296, 1958.

40. Reiches, A.J., and Lane, C.W.: Temporary baldness due to cold wave thyroglycolate preparations. JAMA, *144:* 305, 1950.

41. Rudolph, R.I., Klein, A.W., and Decherd, J.W.: Corn row alopecia. Arch. Dermatol., *103:* 134, 1973.

42. Altman, J., and Stroud, J.: Netherton's syndrome and ichthyosis lineares circumflexa. Psoriasiform ichthyosis. Arch. Dermatol., *100:* 550, 1969.

43. Chernosky, M.E., and Owens, D.M.: Trichorrhexis nodosa: clinical and investigative studies. Arch. Dermatol., *94:* 577, 1966.

44. Hersle, K.: Netherton's disease and ichthyosis circumflexa. Report of a case and a review of the literature. Acta Derm. Venereol., *52:* 298, 1972.

45. Malt, R.A.: Keratin in monilethrix. J. Invest. Dermatol., *44:* 364, 1968.

46. Muller, S.A.: Alopecia: syndrome of generic significance. J. Invest. Dermatol., *60:* 475, 1973.

47. Orentreich, N.: Disorders of the hair and scalp in childhood. Pediatr. Clin. N. Am., *18:* 953, 1971.

48. Papa, C., Mills, O.H., and Hansahw, E.M.: Trichorrhexis nodosa. Arch. Dermatol., *106:* 88, 1972.

49. Porter, P.S., and Lobitz, W.B.Q., Jr.: Human hair: a genetic marker. Br. J. Dermatol., *83:* 225, 1970.

50. Price, V.H., Thomas, R.S., and Jones, F.T.: Microscopic studies of pili annulati. In *Proceedings of XII International Congress of Dermatology*, p. 786. Munich, 1967; Berlin, 1968.

51. Price, V.H., Thomas, R.S., and Jones, F.T.: Pseudo pili annulati. An unusual variant of normal hair. Arch. Dermatol., *102:* 354, 1970.

52. Solomon, I.L., and Green, O.C.: Monilethrix. N. Engl. J. Med., *269:* 1279, 1963.

53. Stelly, W.B., and Rawnsley, H.M.: Aminogenic alopecia: loss of hair associated with argininosuccinic aciduria. Lancet *2:* 1327, 1965.

54. Altman, J., and Perry, H.O.: The variations and course of lichen planus. Arch. Dermatol., *84:* 179, 1961.

55. Burnham, T.K., Fine, G., and Neblett, T.R.: Immunofluorescent "Band" test for lupus erythematosus. Arch. Dermatol., *102:* 42, 1970.

56. Gay, P.J.: Pseudopelade of Brocq: its relationship to some forms of cicatricial alopecia and to lichen planus. J. Invest. Dermatol., *24:* 323, 1958.

57. O'Leary, P.A., Montgomery, H., and Ragsdale, W.E.: Dermatohistopathology of various types of scleroderma. Arch. Dermatol., *75:* 78, 1957.

58. Michel B., Sy, E.K., David, K., and Haserick, J.R.: Immunofluorescent patterns in lichen planus (Abst). J. Invest. Dermatol., *54:* 428, 1970.

59. Scher, W.F., Swanson, P.M., Gomez, F., and Reyes, C.N.: Alopecia neoplastica. JAMA, *213:* 1335, 1970.

60. Golitz, L.E., Shapario, L., Hurwitz, T.I.: Cicatricial alopecia of sarcoidosis. Arch. Dermatol., *107:* 758, 1973.

INDEX